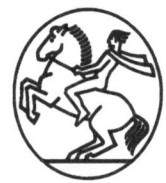

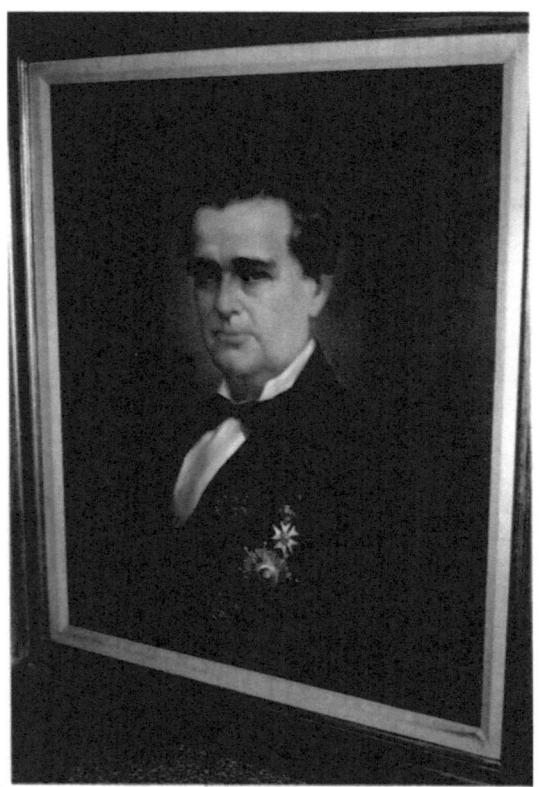

James Marion Sims M.D.-c. 1874

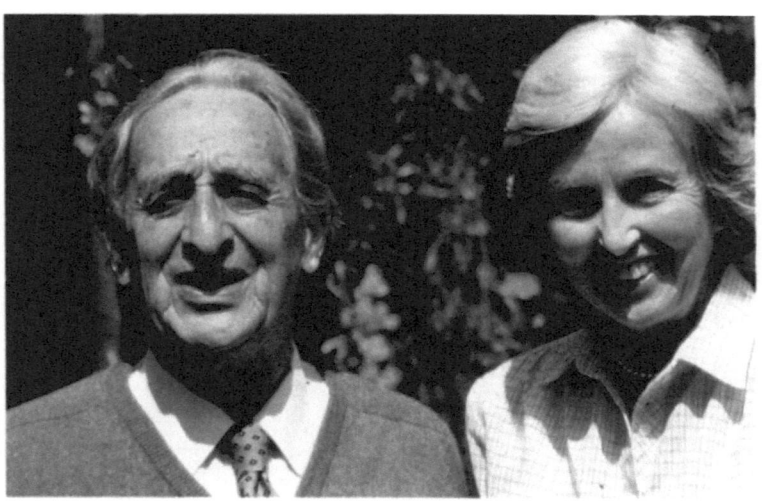

Reg and Catherine Hamlin

Robert F. Zacharin

Obstetric Fistula

With a Foreword by
Professor Otto Käser
University of Basel, Switzerland

Springer-Verlag Wien New York

Robert F. Zacharin,
M.G.O. (Melb.), F.R.C.S. (Eng.), F.R.C.O.G., F.R.A.C.S.,
F.R.A.C.O.G.
M.D. (Melb.), Consultant Gynecologist, Alfred Hospital, Melbourne, Australia

With 136 partly coloured Figures

Library of Congress Cataloging-in-Publication Data: Zacharin, Robert Fyfe. Obstetric fistula. Bibliography: p. Includes index. 1. Fistula, Vesico-vaginal — Surgery — History. 2. Gynecology, Operative — History. I. Title. [DNLM: 1. Fistula — history. 2. Rectovaginal Fistula — surgery. 3. Surgery, Operative — history. 4. Urinary Fistula — surgery. 5. Vesico-vaginal Fistula — surgery. WP 180 Z160] RG104.3.Z33 1988. 618.1'5. 87-32358

ISBN-13: 978-3-7091-8923-8   e-ISBN-13: 978-3-7091-8921-4
DOI: 10.1007/978-3-7091-8921-4

Foreword

Obstetric fistula is as old as mankind. While the incidence has diminished progressively with better health care in Western societies, the situation has changed little in many developing countries. Fistulae of pelvic organs, often monstrous defects, still are a major complication of child-birth causing misery to uncounted young women, and if they cannot find help in one of the very few hospitals with trained specialists, they became urological cripples losing everything: family, home and job. The magnitude of the problem is illustrated by some figures given by Reginald and Catherine Hamlin—about 700 fistula patients treated each year—a total of over 10,000 cases operated upon in their fistula hospital in Addis Ababa, Ethiopia. Most of these injuries could be prevented by better health care at the village level as some studies have shown conclusively. The incidence of fistula is an indicator of the standard of health and obstetrical care.

The author of this book—Obstetric Fistula—is an internationally known Australian gynaecologist who for many years has been interested in all aspects of gynaecological urology, especially urinary stress incontinence, other forms of involuntary loss of urine, and associated gynaecological conditions. He has devised a number of new operations to treat pelvic defects. Robert Zacharin's interest in obstetric fistula was a consequence of his surgical activity in developing countries. The history of fistula management related in this monograph shows a number of relatively well-defined periods, the first from antiquity to the middle of the 17th century when the treatment of fistulae was palliative at best, and the second, characterized by the beginning of modern repair technique. The pioneer was Hendrick von Roonhuyze of Amsterdam, the acknowledged father of fistula surgery. His name and technique went into oblivion, with few attempts at surgical repair in the next one and a half centuries. In the third period—19th and first half of the 20th century—Roonhuyze's technique was rediscovered, other approaches were tested, the vaginal operation was perfected and cure rates improved. Many of the well-known and some of the less well-known surgeons and gynaecologists of the period tried their hands at fistula repair, often suggesting a new modification in surgical

To

James Marion Sims
Founder of the First Fistula Hospital,
Madison Avenue, New York. 1855,

and

Reginald and *Catherine Hamlin*
Founders of the Second Fistula Hospital,
Addis Ababa, Ethiopia. 1975.

"Unhouse'd, unfriended, solitary, slow,
on Tigris Banks I wander to and fro
and with my tears that flowing never cease,
the torrent of the rapid stream increase"

Jami
817–892 AD
Translated by Stephen Weston
1747–1830

technique or inventing a new surgical instrument. Two names became famous among many others, James Marion Sims, who founded the first fistula hospital in New York, and Howard Kelly, the promotor of an individual vaginal or suprapubic approach. The fourth period might be called the era of fistula specialists—Mahfouz, Chassar Moir, the Hamlins, and Lawson—and others who because of better preoperative care and better technique with the addition of grafting, were able to cure the large majority of even the worst fistulae.

Robert Zacharin's book, based on a detailed study of the literature, offers a wealth of information about the history of fistulae and fistula repair priorities together with graphical details of many a famous fistula surgeon. It deals with all aspects of obstetric fistulae involving the pelvic organs: incidence, pathology, diagnosis, prevention, complications and treatment. The book is well-written, easy to read and profusely illustrated. It should be in every gynaecologist's library and read by everybody interested in pelvic surgery.

Otto Käser, M.D., FACOG, FAGOS
Dr. h.c.
Professor and Chairman emeritus
University of Basel
Switzerland

Preface

Undoubtedly this book should have been written by Reginald and Catherine Hamlin, whose contributions to the practical management of obstetric fistula have been recognized throughout the world. On many occasions during visits to Ethiopia, the possibility of such an undertaking was mentioned; but always the continual work load at their Fistula Hospital was adequate reason why such a book never could have eventuated. My wife and I met the Hamlins in Addis Ababa first in 1967 after correspondence about management of urinary incontinence which sometimes followed successful vesico-vaginal fistula closure. Until 1967, in company with most of my colleagues in Australia, exposure to fistula surgery had been minimal and viewed always with some apprehension because of their rarity, so counting 54 vesico-vaginal fistulae during that first visit to Princess Tsahai Hospital was absolutely unbelievable and during succeeding days, this feeling was reinforced repeatedly when the avalanche of new fistula patients continued. Nevertheless, far more impressive than the large number of patients was the meticulous care with which these ghastly defects were repaired by the Hamlins and it was quite usual to have 4 or 5 fistula patients on each operating list. Soon it became very clear that the major cause of the urinary incontinence following closure was a true incontinence due to the terrible bladder injury and for which regrettably I had nothing to contribute; but this first exposure was so memorable and challenging that we have returned many times to Addis Ababa, to work with the Hamlins, slowly absorbing their "tricks of the trade" and learning finer technical details by operating with their assistance and watching them at work. They are most generous with their time and expertise, also extremely patient!

In terms of patient numbers, there would be but a handful of western world gynaecologists with even a moderate experience in dealing with genital fistulae, whereas in other parts of the world, where fistulae still abound, many surgeons have managed several thousand patients. So the occasional fistula surgeon usually prefers to refer urinary fistulae to a urologist rather than attempting to deal with the problem because of a lack of personal experience and also being well-aware of the many technical difficulties involved. The urologist, an expert within the bladder will advocate a suprapubic approach almost uniformly, although on occasion the gynaecologist joins forces with him to tackle the problem by a combined abdomino-vaginal approach. This common clinical situation ignores completely the fact that a majority of vesico-vaginal fistulae are managed best by vaginal surgery and for many reasons.

At the Alfred Hospital, Melbourne, the Gynaecology Department is well-known for its interest in fistula surgery, and since 1967 has had experience with the management of more than 100 genital fistulae—most of surgical origin—referred from many parts of Australia and also from Indonesia. In addition, several visits to Padang and Ujung Padang in Indonesia have increased this experience. More recently, armed with 35 mm slides prepared in Addis Ababa, Khartoum and Indonesia, lectures given in Australia, Europe and the United Sates of America have evoked wide interest from gynaecologists never previously exposed to obstetric fistulae and the problems of their surgical management. For all these reasons it seemed wrong that the work of the Hamlins and other eminent fistula surgeons had not been recorded in book form, especially since the fistula problem is unchanged in many areas of the world and also, few Western gynaecologists may have an opportunity to visit such centres and learn at first hand from the masters of this art. Finally, the principles involved in successful obstetric fistula surgery differ in no way from those employed in the correction of surgically produced fistulae and with such small numbers of referred cases being seen, many principles of management are not well-known nor is their importance fully appreciated. Accordingly, during a recent visit to Addis Ababa, the Hamlins agreed to the suggestion that I should attempt such a book, which in general terms would deal with the historical aspects of the problem and then the technical details of present-day fistula surgery. In any discussion about obstetric fistula, the historical approach is exceedingly important and the vast associated bibliography needs assimilation before any thoughts of proceeding to present day details can be entertained.

To assess recent trends in fistula incidence and management, Egypt, Jordan and the Sudan were visited in September 1985. In Cairo, discussions with Professor Sherbani of Kasr el Aini Hospital about past and present fistula problems in Egypt were wide-ranging, and additionally the facilities of the Mahfouz Obstetrical and Gynaecological Museum were made available. After leaving Cairo I corresponded with Professor Mahran of Ain Shams University. In Amman, Dr Farid Akasheh the doyen of Jordanian gynaecologists made the visit memorable and opened all the necessary doors, while in Khartoum, Professor Hadad Karoum and his staff at the University and the General Hospital arranged visits to outpatient clinics and operating sessions where much valuable information was collected.

With certain historical aspects, especially Queen Henhenit and the New York activities of James Marion Sims, Harold Tovell of St Luke's Hospital New York has been an enthusiastic and valuable ally. In November 1986 a visit to Birmingham, Alabama was arranged by Hugh Shingleton known widely for his knowledge of the life and time of Sims. This included access to the Reynolds Historical Library and an excellent historical excursion to Montgomery where Felix Tankersley was so helpful. So much additional information was gained about Sims and Alabama that the chapter concerning him was expanded greatly. I am indebted to Edwin Bridges the Director of the Alabama Department of Archives and History at Montgomery and to Miss Mary Claire Britt, Curator of the Reynolds Historical Library in the University of Alabama at Birmingham for their assistance.

Many friends and colleagues have offered helpful opinions and constructive criticism of the preliminary manuscript and I am grateful to Harold Tovell of New York, James Ingram of Tampa, Robert Marshall, James Mortensen, Keith Layton and Norman Beischer of Melbourne, John Lawson of Newcastle-on-Tyne, U.K., John Kelly of Birmingham, U.K. and finally Reginald and Catherine Hamlin of Ethiopia.

Up to date information about the present fistula situation in West Africa has been obtained by discussions in London with John Lawson and Una Lister, and from correspondence with Sister Ann Ward of St Luke's Hospital in Cross River State, Nigeria.

Checking the bibliography and obtaining photostats particularly of older papers has been a long and tiresome job, and without the dedicated help of Enid Meldrum and Kathy Hutton from the Medical Library at the Alfred Hospital, Melbourne, the list would have been incomplete and contained many errors. Most of the photographs originated in Ethiopia and others came from the Sudan, Indonesia, Nigeria, Australia and the United States of America and the hard work of preparing them for publication and producing the excellent line drawings to illustrate the colour photographs, was effected in the Visual Aids Department at the Alfred Hospital, Melbourne, by Cam Harvey, Caroline Hedt and Sharon Arnott. The stanza by the 8th century Persian lyric poet Jami, which sets the fistula scene so admirably, was suggested by Richard Newing. Finally I offer sincere thanks to my daughter Jane who expertly typed the manuscript so many times.

Robert F. Zacharin
Melbourne, 1987

Contents

Acknowledgements

(i) Figure 36: reprinted with permission of American Journal of Surgery, "Postoperative vesico-vaginal fistulas: genesis and therapy." W. Latzko. *58*, 211 (1942).

(ii) Figures 54 and 55: reprinted with permission of Grune & Stratton, New York. "Surgical treatment of cancer of the cervix." J. V. Meigs (1954).

(iii) Figures 56–58: reprinted with permission of Journal of Urology, "The repair of extensive vesico-vaginal fistula with pedicled omentum: a review of 27 cases." I. Kiricuta and A. M. B. Goldstein. *108*, 724 (1972).

(iv) Figures 59 a–c and 113 a–c: reprinted with permission of Clinical Obstetrics and Gynecology, "Incontinence: Vesical and urethral fistulas." R. E. Symmonds. *27*, 499 (1984).

(v) Figure 60: reprinted with permission of Churchill-Livingstone, Edinburgh, "The life of an Egyptian doctor." N. Mahfouz (1966).

(vi) Figures 85 and 86: reprinted with permission of Surgery, Gynecology and Obstetrics, "Vesico-vaginal fistula and its management." L. E. Phaneuf and R. C. Graves. *88*, 155 (1949).

(vii) Figures 87 a–d: reprinted with permission of Journal of Urology, "The repair of vesico-vaginal fistula by the transperitoneal transvesical approach." J. W. Dorsey. *83*, 404 (1960).

(viii) Figures 88 a, b: reprinted with permission of Charles C. Thomas, Springfield, Illinois, "Suprapubic closure of vesico-vaginal fistula." V. J. O'Conor (1957).

(ix) Figures 89 a–c: reprinted with permission of Journal of Urology, "A flap technique for repair of vesico-vaginal fistula." C. T. Su. *102*, 56 (1968).

(x) Figures 90 a, b: reprinted with permission of British Medical Journal, "The repair of vesico-vaginal fistula by a new technique." J. B. Macalpine. *2*, 778 (1940).

(xi) Figure 91: reprinted with permission of Journal of Urology, "Vesico-vaginal fistulas on one gynecological service." V. F. Marshall. *121*, 25 (1979).

(xii) Figures 92 a–c: reprinted with permission of Australian and New Zealand Journal of Surgery, "Vesico-vaginal fistula–a method of repair." N. F. Greenslade. *38*, 283 (1969).

(xiii) Figures 111 a, b: reprinted with permission of Journal of Obstetrics and Gynaecology of the British Empire, "Treatment of a type of juxta-urethral vesico-vaginal fistula." G. B. Thomas. *54*, 665 (1947).

(xiv) Figure 112: reprinted with permission of Urological and Cutaneous Review, "Reconstruction of the urethra with a tube from bladder flap." R. W. Barnes and W. Wilson. *53*, 604 (1949).

(xv) Figure 117: reprinted with permission of Journal of Obstetrics and Gynaecology, "Evaluation of methods of treatment of urinary fistulae in women." M. Foda. *66*, 372 (1959).

(xvi) Figure 118: reprinted with permission of South African Medical Journal, "Vaginoplasty following vesico-vaginal fistula repair: a preliminary report." J. S. Dick and P. M. Strover. *45*, 617 (1971).

(xvii) Figures 119, 124 a, b, and 136: reprinted with permission of Proceedings of the Royal Society of Medicine, "Recto-vaginal fistula following difficult labour." J. B. Lawson. *65* (3), 283 (1972).

(xviii) Figures 120 a–c and 125 a–g: reprinted with permission of American Journal of Obstetrics and Gynecology, "The surgical treatment of complete perineal tears in the female." F. Miller and W. Brown. *34*, 196 (1937)

(xix) Figure 126: reprinted with permission of Obstetrics and Gynecology, "Anterior rectal wall advancement." F. Mengert and S. A. Fish. *5*, 262 (1955).

(xx) Figure 127: reprinted with permission of Surgery, Gynecology and Obstetrics, "Repair of recto-vaginal fistulas." J. Greenwald and B. Hoexter. *146*, 443 (1978)

(xxi) Figures 128 a, b: reprinted with permission of Surgical Clinics of North America. "The management of recto-vaginal fistulae." D. A. Rothenberger and S. M. Goldberg. *63*, 61 (1983)

Key to Diagrams

AC   Anal canal
AF   Allis forceps
AN   Aneurysm needle
AS   Anchor suture
BL   Bladder
CAF   Curved artery forceps
CX   Cervix
CCG   Chromic catgut
DS   Donor site
DT   Drain tube
Fc   Foley catheter
Gp   Gauze pad
GS   Guy suture
Mc   Metal catheter
MFG   Martius fat graft
NS   Nylon suture
Nu   Neourethra
P   Pointer
PCGS   Plain catgut suture
Pr   Probe
PS   Perineal suture
RAS   Reconstituted anal sphincter
S   Swab
SAF   Straight artery forcep
Sc   Scissors
SpS   Sphincter suture

SS   Stabilizing suture
ST   Scar tissue
TDF Toothed dissecting forceps
UC   Ureteric catheter
V   Vagina
VS   Vaginal speculum
Vu   Vulva

1

Historical Introduction

The Era Before James Marion Sims

There is a commonly held yet erroneous belief, that James Marion Sims, the father of American gynecology, was first to close a vesico-vaginal fistula, similar entirely to the statement, that Captain James Cook discovered Australia. The history of both endeavors shows that the real story is very different and in the case of both these great men, there were many who went before them.

Earliest recorded medical references and particularly in gynecology, have been found scattered through ancient Egyptian documents known as the papyri. Rare medical engravings, even antedating papyral sources were found on the doorpost of a tomb excavated in the necropolis of Saqquarah, Egypt. The tomb was that of an unknown physician who lived during the reign of King Atoty, the first king of the 6th dynasty, and the pictures represent incision of a boil on the neck and circumcision.

There are 7 papyri in all and gynecological references occur in the first two, the Kahun and the Ebers. Their translation became possible with the discovery of the Rosetta stone in 1799, which when deciphered, supplied the key to those ancient Egyptian scripts.

One of the oldest, the Kahun papyrus dates probably to about 2000 BC and was discovered in April 1889, by Flinders Petrie, an English archeologist at Kahun in the Fayyum area, south of Cairo. Painstakingly, scores of fragments were pieced together to reconstruct 3 registers of hieratic text, however many fragments were missing. In 1898, the document was deciphered by Francis Griffith, but although the gynecological portion was written in a clear script, the fragmentary condition of the document rendered the translation imperfect. A true perspective of the antiquity of the Kahun papyrus may be appreciated by realizing that oldest comparable texts from Babylon date from about 700 BC, old Chinese texts are certainly later than 200 BC whilst those from India intrude into the Christian era. Purchased by George Ebers, a German Egyptologist wintering in Egypt in 1872, the Ebers papyrus was discovered allegedly between the knees of a mummy from the Theban acropolis. This papyrus which now is in the library at the University of Leipzig, is 65 feet long and 14 inches wide and consists of 108 columns each of about 20 lines, and dates to 1550 BC The gynecological reference in this papyrus deals with uterine prolapse, but at the end of page 3, two fragmentary prescriptions occur, one a cure for toothache, and the other relates possibly to vesico-vaginal fistula and warns the physician against attempting to cure it. "Prescription for a woman whose urine is in an irksome place: if the urine keeps coming and she distinguishes it, she will be like this forever." Certainly this is the oldest reference to vesico-vaginal fistula and indicates with clarity, the antiquity of the problem.

Maughs (1884) discussed "what the ancients knew concerning obstetrics and gynecology" and presented the contributions of Archigeres, 1st century AD, Philumenus, 2nd century, Oribasius, 4th century and Aetius, the most learned able, experienced and honest of all Greek compilers who practiced and wrote at Alexandria in the 6th century. While a remarkable range of knowledge was presented including mention by Archigeres of the dioptra or speculum vaginae, remarkably there was no reference to urinary incontinence or fistula.

Avicenna the renowned Arabo-Persian physician who died in 1037 AD, first recognized that urinary incontinence in the female may be due to a fistula following difficult labor. His textbook "Al Kanoun" one of the most famous medical books ever written, was used in medical schools both in Asia and Europe for more than five centuries. In the chapter on pregnancy prevention he gave the following advice and warning: "In cases in which women are married too young, and in patients who have weak bladders, the physician should instruct the patient in the ways of prevention of pregnancy. In these patients the bulk of foetus may cause a tear in the bladder which results in incontinence of urine. The condition is incurable and remains so till death."

Remarkably, no further reference to fistula appeared until the end of the 16th century, when several clear descriptions appeared simultaneously. Felix Platter, Basle (1597) in Israel Spach's great work (Fig. 1) "Gynaecorum" gave the following description: "As a sequence of a difficult first labour, the young country girl had the opening of the bladder rent to such a degree that there was a long gaping furrow in its place, and the open bladder could be seen. I have twice inspected it myself and discovered that it was so by using a probe. On account of this injury, there is a constant involuntary discharge of urine, and the surrounding parts become exco-

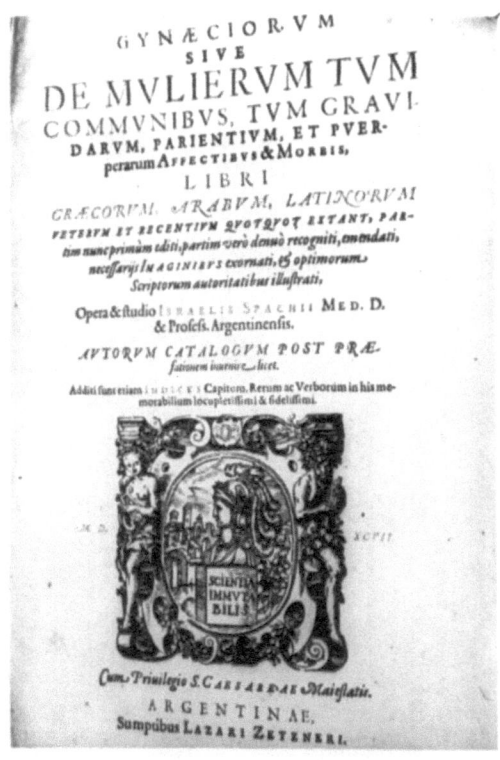

Figure 1. Title page of Israel Spachs "Gynaecorum"

riated and inflamed." Luiz de Mercado (1597) a physician of Valladolid seems first to have used the term "fistula" rather than the usual word "ruptura" when he wrote, "what an empty and tragic life is led by the affected victims and how great are their embarrassments—uncontrolled urine runs from the fistula with ease" (Shorter 1984).

Professor D. E. Derry (1935) described the pelves of five women of the 11th dynasty in Egypt, and Queen Henhenit (circa 2050 BC) one of the wives of King Mentuhotep II was of special interest. Her mummy had been buried in chambers below the terraces surrounding the pyramid of King Mentuhotep II at Deir-el-Bahri, at Thebes. The funerary temple of Mentuhotep II was discovered by Edouard Naville, and both sarcophagus and mummy were sent to the Metropolitan Museum of Art in New York, in 1907, in acknowledgement of financial support for his archeological

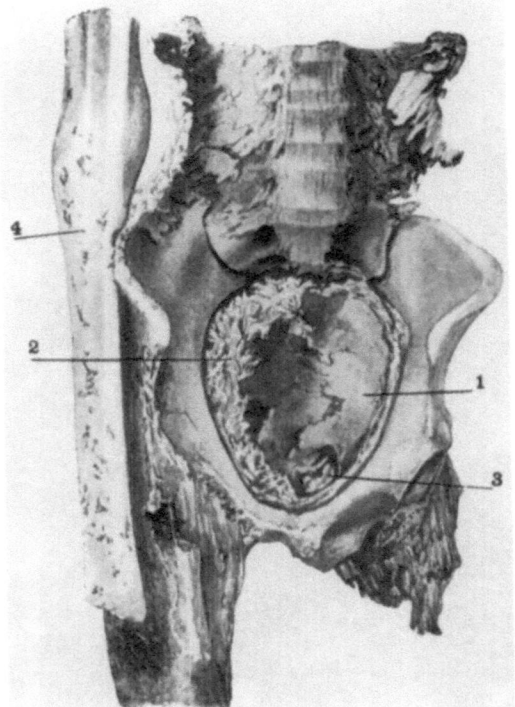
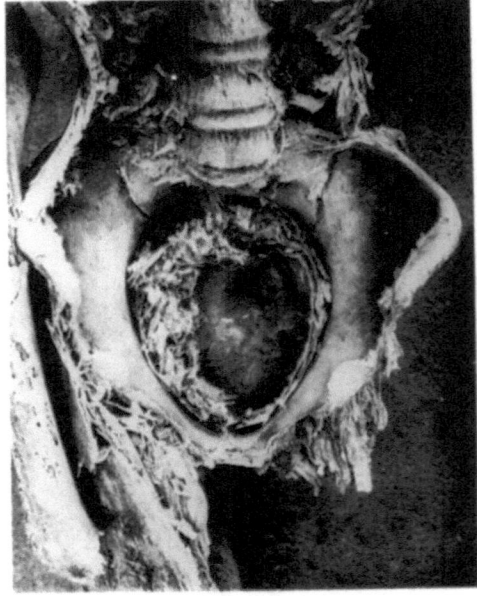

Figure 2 a   Figure 2 b

Figure 2 a. Pelvic cavity of Henhenit showing excessive anteroposterior pelvic diameter and rupture of the vagina into the bladder; *1* bladder cavity enormously dilated; *2* thickened, infected bladder mucosa; *3* large vesico-vaginal fistula; *4* right arm

Figure 2 b. Details of pelvis in 2 a. (From Derry)

work. Henhenit's mummy was examined in New York and whilst the vagina appeared normal, a mass of tissue 10 cm long, probably intestine, protruded through the anus. In 1923, the trustees of the Metropolitan Museum generously returned the mummy to the Cairo School of Medicine for detailed examination (Englebach and Derry 1942).

The body was extremely well preserved and in particular there was no abdominal incision. In all mummies of this period no attempt was made to open the abdomen through the customary left flank incision for the purpose of removing the viscera. The body showed a widely dilated vagina

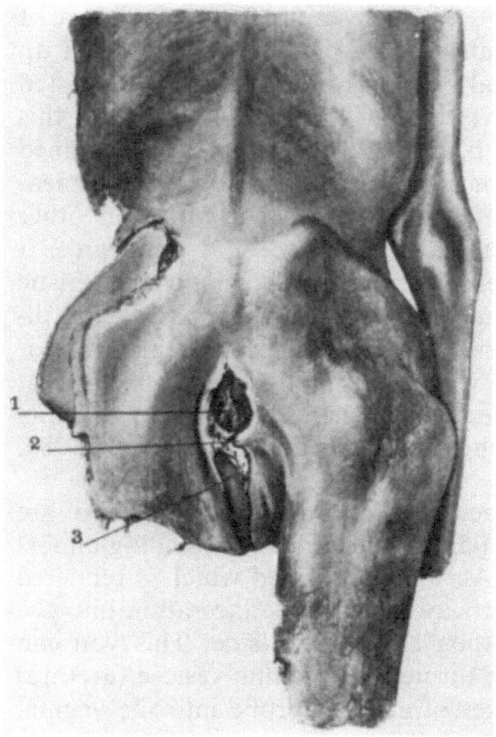

Figure 3. Posterior surface of mummy of Henhenit showing a complete perineal tear. *1* Anus; *2* perineal tear; *3* vagina. (From Derry)

and rectum, with shiny particles of resin on the inner rectal surface indicating that an oleo-resin, turpentine had been injected. When the abdominal cavity was opened, Derry discovered a rent in the bladder communicating directly with the vagina and so the exterior, and what had appeared as dilated vagina when seen through the vulva, in reality was the bladder. In addition the pelvis was an abnormal shape with a much reduced transverse diameter and the antero-posterior, exceptionally long. The pelvic brim index approximated that of apes and the pelvis illustrated a further ape-like condition, namely a high standing sacral promontory. Also, there were only four lumbar vertebrae, and six sacral (Figs. 2 a, b and 3). Even allowing for the present dried up tissues, Derry believed it would have been difficult for a fetal head to pass, and that the severe damage discovered, probably occurred at the time of parturition resulting in Henhenit's death. The injury was considered to be a tear from the vagina into the bladder due to the abnormally narrow pelvis through which the child had to be dragged by force. The vagina was discovered crushed between the distended bladder and rectum, which itself was obliterated by descent of the lower part of the large bowel which protruded outside. The presence of this dried up intestine protruding through the anal orifice outside the body, suggested an attempt had been made to remove some of the organs at least by this route. It is likely Henhenit was Nubian, and if her pelvis had been examined in isolation, it would have been considered grossly deformed the measurements corresponding to those of a chimpanzee, but with four other mummies exhibiting similar characteristics although of lesser degree, it seemed her pelvis was only an extreme example of a racial characteristic common to all five women. Only one pelvis even approximated brim diameters common in Europe. To Queen Henhenit belongs the dubious honor of having suffered the most antique vesico-vaginal fistula documented. It has not been possible to discover the present whereabouts of her mummy but presumably it is at the Cairo School of Medicine still (Dorman 1985, Harer 1986).

Pinaeus (1650) wrote: "Among accidents not rare in difficult labor are a loss of substance of the posterior part of the bladder, extending almost to the implantation of the ureters. An ulcer is formed which is rendered callous by the urine running straightway through the laceration into the sinus pudoris (upper vagina) and then escaping outside. This you can recognize by inserting a silver probe through the collum vesicae (urethra) into the bladder and the index finger of another probe into the vagina, when the two probes are made to touch."

In 1663 Hendrick van Roonhuyze of Amsterdam, published a book often referred to as the first text on operative gynecology and in 1676 it was translated into English (Figs. 4a, b). The first section entitled rupture of the bladder, gave a remarkably clear description of vesico-vaginal fistula and probably he was first to have proposed a scientific method of therapy. His innovations were:

1. Proper exposure of the fistula with a speculum.
2. Denudation exclusive of the bladder wall.
3. Approximation of the denuded edges by means of "stitching needles made of stiff swans's quill".

He proposed a method of railroading with two catheters to diagnose the fistula accurately, and described "conveying one into the ordinary urinal passage of the bladder and the other through the vagina into the rupture and bringing both together so as to perceive them by contact and sound. Also by applying the speculum so as you may see plainly with your eyes and then feel with your fingers, the rupture". He suggested that the child striving with great force to come into the world, thereby endangered the

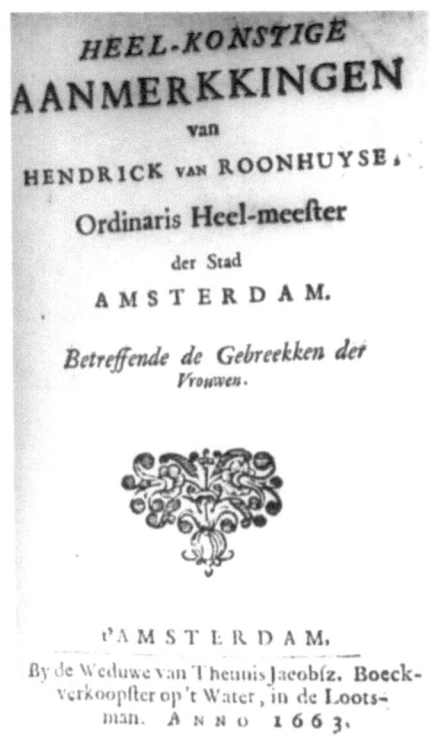

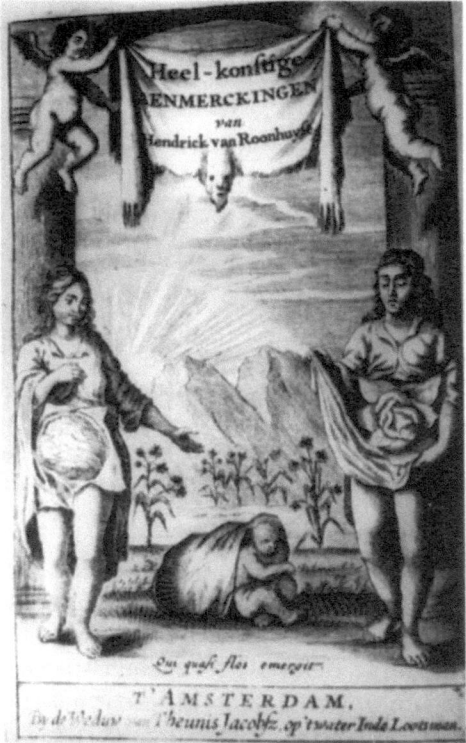

Figure 4 a   Figure 4 b

Figures 4 a, b. Title page and frontispiece of Hendrick van Roonhuyse's "Operative Gynaecology"

bladder and especially so if "diureticks" had been used to hasten the birth. The operation should be performed in the following manner: "Patient is placed on a table toward a good light with the upper part of the body covered, and the lower secured with swathing bands as is usual in the case of cutting persons of the stone." He detailed correct surgical principles and described the operation clearly: Lithotomy position, use of the speculum for proper fistula exposure, denudation of the fistulous opening with finally an approximation of the vivified edges by sharpened swan's quill pins. He preferred the swans quill pins rather than the silver or golden needles used at that time in the repair of cleft palate (Fig. 5). Following fistula closure a healing salve was applied consisting of two or three large flat wicks moistened with warm balsam oil, and the vagina was filled with suitable

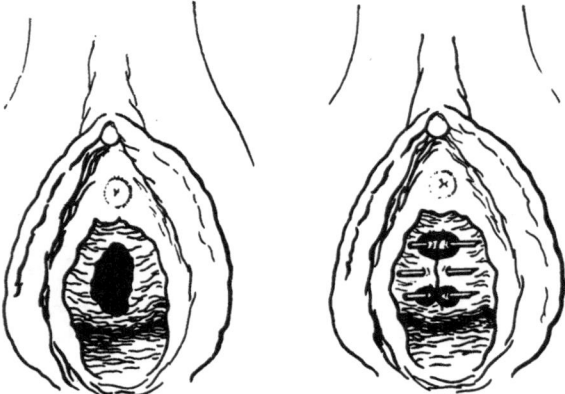

Figure 5. Van Roonhuyse's use of sharpened swan's quills was the earliest attempt at operative closure of vesico-vaginal fistula. (From Miller)

moistened sponges which swelled and exerted some pressure. "Upon removal of these compresses, the patient can void carefully but must lie still in bed on her back with the lower body elevated until cure is complete." With large defects he believed surgical cure was impossible, and devised linen compresses and "different instruments of copper or silver to be worn bandaged to the body, to catch the urine on walking or standing; but the women could not sit down with them." Undoubtedly, with such a clear and positive description, van Roonhuyze must have operated upon some patients yet much discussion was aroused by his claims, some believing the conception utterly impracticable, whilst Naegele considered the technique could be applied only to urethral injuries. Clearly this brilliant Dutch gynecologist in enunciating these important prinicples laid the foundations for future management of genital tract fistula, and although later writers modified some of these principles then added details of their own ideas of surgical correction, nevertheless the truth of his basic principles has stood the test of time.

Christoph Voelter (1679) believed excessive food and fluid intake during labor distended the rectum and vagina contributing to injury from pressure by the fetal head and advised frequent catherization during labor. To diagnose a fistula, he injected barley water into the urethra and observed whether or not fluid appeared in the vagina. He advocated immediate repair using van Roonhuyze's method and employed a retention catheter, the first reference to catheter drainage after fistula repair. Also, he first

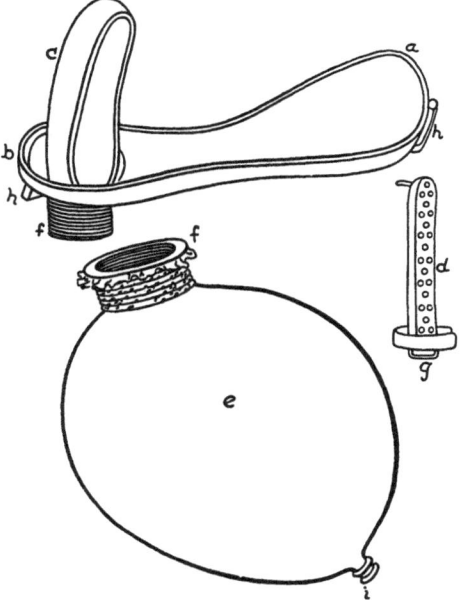

Figure 6. An early type of urinal with an intravaginal extension to fit over the fistula. (From Miller)

suggested the use of a needle holder to insert interrupted sutures of either hemp or silk.

Mauriceau (1712) who gave detailed descriptions of labor mechanisms and first described brow presentation, regarded vesico-vaginal fistula as incurable. He did not suggest surgery but hoped for spontaneous cure.

Johann Daniel Mittelhaeuser (1716) from the University of Jena, described both position and structure of the bladder and the pressure exerted by a fetal head during prolonged and difficult labor with production of bladder necrosis. To control the incontinence he suggested a wooden pessary which filled the vagina snugly. In the late 1700's, three French surgeons, Desault, Chopart and Petit, all favored conservative managment and devised various types of catheters, absorbent tampons, and urinary receptacles (Fig. 6).

Published in 1752, a posthumous text written by Swiss physician Johann Fatio, contained details of two successful bladder fistula repairs performed in 1675 and 1684 using the van Roonhuyze technique.

Many of the historical references in this chapter are taken from Howard A. Kelly (1912) "The History of Vesico-Vaginal Fistula", Norman F. Miller (1935) "Treatment of Vesico-Vaginal Fistulas" and Harvey Graham (1950) "Eternal Eve".

He spoke of "the crushing rupture of the neck of the bladder in difficult labors by which it came to pass that women could not hold their urine and must endure this wretched condition throughout life". He believed the chief cause was excessive fluid intake which greatly distended the bladder and when a difficult labor followed or if the head impacted in the pelvis, rupture or imflammation of the bladder neck occurred producing ulcerations and fistula. An inexperienced pitiless midwife could cause this injury especially by urging the birth before the bladder had been emptied or relieved by catheter. In reviewing various types of medication suggested, including pulverizing a living toad inside a new pot, with the powdered toad being carried in a little bag over the pit of the stomach, he said: "I readily grant such cures their fame and credit the statements of such distinguished men. I must, however, beg pardon when I declare that for myself I prefer to resort to surgical procedures in a recent fistula at the neck of the bladder." The patients, one aged 15 and the other 28, were placed in lithotomy position, the fistula exposed with a suitable speculum and the margins denuded with delicate sharp scissors. He used sharpened quills and linen sutures to hold the coapted raw edges together. Then the parts were dressed with balsam, protected with a pledget, and the vagina filled with an absorbent dressing. The dressings were renewed whenever the patient urinated, and both cases had healed within 14 days. So did the brilliant suggestions of van Roonhuyze bear fruit within 13 years, but for the next century and a half these precious observations were forgotten.

Levret (1766) realizing that fistula followed delayed labor which caused slough, recommended lotions and injections as soon as the slough had separated in order to secure an abundance of fresh granulations to facilitate "obturation" of the opening. Should the patient be seen later after the fistula had formed, he advocated scarification of the edges of the ulcer with a curved bistoury, using a "speculum uteri". To do this he suggested placing the patient on her knees and elbows, supported by a large pillow under the stomach, then operating from the rear.

William Smellie (1776) although he described an operation for fistula, perhaps never performed such an operation himself nor witnessed it since he added "I wish the operation may not be found impracticable."

François Deleurye (1777) favored suturing and the application of agglutinating ointment but in the event of failure, inserted a reservoir made from tin and containing a vaginal sponge, into the vagina. In 1779, Mitchell a surgeon from Wopping near London, reported spontaneous healing of a fistula to the London Medical Society. The fistula occurred 12 days after a difficult delivery, and was confirmed by injecting oil into the bladder then observing its appearance in the vagina near the bladder neck. Also, a probe introduced into the urethra passed readily into the vagina. Treatment was solely by means of a flexible retention catheter. After 3 weeks the patient was improved and cured completely by 6 months.

At the beginning of the 19th century, fresh ideas regarding treatment of vesico-vaginal fistula began to appear, and reached their zenith half a century later with the great contributions of de Lamballe, Wützer, Simon, Sims, Emmet and Bozeman. Possibly the first important step was that of Lewinski (1802) who devised a cannula which carried a concealed needle. Introduced through the urethra the cannula was held against the fistula margin so allowing the needle to be thrust through and threaded, then by withdrawing the needle, the thread was placed in position. Passing the needle through the opposite side and disengaging the thread, completed the suture. Although not put into practice, this method demonstrates the technical diversity which surgeons employed in efforts to handle this apparently hopeless malady. Desault (1804) suggested obstructing the opening of the fistula with a plug, and used a sphere of gum elastic or valve covered with wax together with a large catheter retained by means of a truss. Naegele (1812) made an extensive study of fistula, beginning with cadaver dissection and endeavored to freshen the fistula edges with scissors or bistoury without using a speculum relying on his sense of touch, a method described by Lawson Tait. Also he tried curved silver or gilt covered needles with a twisted suture. James (1813) in his "System of Midwifery" suggested the use of an elastic catheter to aid spontaneous healing and advised the application of caustic when the opening was small and freshening the edges should it be large.

Schreger (1817) appeared successful when he denuded and sutured the fistula margins with interrupted silk sutures. On the other hand, l'Allemand (1825) used silver nitrate to produce a slough and following its separation attempted to draw the eges of the fistula together with an instrument called a "hook sound". Although useless and dangerous, the method attained an undue celebrity. Samuel Hobart of Cork reported a solitary cure in 1825 and used the knee-elbow position with a special vaginal speculum. In 1829 Henry Levert of Mobile, Alabama experimented with metal ligatures "as applied to arteries" using lead, gold silver and platinum to find "not the slightest trace of inflammation existed in the neighbouring parts, on the contrary, they seemed perfectly natural". He concluded that arterial ligation with lead and other metals was free from danger and may have some peculiar advantages. In that same year, Malagodi from Bologna, Italy, cured a patient first hooking the fistula down with his finger and prepared the margins by using first the index of the right hand and then the left. He united the edges with braided sutures passed on small needles, drained the bladder through the urethra and when the opening was almost closed, it healed completely following application of caustic. Again in 1829, Roux proposed the knee-elbow position for better exposure, although this position and a gutter speculum had been used already by Levret (1766) and Schreger (1817).

When the fistula was small, Baron Dupuytren (1829) recommended that cautery should be applied yet though it succeeded occasionally in his hands, with others it failed almost uniformly. He employed lithotomy position, then introducing a large bougie into the urethra, passed it back to the fistula, enabling him to push the bladder down and forwards, bringing the fistula into view. He incised around the fistula margin, removed the whole circumference, then freed the vagina from the bladder right around the opening. This was done to increase the likelihood of union with the larger surface, and also to avoid the necessity of passing the needle through the bladder. He introduced the needle one third of an inch from the edge of the vaginal wound, and brought it out on the opposite side at the same distance. He used three sutures sufficient to close the orifice, then the threads were tied tightly. A short silver catheter was introduced into the bladder and the patient lay on her right side to prevent urine coming into contact with the repair. The patient suffered a diet of thin arrowroot, milk, water and a solution of gum arabic and the catheter was removed the following morning to prevent obstruction. After cleansing it was replaced, then removed daily for 5 days when speculum examination showed the sutures to be quite firm. The wound seemed healed with no leakage and after removing the sutures with minor difficulty, intermittent catherization was employed for a further 17 days, when she was re-examined. Finally the catheter was used 2 or 3 times each day for some weeks. Gooch (1831) alluded to a patient who recovered after a gum-elastic bottle with a sponge attached was pressed into the vagina and kept opposite the opening; but this must be regarded as a most unusual and extraordinary event. Duges of Montpellier (1831) treated a case where l'Allemand had previously failed. The fistula was situated at the bladder neck and exposure was effected with a gutter-shaped speculum then a male bladder sound brought the fistula down and into view. He seized the margin of the upper lip of the fistula with museaux forceps or a hook, freshened the edges with scissors

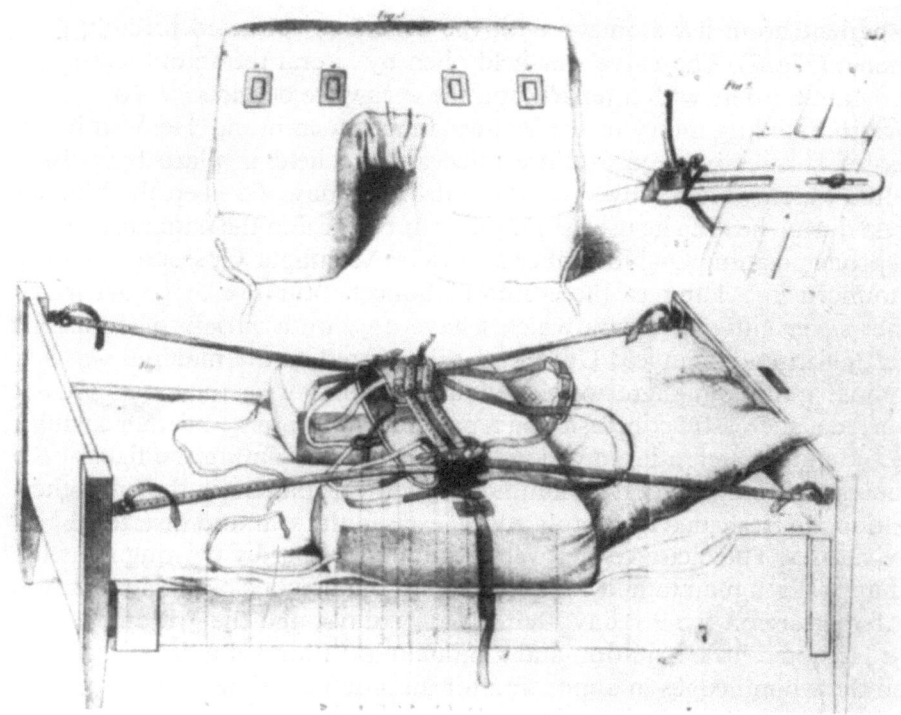

Figure 7. Wützer's bed and harness maintained the knee-chest position during prolonged vaginal surgery. (From Miller)

curved on the flat, then denuded the posterior lip by catching it with a double hook and transfixing the margins with a bistoury. A double waxed thread was passed through both fistulous margins in the direction from vesical to vaginal surface and tied. A sound was inserted and the bladder drained, but on the 3rd day, the threads were removed because of hemorrhage with consequent failure of the procedure. William Campbell (1833) of Edinburgh described a bladder neck fistula very clearly, and his experience indicated that catheter drainage with the recumbent position employed perseveringly, permanently relieved cases even when others had pronounced the patient as hopeless. Such phraseology of course does not allow the conclusion that his patients were cured.

Up until 1852 Wützer of Bonn, had obtained the signal success of curing 11 of 35 cases. In one patient he succeeded at the 33rd procedure and the name of Lucie Stich has been perpetuated as heroine and martyr in the cause of science. He chose not to use lithotomy position but preferred the patient upon her stomach with the perineum retracted forcibly by a crotchet (Fig. 7). The vulva was held open by lateral retractors. Grasping the fistula borders with a tenaculum, the eges were denuded $^1/_4$ to $^1/_3$ inch in width avoiding injury to the bladder mucus membrane. He used insect pins for sutures inserted at close intervals and held in place by twisted sutures which were removed on the 3rd or 4th day. To keep the bladder at rest during healing he used suprapubic drainage and the patient strapped in a prone position. On November 21st 1834, Montague Gosset of London, announced in a letter to the editor of Lancet, "the use of gold wire or rather silver gilt-wire suture which I have used on a variety of occasions with uniform advantage". Until then the favored suture material was silk or goose quill; but there were obvious problems with their use. Gosset reported a successful conclusion in a patient who presented with a calculus protruding through a large vesico-vaginal fistula. Dilating the fistula, the calculus was removed and 4 months later with the patient in the knee-chest position, he freshened the fistula edges, excised the scar and inserted 3 gilt-wire sutures. The incised edges were brought together by twisting the wire, and apposition maintained completely until the fistula closed. He removed the 1st suture on the 9th day, the 2nd at 12 days, and the 3rd on the 21st day. He noted little irritation and minimal ulceration yet a great ability to keep the wound edges in apposition for an indefinite time, thus increasing the chance of union. He concluded that it was in a minute and delicate operation such as closure of fistulous openings, where success depended upon speedy union of the parts, that the advantages of gilt-wire were most manifest. This then was the first description of the use of a wire suture, later to be popularized and extended by James Marion Sims. Also in 1834, Wagner of Danzig described splitting the posterior edge of the fistulous opening then placing the bevilled anterior edge into this cleft.

In 1834 Jobert de Lamballe of Paris working at about the same time and along similar lines to Sims, Emmet, and Bozeman in the United States of America, began by attempting to plug the fistula with transplanted flaps taken from the vulva, detached then twisted and sutured into place, but with few successes. In 1845, he described a most important principle called "autoplastie par glissement", wherein he detached the upper border of the fistula from the cervix in order to reduce tension when uniting the fistula and by 1849 had 13 cures but 2 deaths, due in part to the highly infected surgical wards of Parisian hospitals. Alfred Velpeau (1839) the famed professor of clinical surgery in Paris, voiced the problems that fistula surgeons were experiencing when he declared, "To abrade the borders of an opening when we do not know where to grasp them, to shut it up by means of needle and thread when we have no point apparently to which to secure them: to act upon a moveable partition placed between two cavities hidden from our sight, and upon which we can scarcely find any purchase, seems to be calculated to yield no other result than to cause unnecessary pain to the patient." Furthermore he asserted that of all cases reported as cured, there were few free from doubt.

John Peter Mettauer of Virginia, in a letter to the editor of the Boston Medical and Surgical Journal, stated that he had successfully operated upon a vesico-vaginal fistula in August 1838, a year before the case reported by Hayward. The fistula was the size of a half dollar and he performed the operation through "a hollow conoidal speculum of proper size and length." Six leaden wire sutures were used and they were tightened once only after the procedure. Following their removal in three weeks, union was firm. He claimed this to be the first successful fistula closure in the United States of America and requested the editor to confirm this fact. Furthermore, he advocated wide publicity if necessary via the newspapers for every case cured, so that the availability of cure should "be presented to individuals too delicate and modest to make known their situations, believing them incurable; and preferring concealment and seclusion from society rather than expose an incurable and disgusting infirmity". Mettauer confirmed the relationship between unrelieved obstructed labor and vesico-vaginal fistula, then described his experiences with 6 cases using the following technique: the vagina was dilated with two broad spatulae pressed firmly against the opposing sides of the passage walls and held steadily by two assistants. Denudation of the fistulous margin was the first step, whilst the wound surface was washed frequently with cold water which served to remove adhering clot and arrest blood flow. He closed the fistula with 8 metallic sutures tightened progressively by traction and twisting their free ends together. During the tightening process, a probe adjusted the fistula margins from time to time, ensuring accurate approximation without puckering or folding. The cut wires projected just beyond the vulval verge, sheathed in oiled silk to minimize irritation. A silver catheter was retained by tapes attached to a circular body bandage and on the 3rd day the wires were tightened further, again on the 7th then removed on the 13th day. Perfect union had occurred and the catheter was discarded finally after 4 weeks. One patient had had two children since, without any fistula recurrence and Mettauer believed, from his reported experience, that every vesico-vaginal fistula was curable.

Few surgeons surpassed Mettauer in daring and originality; he was amongst the foremost educators of his day; and his contributions to medical literature alone should have saved his name from oblivion. In spite of this, Mettauer is unmentioned by many medical biographers; whilst those who refer to his work do so in a very casual manner. "Sic transit gloria mundi." Mettauer's father, a young Fench surgeon named Francis Joseph Mettauer accompanied Lafayette's American expedition, and after the battle of York-town settled in Prince Edward county, Virginia, where he married Elizabeth Gaulding. John Peter Mettauer was born in 1787. Receiving his medical degree, John Mettauer returned to his native state settling in Prince Edward county near Farmville, Virginia with the resolution "though doomed to labor in the country as a practitioner, to continue my studious habits." Such was his surgical skill that patients came to him from far and wide, from the most remote regions of America and even from abroad, and at the height of his career it was not unusual for him to have as many as sixty patients under his care at any one time, with every suitable house in the neighborhood sheltering at least one patient convalescing from an operation or one awaiting his turn at the master's hands. Mettauer's operations were characterized not only by skill; but daring and originality. Undoubtedly, he was the first western surgeon to operate for cleft palate and certainly was amongst the first to undertake such operations as amputations at the shoulder, ligation of the carotid artery and resection of the superior maxilla. Probably his greatest claim to fame rested upon his being the first surgeon in the USA to operate successfully for vesico-vaginal fistula (Fig. 8).

On may 10th 1839, George Hayward a surgeon at Massachussetts General Hospital Boston, closed a vesico-vaginal fistula present for 15 years. It had occurred ten days following forceps delivery of a stillborn child which died during a three day labor, and during the entire time the patient had been unable to void. Hayward reviewed the present state of knowledge, and stated: "Such a patient has no power for retaining urine, and is rendered miserable by the excoriation and soreness thus produced and loathsome to herself by the foetor of the urine." He quoted Diffenbach who had said: "Such unhappy beings are forced to exclude themselves from society; the very atmosphere surrounding them is polluted by their presence, and even their children shun them; thus rendered miserable both morally and physically, they yield themselves a prey to apathy; or a pious resignation alone saves them from self destruction." Hayward noted that the degree of suffering however was not the same in all patients, but depended upon the site of the fistula. His technique included lithotomy position and introducing a large whalebone bougie through the urethra

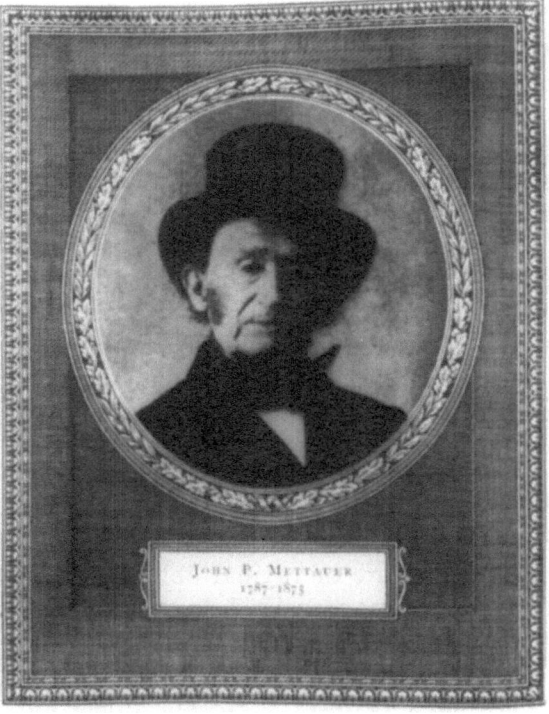

Figure 8. John Peter Mettauer. (From Willis)

into the bladder to force the fistula down so it could be seen and handled. Dissection began with the removal of a narrow margin from the whole circumference of the fistula orifice, then the vaginal wall was freed from the bladder all around the opening, partly to improve the likelihood of union by presenting a larger surface, but also to avoid the necessity of passing the needle through the bladder. The needle was introduced $^1/_3$ inch from the wound edge and passed through "the membrane of the vagina and cellular membrane beneath and brought out at the opposite side at about an equal distance". He used as many sutures as necessary to close the fistula orifice, and they were tied tightly. A short silver catheter was left in the bladder. It is important to note that Dupuytren (1829) and Hayward (1839) detached the bladder from the vagina many years before the layered technique described and attributed to Mackenrodt. Hayward recognized that obstacles to success in fistula surgery were numerous, in particular, "the narrow space in which the operation is to be performed, the disposition of urine to pass between the lips of the wound, the proximity of the ureters, the great secretion of mucus by the inner coat of the bladder wall calculated to interfere with the union of the parts and the want of readiness with which mucus surfaces take an adhesive inflammation, are all factors likely to defect any operation however well it may be done".

Vidal de Cassis (1841), who invented a spring forceps for approximating the fistula edges said operations for closing a fistula were numerous which proved their difficulty in succeeding. He divided available methods into direct and indirect, the direct attempting to obliterate the opening by compression, cauterization or suture, whilst the indirect operated on surrounding parts, ignoring the fistula. He believed only a very small recently formed fistula would respond to the direct method and his experience of the indirect method involved partial colpocleisis performed in 1813 following accidental cauterization of the posterior vaginal wall with silver nitrate, causing enormous vaginal swelling and adhesion between the anterior and posterior vaginal walls, yet it succeeded for only 15 days. Nevertheless in 1832 he demonstrated his procedure of vaginal obliteration in public, upon a menopausal patient. Furthermore in 1844 Auguste Berard repeated the Vidal operation for vesico-vaginal fistula upon a 30-year-old female with a very large fistula and although the result was encouraging initially, the patient died from peritonitis 17 days later. The operation raised a tempest. Later, Sims condemned the technique in which "the bladder and vagina became a grand compound receptacle of urine and menstrual secretions".

Blasius (1841) in his Handbuch der Chirurgie (2nd edition) gave an excellent historical outline of methods of treatment to date, the present situation indicating that successes were few and failures frequent. No well-defined rules for operative procedure could be laid down. Accordingly, he described methods in use which involved denudation of the fistula margin and union by suture, including the dovetailed suture very similar to that recommended by Pancoast of Philadelphia. Blasius's account was described by Howard Kelly (1912) as "a model of clearness in stating a difficult problem."

Diffenbach (1845) belongs with the history of fistula due to the imperishable classic description he wrote in his despair, picturing the wretched condition of these abandoned sufferers. He tried all methods of treatment including cautery, freshening the flaps, transplantation and purse-string sutures. He made a classical denudation, united the wound margins using silk sutures 6 to the inch and drained the bladder by catheter for 8 days.

In spite of his best efforts, he was never able to cure a large fistula, and exclaimed: "I have operated on one woman 18 times and discharged her unrelieved. I have filled entire wards with these wretched women gathered from all countries; I have exhausted every measure and I have been able to cure but few of them."

Metzler of Prague (1846) described an instrument like the Sims speculum used to retract the posterior vaginal wall, in order to expose the anterior. He used the knee-elbow position, lifted the posterior vaginal wall with the speculum and freshening the fistula edges with curved scissors, approximated them with gilded needles held in place by clamps of shot. In 1847 Joseph Pancoast professor of anatomy in Jefferson Medical College, Philadelphia, reported two cases cured by a tongue and grooved incision, known as the split flap method, and the wound was adjusted by silk thread plastic sutures.

Maisoneuve of Paris (1848) reported a cure where the whole anterior vaginal wall had disappeared, using the relaxation incision of Jobert de Lamballe at the vaginal vault, and another which he called the urethro-pubic incision by which the urethra was loosened from the under surface of the pubis. In 1851 he used and described accurately a procedure very similar to the Schuchardt parasacral incision in which levator and coccygeus muscles were divided into the ischiorectal fossa and opened widely, so that when the rectum had been forced back, the operative field in the pelvis became almost superficial, thereby making a difficult fistula accessible. In 1864 he wrote: "I then cut the perineum in its whole extent at the left side of the rectum which I pushed back and I prolonged the incision towards the ischiadic incisure; by that large opening I could easily advance to the ground of the vaginal cul-de-sac." Also, it should be mentioned that far too little credit has been given to Maisoneuve who, following on bladder mobilization described by Dupuytren and Hayward, first carried out complete mobilization of the bladder in the manner advocated later by Mackenrodt.

In 1852 James Marion Sims published his classical article on the treatment of vesico-vaginal fistula, ushering in an era of great interest in the problem together with great controversy in management.

The antiquity of obstetric fistula is well-documented, and ancient physicians while being well aware of its cause, admitted the impossibility of cure. The anatomical defect was proven first by Felix Platter (1597) who passed a probe through the fistula, and this situation remained until the momentous work of Hendrick van Roonhuyze, the acknowledged father of present day fistula surgery. His genius began the change from hope-

lessness of the past to an optimism for the future by describing diagnostic
features of bladder fistula, and enumerating some of the principles involved
in surgical correction, especially adequate exposure, freshening fistula edges
then their accurate coaption. Nevertheless he believed larger defects were
incurable. These surgical principles were put to the test successfully by
both Johann Fatio and Christoph Voelter but then the mists of time closed
over and blotted out this illumination, and much like Briar Rose in the
fairy tale, these great advances lay forgotten for nearly a hundred and fifty
years. During this time, contributions from eminent surgeons consisted
only of a series of statements of despair and futility in their inability to
cope with the problem, the only practical offerings being symptomatic
treatment in the form of receptacles and plugs designed merely to soak up
urine or staunch the continual leakage. Following these nonproductive
years slowly the principles began to emerge once more. Catheter drainage
originally proposed by Voelter came to be mentioned more and more,
access to the fistula both for diagnosis and therapy was improved by the
knee-elbow, knee-chest, lithotomy and prone positions, and various ma-
noeuvers to bring the fistula into view and down to the surgeon were
described. For this purpose a variety of vaginal speculums, retractors,
hooks, tenacula, sounds and bougies were devised and in addition, suture
materials changed from birds' quills to linen, silk and eventually non-reactive
metal. Bladder mobilization truly commenced with the "autoplastie par
glissement" of Lamballe (1834) enhanced by the work of Dupuytren, Hayward, Maisoneuve and eventually Mackenrodt (1894) upon whose shoulder
the honor for the idea has fallen. Prior to this advance, scar excision and
freshening the fistula circumference had been well-tried by many surgeons.
Vidal de Cassis (1813) attempted colpocleisis as a method of dealing with
the large fistula.

All these attempts played a role in helping establish a complete picture
of the many facets concerned in fistula diagnosis and managment and most
importantly, to firm up the principles of surgical attack as accepted today.

In 1838, John Mettauer, Virginia reported closure of a vesico-vaginal
fistula to the editor of the Boston Medical Journal and this has been
accepted as the first successful case in the United States of America. In
addition to his surgical skills he employed irrigation of the surgical area
to facilitate dissection and accuracy of mucosal inversion during bladder
closure.

Thus the stage was set with most of the surgical principles defined
awaiting the master touch of Sims and his associates. Prior to Sims only
an occasional succcess had been reported, and there was an evident inability

to repeat this in a series of patients. It was Sims' genius which enabled him to utilize all the important surgical principles already enunciated, together with a well-defined meticulous technique which included painstaking care before, during, and after the surgery. Accordingly the contributions of Sims, Emmet and Bozeman need to be seen against this historical backdrop since their skills, for the first time, put the technique of fistula surgery on a plane never before realized or even anticipated, so success became much more predictable.

2

James Marion Sims (1813–1883) and the First Fistula Hospital

C. Lee Buxton (1968) wrote: "Dynamic, vital, imaginative, sometimes contentious, always filled with dedication to a burning mission, this ever gentlemany physician by professional and personal attributes of permanent quality, helped create gynaecology as a speciality. His dramatic surgical success with vesico-vaginal fistula is the accomplishment for which he is best known, but the qualities of stubborn dedication and persistence revealed in his quest for success in this operation, are a more profound revelation of the man than the operation itself."

It is difficult for the modern generation of gynecologists to realize how great an influence James Marion Sims exerted upon the world of surgery. In 1883, a formal assessment of his importance in the development of gynecology appeared in the British Medical Journal: "On November 13 last there died at New York a man who bears a name that will ever be identified with gynaecology; indeed Dr. J. Marion Sims must be considered as the establisher of that branch of medical science which before his day had been looked upon as a mere accessory of obstetrics." "The life and work of Sims should give heart to the young surgeon. By patience, sheer industry and a tenacious purpose, he rose from an obscure existence in a remote country district to be the most renowned figure in the surgical profession, loved and honoured at home and abroad. To take infinite pains; to develop the capacity for hard work; to keep everlastingly at it; to do one thing well; not merely to win success, but to deserve it—these are attributes of genius. And James Marion Sims was the surgical genius of his age (Royster 1922)."

No surgeon has achieved so wide a distinction nor such universal acclaim as Sims, whose name and fame were known throughout the civilized world. Heralded in all the countries of Europe, he received decorations from the governments of France, Portugal, Spain, Belgium and Italy, and through him American surgery was carried to the four corners of the earth.

Born on January 25th, 1813 near Hanging Rock Creek, Lancaster County, South Carolina, James Marion Sims was the eldest in a family of eight. Descended from English and Scottish forbears, his paternal great-grandfather, Sherrod Sims was born in Virginia in 1730, the son of a colonist who had arrived some years earlier from England. Sims' father John was orphaned aged 14 but overcame the handicap of an absent education later to become storekeeper, tavern proprietor, county sheriff, surveyor and farmer. Marion Sims grew to manhood in Lancaster, his first school being a primitive log cabin, where flogging was an accepted form of discipline. Later he attended the Franklin Academy and prepared for admission to the College of South Carolina, at Columbia. Aged 19, Sims was not remarkable for character traits which might have distinguished him from his peers, but his scholastic standing was fairly high. He was described as having a handsomely chiselled face, a small and delicate physique with a genial smile and buoyant disposition. Not wishing either to follow his mother's preference for the church, or his father's for the law, he chose medicine, a decision made without real enthusiasm, and began the study of anatomy and surgery as an apprentice to Dr. B. C. Jones, a practitioner of Lancaster. He registered for a course of lectures at the Medical College in Charleston, South Carolina, and graduated in 1834 aged 21. In 1835 he gained an M.D. from Jefferson Medical College, but confessed he had learned very little medicine. He entered practice in Lancaster with a set of surgical instruments, seven books and a chest full of medicines. After two months he had two patients and two deaths, both infants, who succumbed to "cholera infantum" and so discouraged was Sims that he moved to Mt. Meigs, Alabama in October 1835, switching his practice from pediatrics to obstetrics by accepting a Mrs. Fitzgreene who had given birth to a daughter several days before and now suffered puerperal sepsis. This patient also died; but from then his practice blossomed and in 1836 he married his childhood sweetheart Theresa Jones daughter of the Dr. Jones with whom he had served his early clerkship. A recent visit to Mt. Meigs with Dr Felix Tankersley showed a pleasant rural area, swampy in places and a delightful old church perhaps near to the house occupied by the Sims family; but of which, regrettably there is now no trace (Fig. 9 a). One year later he moved to Cubahatchee, 10 miles east of Mt. Meigs to practice with Dr. Blakney and admitted to an annual income of $ 3,000. During 1838 he received an offer from a Philadelphia business man to become a clothing merchant in Vicksburg, Mississippi which he accepted, quickly selling his home, however the venture fell through, so buying another house he returned to medical practice with Dr. Blackney. The malarial-ridden

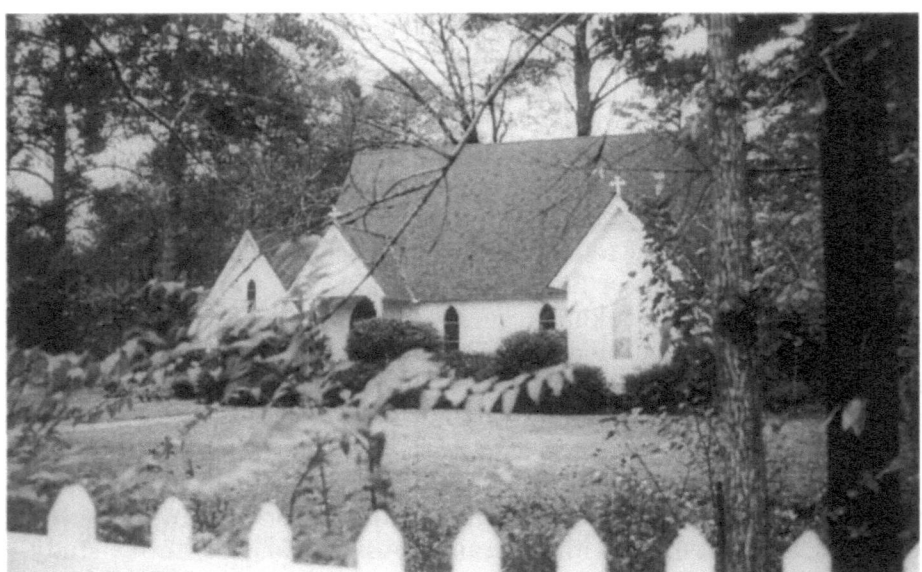

Figure 9 a. The church at Mt.Meigs

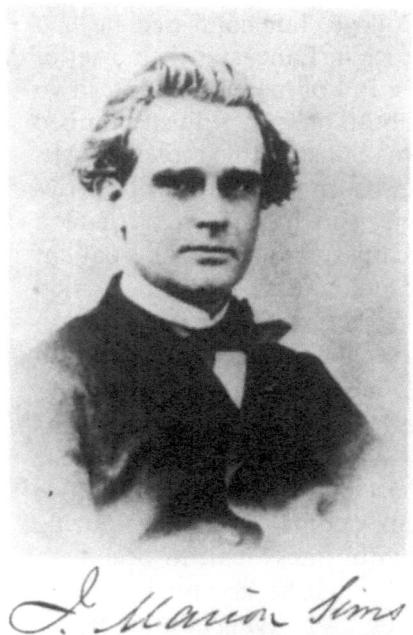

Figure 9 b. The young James Marion Sims

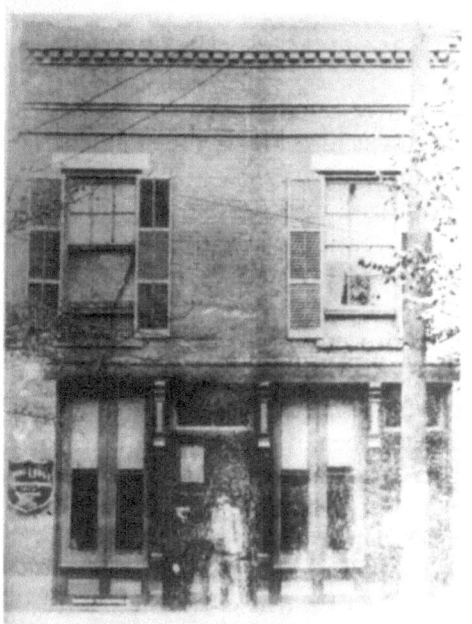

Figure 10 a

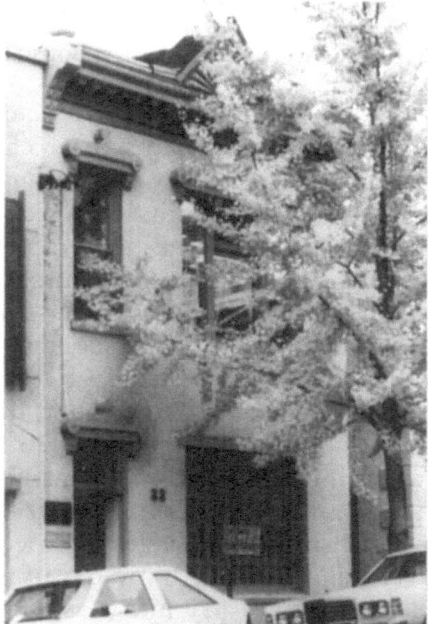

Figure 10 b

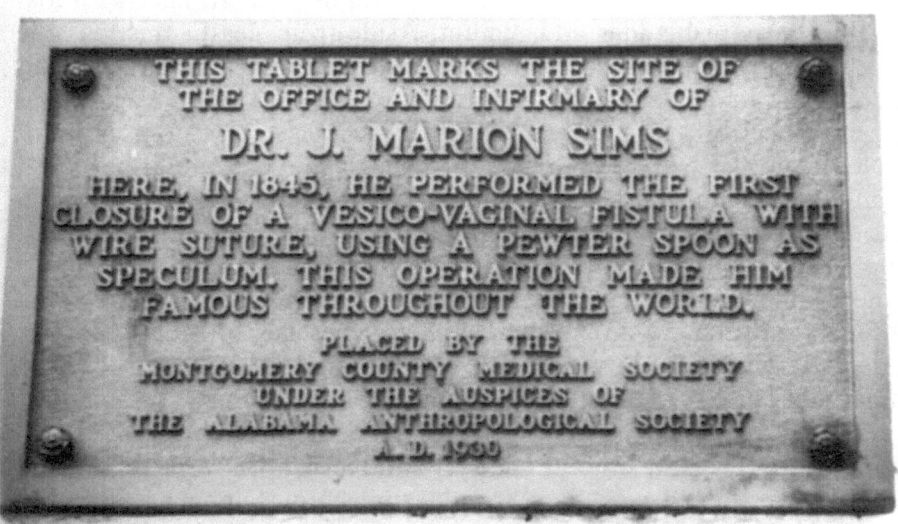

Figure 10 c

Figure 10 a–c. a The Perry Street Office as it was about 1890 and photographed by Dr. Thigpen. The building was occupied by a plumber but had been identified by Dr. Henry who was still living in Montgomery and was Sims' last surviving student, and instructed in that very office. – **b** The office now. – **c** The wall plaque which marks the site of Sims' hospital

swamps about Cubahatchee affected the entire Sims family and in 1840 following a malaria epidemic which nearly cost him his life, he moved to Montgomery, Alabama—a thriving metropolis of 4,000—where he enhanced his reputation as a surgeon by performing the first operation in the south for strabismus, the first successful treatment of club foot in that region, as well as a bold venture in plastic surgery to improve a young woman's hare lip. He used a four-wheeled vehicle to make his rounds, with a small negro boy at his side, and a medicine box and case of surgical instruments at his feet (Fig. 9 b). In corner of the yard behind his office, which still stands in Perry Street, Montgomery, he erected a single storey eight bed hospital later increased to 16 and here began experiments directed towards the cure of vesico-vaginal fistula, a condition considered incurable (Figs. 10 a, b, c). Early in June 1845 he had encountered his first vesico-vaginal fistula when called by a colleague, Dr. Henry, to a 17-year-old slave, Anarcha, in her third day of labor. He described it in his own words in "The Story of My Life" (1884), "The child's head was so impacted in the pelvis, that the labor pains had almost entirely ceased yet without any great efforts the child was brought away with forceps. The patient rallied from the confinement and seemed to be recovering until five days following delivery when there was an extensive sloughing of the soft parts with loss of control of both bladder and rectum. Aside from death, this was the worst accident that could have happened to the poor young girl. I found an enormous slough spreading from the posterior wall of the vagina and another thrown off from the anterior wall—the case was hopelessly incurable. I told her employer that she would not die but would never get well and that he should take good care of her as long as she lives. Although I had now practiced medicine for ten years I had never yet before seen a case of vesico-vaginal fistula and I looked upon it as a surgical curiosity although a most unfortunate one. Within the next two months I had seen both Betsy and Lucy, young women with large fistulae." In July 1845, Dr. Harris of Lowndes County sent Betsy to him and in August, Mr. Tom Zimmerman, an old friend of Cubahatchee days sent Lucy.

At about this time he answered an emergency call from a woman complaining of pressure on both bladder and rectum following a fall from a horse. Mrs. Merrill was 46 years old and stout weighing nearly 200 pounds and earned a living for herself and ne'er do well husband by taking in laundry. While returning home by pony, clutching a bundle of clothes, the horse was frightened by a hog when passing a pig sty and jumped sideways unseating his rider who landed flat on her buttocks. She had no broken bones yet lay in bed complaining of a sense of tenesmus in both

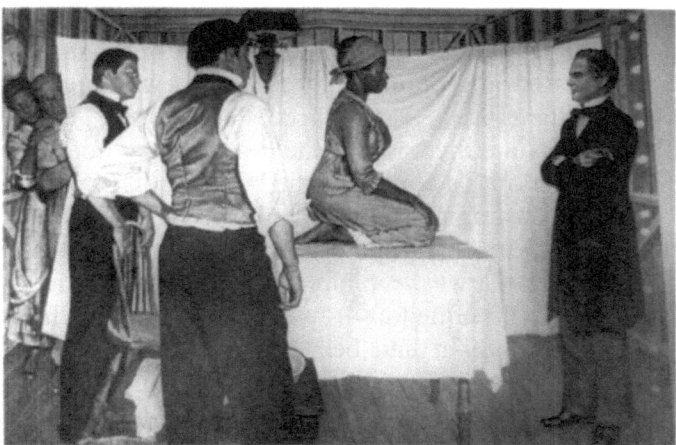

Figure 11. Painting depicting the scene at the hospital with Sims about to examine Betsy with the pewter spoon, aided by two medical students. Presumably the other two patients are Lucy and Anarcha

bladder and rectum. He wrote: "By digital examination I discovered a retroverted uterus and remembering what Dr. Prioleau at Charleston Medical College had told me, I placed the patient in the genu-pectoral position and rather than introduce one finger into the rectum and the other into the vagina, I introduced both middle and index fingers into the vagina, and immediately touched the uterus. I commenced making strong efforts to push it back and thus I turned my hand with the palm upward, then downward, and pushing with all my might, when suddenly I could not feel the womb or the wall of the vagina. I could touch nothing at all and wondered what it all meant. It was as if I had put my two fingers into a hat and worked them around without touching the substance of it. Whilst I was wondering what it all meant, the patient Mrs. Merrill said: "Why Doctor I am relieved." Suddenly there was an explosion as though there had been an escape of air from the bowel, and she was extremely mortified and began to apologize, but I said that it was not from the bowel but from the vagina and it has explained now what I did not understand before. I said to myself if I can place the patient in that position and distend the vagina by the pressure of air so as to produce such a wonderful result as this, why can I not take the incurable case of vesico-vaginal fistula which now seems so incomprehensible and put the girl into this position so as to be able to see exactly the relations of the surrounding tissues."

Sim's observation that in the knee-chest position air would rush into and balloon the vagina as soon as the vulval orifice was open, was vital to his further development of fistula surgery. Fired with enthusiasm he hastened back to his hospital stopping only to buy a large pewter spoon and collect two medical students (Fig. 11). He placed Betsy in the genu-pectoral position with a student on either side of the pelvis to lay hold of the nates and pull them open. Before he could get the bent spoon into the vagina, the air rushed in with a puffing noise dilating the vagina to its full extent. "Introducing the bent handle of the spoon, I saw everything as no man had ever seen before. The fistula was as plain as the nose on a man's face. The edges were clear and well-defined and distinct, and the opening could be measured as accurately as if it had been cut out of a piece of plain paper. I said at once why cannot these things be cured. It seems to me there is nothing to do but pare the edges of the fistula, bring it together nicely, introduce a catheter in the neck of the bladder, and drain the urine continually and the case will be cured." He increased the hospital to 16 beds, then made a proposition to the owners of the negro slaves, that he would agree not to perform any experiment or surgery on either of them which might endanger their lives. He offered this free, but the owners had to pay their taxes and clothe them. It took Sims three months to have necessary instruments made and gather the patients together. Surgery was performed first on Lucy without anesthesia of course, but the poor girl on her knees bore the operation with great heroism and bravery. In front of a dozen doctors who came to observe, Sims succeeded in closing the fistula in about one hour. To drain urine from the bladder, he used a piece of sponge in the bladder neck with a silk string acting as a capillary tube. Five days later, the patient was very ill and everything had to be removed, so cutting all the sutures loose, he attempted to remove the sponge from the bladder; but it was impacted due to infiltration with calcareous matter, and there was no choice but to pull it out by force. Ten days later Lucy was fully recovered and reexamination showed the enormous fistula had disappeared, replaced by two little openings in the line of union across the vagina.

A common stumbling block to successful fistula surgery had been difficulty with visual examination but Sims had now achieved this with the genu-pectoral position and pewter spoon. The next step to success was an appropriate suture material together with the ability to tie the suture firmly, and his experiments in this regard dragged on for over four years. The idea of clamping a small lead shot onto the suture came to him whilst pondering on the problem in the early hours of the morning, when as a boy, he recalled fixing sinkers to his fishing line in this fashion. The technique was tried first in November 1848 and allowed him to fix the sutures securely at a much high level than his fingers could reach, but still success eluded him until he began to use silver wire sutures. Unaware of the work of Levert or Gosset, he was walking from his house to the hospital when he noticed "a little bit of brass wire in the yard, very fine and such as was formerly used as springs in suspenders before the days of India-rubber". His jeweller made a similar wire of silver for him and he used this in the successful operation on Anarcha. Anarcha alone had undergone 29 operative procedures. Gradually he changed from silk to lead and finally silver wire drawn as fine as horse hair and at the 30th operation on Anarcha on the 21st June 1849 the fistula was sealed completely. He wrote: "On the 21st June 1849, it was done. A young colored woman who had never murmured at the preceding failures was placed on the operating table for the 30th time and the silver wire sutures were applied with the leaden bars and perforated shot ... and on the 8th day the parts were perfectly healed. I shall not dwell upon my feelings at this time."

Sims was aware others had been successful with fistula surgery, quoting Hayward, Pancoast, Mettauer and Lamballe who had operated many times but with few successes. Although Hayward reported a cure in 1839, by 1951, he had performed a further 19 operations but with only two successes. Sims operated 50 times in four years without success, but following the first success he uniformly closed vesico-vaginal fistulae, whereas with other surgeons succcess had been more or less accidental when cure was achieved (Burford Word 1972).

Sims' great achievement was not priority in curing vesico-vaginal fistula, but in perfecting and popularizing a technique simple in principle and more nearly universally applicable than any other previously devised, and both speculum and the silver wires were very important features. Repeat success indicated that when this technique was used correctly, primary union became the rule and not the exception. Emmet (1884) wrote: "What had been done, fell on barren soil, bore no fruit, was not appreciated and was destined to be forgotten. From Dr. Sims' hand the operation was accepted by the profession; it was immediately put into successful practice, and to the present day it has not been materially modified for the better in either its principles or its mode of execution." Within weeks after success with Anarcha, he utilized the same technique to cure all patients in his hospital. In January 1852 his classic paper "The Treatment of Vesico-Vaginal Fistula" was published in the American Journal of Medical Sciences and in this paper Sims summarized his views on management enunciating the principles of surgical correction for which he is remembered.

"Vesico-vaginal fistula" he said, "was produced generally by tedious labur, the impacted fetal head jamming the anterior vaginal parieties against the pubic symphysis, to obstruct the circulation of the parts and result in a slough of greater or lesser extent, according to the degree and duration of the impaction. Also fistula may follow prolonged retention of a vaginal pessary, a calculus, abscesses and venereal ulcerations. Incontinence of urine following tedious labor after a lapse of 1–15 days always will prove its existence, the clothes and bedding of the unfortunate patient being constantly saturated with the discharge exhaling a disagreeable effluvium alike disgusting to herself and repulsive to others. The accident is never fatal; but it might well be imagined that a lady of keen sensibility so afflicted and excluded from all social enjoyment might prefer death."

He classified fistulae into four distinct types: urethro-vaginal, bladder neck fistulae with destruction of the trigone, those involving the body of the bladder of which Velpeau had said, "there is no fact up to the present time which proves indisputably that they have ever been cured", and finally utero-vesical, the opening communicating with the uterine cavity. In a brief historical survey, he indicated odd cases had been cured; but since they were so few, no general principles of treatment had emerged and certain success in any single instance could not be predicted. The great difficulty had been applying the suture to the fistula, and accordingly a number of clumsy and complicated instrumental apparatuses had been designed. Other surgeons had endeavored to improve different stages of the procedure, and Sanson, even proposed enlarging the urethra by incision, to permit his finger to pass along the urethra into the bladder, merely to depress the fistula towards the vulval opening! Sims agreed that cauterization had little chance of success particularly in fistulae of any size. He was properly scathing about the operation designed by Vidal de Cassis for "obturation of the vulva" whereby the bladder and vagina became a giant compound receptacle for urine and menstrual secretions. Predecessors whom he praised were Mettauer who used "leaden" sutures, and had cured several cases, and Jobert de Lamballe the author of "autoplastie par glissement", who had achieved a greater success than any other surgeon. Sims concluded "that all that is worth knowing on the subject is due to America and France; whilst German and British surgery have done comparatively nothing for the amelioration of this loathsome and troublesome disease." He gave due acknowledgement to Hayward whom he believed had first closed a fistula in the United States of America in 1839 and Pancoast of Philadelphia who had operated successfully on two patients utilizing a tongue and groove principle to draw together the fistula edges.

Sims claimed originality "for the discovery of a method by which the vagina can be thoroughly explored and the operation easily performed: for the introduction of a new suture apparatus, which lies embedded in the tissues for an indefinite period without danger of cutting its way out, as do silk ligatures: and for the invention of a self-retaining catheter which can be worn with greatest comfort by the patient during the whole process of the treatment". However, as mentioned previously, none of these observations or discoveries, although made independently by him could be considered as original. The major portion of his paper dealt with the operative position of the patient, management of the fistula edges, suture apparatus, self-retaining catheter and the postoperative management. The patient knelt on the table with her nates elevated and head and shoulders depressed. The knees were 6–8 inches apart with the thighs at right angles to the table, and all clothing was loosened thoroughly. An assistant on either side retracted the buttocks, their fingers extending to the labia majora and in this position the abdominal and pelvic viscera fell towards the epigastric region, air entered the vagina stretching it to its utmost limits, affording an easy view of the fistula. Exposure was facilitated by introducing the lever speculum into the vagina, lifting the perineum upwards (Figs. 12 a, b). He advised having two or three different sizes of lever speculum and suggested that the speculum should widen a little as it approached its end, making it somewhat in the shape of a duck's bill (Fig. 13). The concavity of the speculum was highly polished to reflect light and in addition a small slightly convex spatula was needed occasionally to press the urethra down towards the symphysis pubis, when endeavoring to detect small fistulae near the trigone. "A delicate tenaculum and a sharp pointed knife alone are necessary, the tenaculum hooking up and elevating the edge of the fistula, while the point of the knife is applied to separate the parts so raised. The process is continued until the edge of the opening is well-vivified all around. The denudation should be $1/4$ to 1 inch wide" and he commented, "that often the common mistake was not removing enough of the callous edge." "There is no point in removing any of the bladder mucosa unless it is much altered in character and projects through the fistula into the vagina. Prolapse of the bladder into the wound can be nullified by passing a curved metal bougie through the urethra to retract the bladder. Alternatively, a piece of soft sponge rubber pushed into the bladder will be effective. A small sponge on the end of a piece of whalebone is useful to mop up blood during the scarification process." He stated: "I cannot lay too much stress on the great necessity in perfecting well this part of the

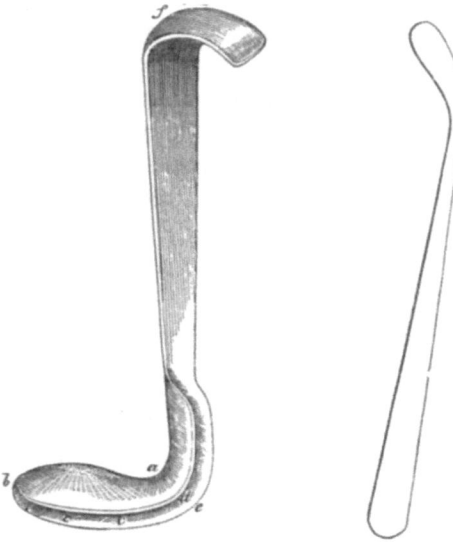

Figure 12 a

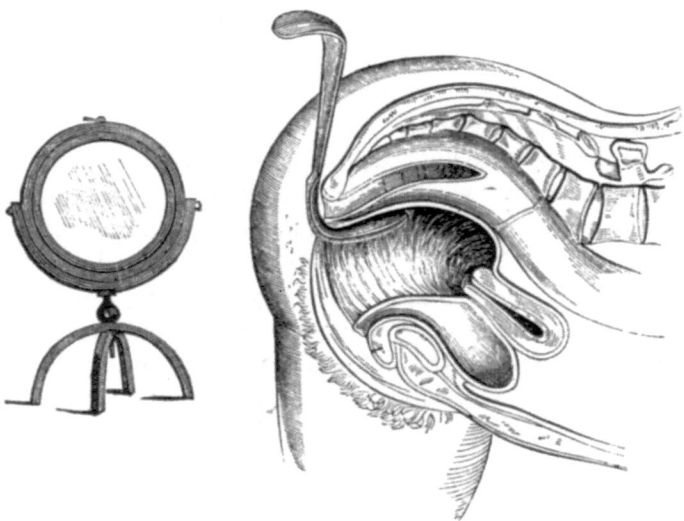

Figure 12 b

Figures 12 a, b. With the patient in the knee-chest position, the lever speculum and spatula were used to display the fistula, illuminated by an 8–10 inch glass placed on a table by the window, and adjusted by the assistant to direct light into the vagina. (From Sims)

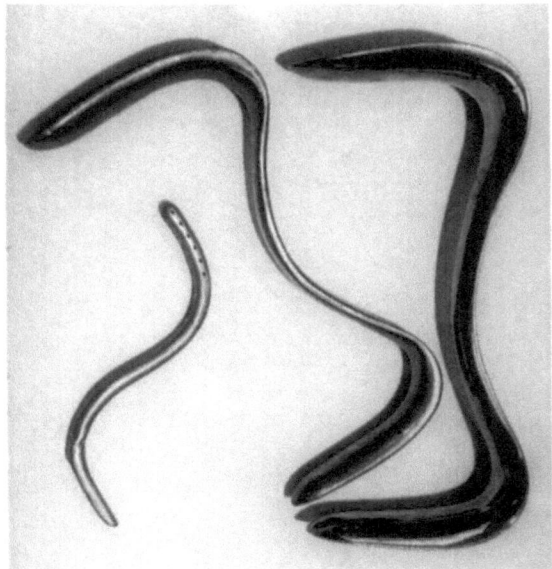

Figure 13. Sims' speculums and sigmoid catheter. (From the Reynolds Historical Library—the University of Alabama at Birmingham)

operation, for upon a proper and free denudation of the fistulous orifice, success or failure will mainly depend."

He termed his suture the "clamp suture", being composed of small annealed silver wire drawn to about the size of horse hair, and fastened to cross bars which acted as clamps, embracing the parts between them in close apposition. He claimed if properly applied, the suture never ulcerated and always could be removed by means of scissors, hooks and forceps. He noted that passage of his L-shaped needle through the anterior edge of the fistulous opening was quite easy; but to facilitate its passage through the yielding nature of the posterior margin, required a special support and he devised a blunt hook placed flatwise just beyond the spot at which the needle was to emerge (Fig. 14a). Initially he passed silk stitches, then replaced them with the silver wire, passing the distal ends of the wire through

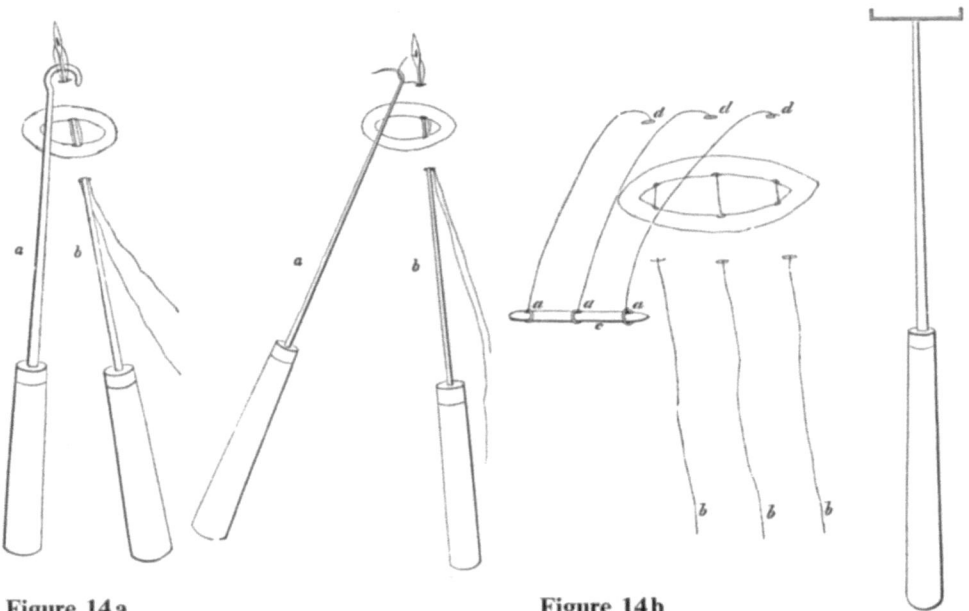

Figure 14a   Figure 14b

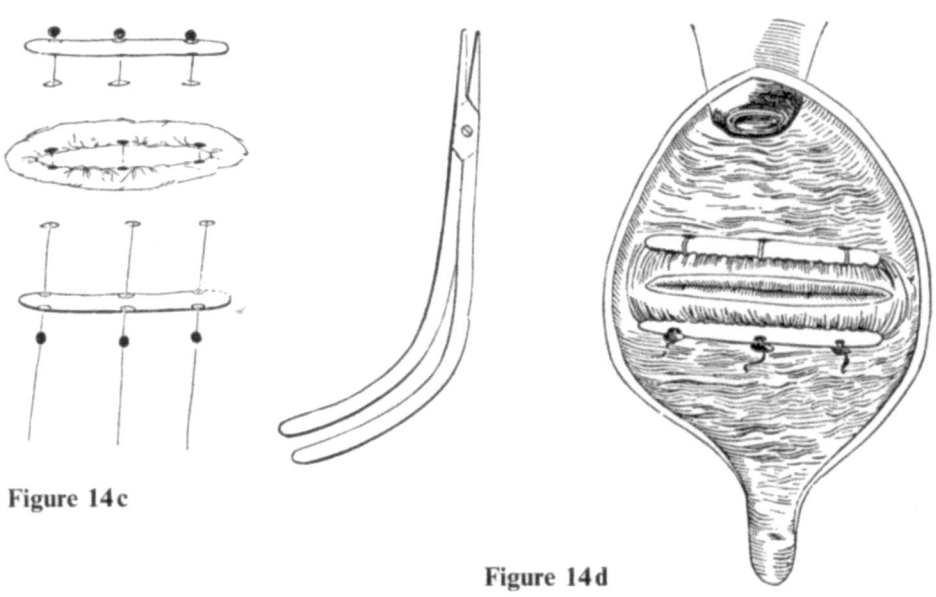

Figure 14c

Figure 14d

small oblong holes in the bar to suit the distances between the points of suture, then the wires were fastened to the bar or clamp by being turned twice about it (Fig. 14 b). The second bar was pressed onto the proximal end of the wires and pushed along them into the vagina until it occupied a position in front of the fistula corresponding exactly to that behind it (Fig. 14 c). Pushing against the proximal clamp brought the denuded edges of the fistula into such close contact that "it would be difficult to enter a common sized probe between them". The force necessary to tighten the clamps depended upon the operator's judgement. A small perforated birdshot was passed along each wire close against the proximal clamps and with the wire held securely the shot was compressed firmly with a long strong pair of forceps and then the excess wire was cut and the ends bent over effectively to prevent their slipping off (Figs. 14 d and 15).

Reviewing previous methods of bladder drainage, Sims remarked that "should a single drop of urine find its way through the fistulous orifice, it would be sure to be followed by more and so eventually a failure". Initially he used a long narrow piece of sponge for drainage, then a gum-elastic bougie but finally settled for a large silver catheter curved in opposite directions to give it a signoid form. "When such a catheter was well-fitted to the patient, it could be worn with great ease and never would turn or slip, and it mattered not whether she lay on her back or side. It was perfectly self-retaining (Fig. 16). He was a great advocate for large doses of pain-killer particularly laudanum. "Old fistula cases were generally quite used to it, and those weren't soon learnt of its beneficial effects. It calmed the nerves, inspired hope, relieved the scalding of the urine, prevented a craving for food, produced constipation, subdued inflammatory action and assisted

---

Figure 14 a–d

a Passage of the needle through anterior and posterior fistula edges, aided by the blunt hook, then a tenaculum hooked up the wire suture and the needle was withdrawn.

b Distal ends of the wire suture passed through the bar, which was then pulled against the vaginal wall and positioned accurately, using the broad fork which acted as a pulley for the sutures.

c Second bar fitted onto the proximal ends of the silver wire sutures and perforated bird shot passed along each suture, and when the bars were sited correctly, the strong forceps compressed the shot.

d The closed fistula with the suturing apparatus. (From Sims)

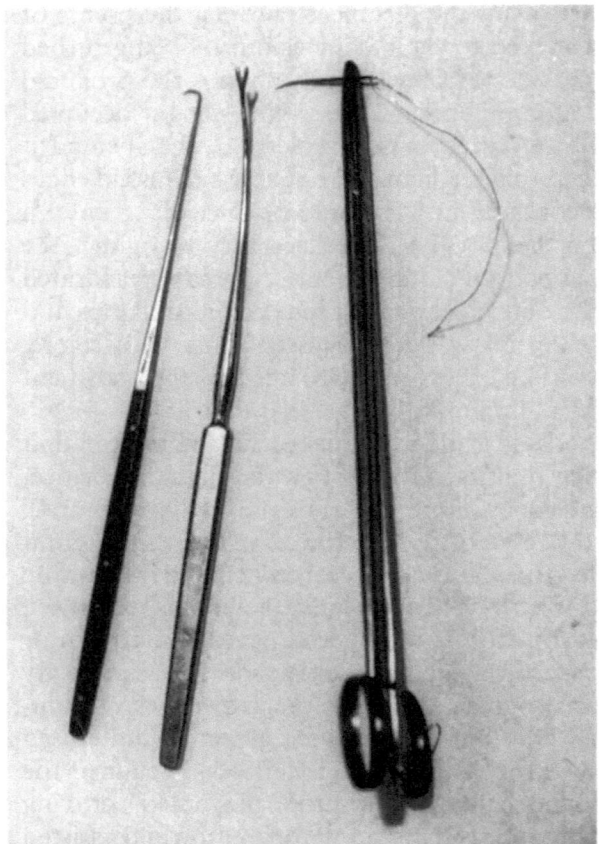

Figure 15. Later development of the Sims needle-holder. L-shaped needle loaded with the silver wire suture, the delicate tenaculum and the blunt hook. (From the Reynolds Historical Library—the University of Alabama at Birmingham)

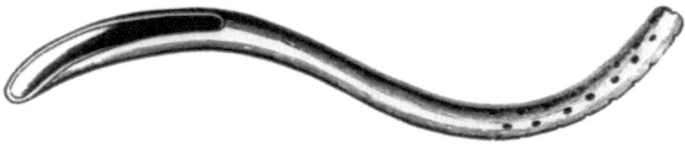

Figure 16. Detail of Sims' sigmoid self-retaining catheter. (From Sims)

the patient doomed to a forthnight's horizontal position to pass the time with pleasant dreams and delightful sensations, instead of painful forebodings and intolerable sufferings." He advocated removal of the catheter once or twice each day to clear it of concretions and mucus and emphasized that it should be watched very carefully indeed, and never should be permitted to remain long enough to become obstructed. Furthermore the patient's comfort was to be promoted greatly by washing the vulval opening once a day or more with warm or cold water and sometimes the water had to be thrown with considerable force to remove the urinary deposits. He advocated suture inspection on the 3rd or 4th day and again on the 6th or 7th and their removal on the 9th or 10th. The flattened shots were clipped off, and the anterior clamp elevated from its bed and removed. Then the posterior one with the wires attached could be hooked up, pushed backwards, disengaged entirely, and lifted out with forceps. The patient was replaced in bed and the use of the catheter coninued for several more days. The total time for the procedure occupied about 15 days.

Later in 1857, he decided the objectives of the knee-chest position could be provided with less discomfort, by lying the patient on her side in what has come to be known as Sims left lateral position. "In this position the thighs are to be flexed at nearly a right angle to the pelvis, the right a little more than the left. The left arm is thrown behind and the chest rotated forwards, bringing the sternum quite closely in contact with the table while the spine is fully extended, with the head resting on the parietal bone. The assistant at her back elevates the right side of her nates with his left hand while the right holds the speculum which draws up the perineum, allowing the pressure of the atmosphere to dilate the vagina so as to bring every part of it into view (Fig. 17)."

In October 1853, Sims sold his medical practice to his assistant Nathan Bozeman of Montgomery, Alabama and moved to New York. His health had improved and he wanted to see founded there "a great hospital to be devoted to the treatment of the diseases peculiar to women". Dr. Bozeman a man with his own ideas about fistula surgery techniques, was destined to be a constant annoyance to Sims who never forgave him for publishing Sims' ideas as his own (Fig. 18). Sims wrote, "notwithstanding the fact that the doctor lived in Montgomery for several years without any professional position until I gave it to him, that he is indebted to me for what he could never have obtained without my aid, he appropriates to himself every step of the operation that resulted from my own individual and unaided effort—even my silver wire and perforated shot, the only things of any real value whatever, and published it as his operation by a New

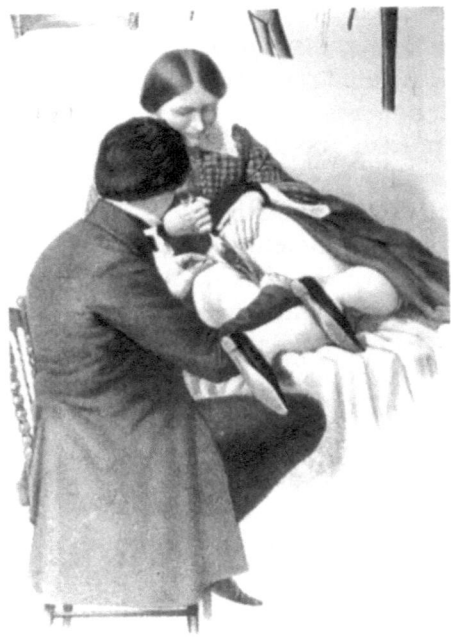

Figure 17. Sims left lateral position. (From Savage)

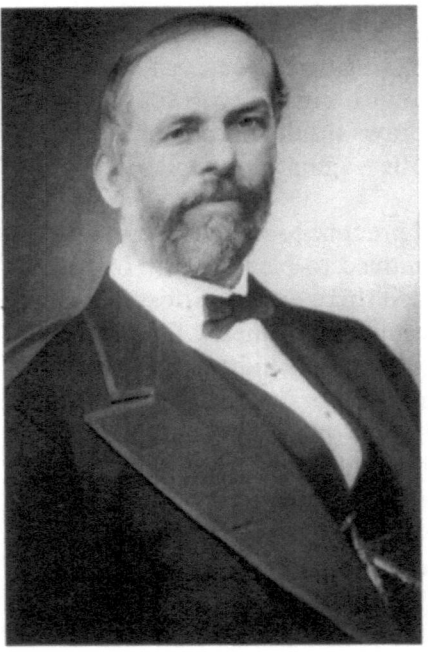

Figure 18. Nathan Bozeman. (From the Alabama Department of Archives and History, Montgomery, Alabama)

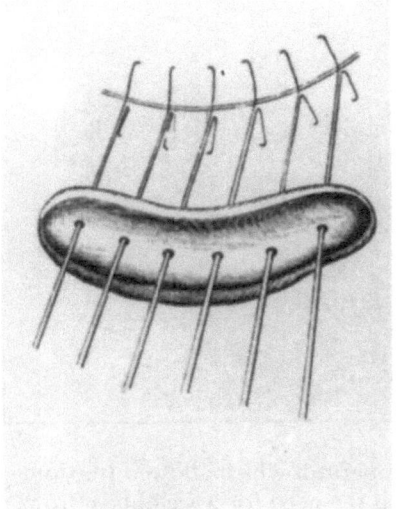 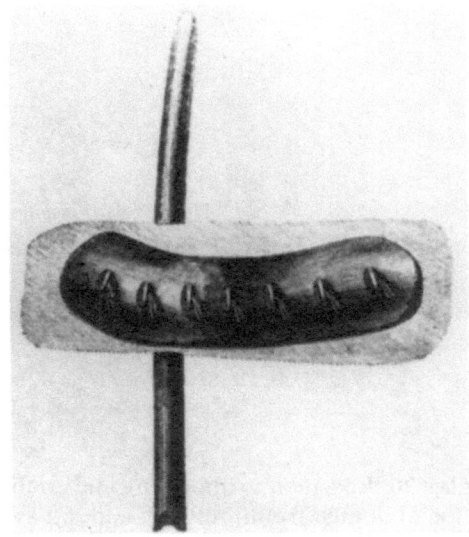

Figure 19 a   **Figure 19 b**

Figure 19 a, b

a Passing the Bozeman button along the double sutures

b Button held in place by shot compressed onto each double suture. The catheter shows diagramatically the relationship of the fistula to the urethra. (From Bozeman)

Mode of Suture, making strenuous efforts to place my labors entirely in the background". At times Sims could be highly excitable, jealous of his rights and keenly alive to any encroachment on his claims to those discoveries, which he thought belonged exclusively to himself and which he considered unjustly invaded. He was to exhibit similar traits in later years during his running battle with the authorities at the Woman's Hospital over certain important matters of principle. Bozeman (1856) extolled the place of the metallic sutures and plates adding various modifications of his own, especially the "Bozeman button". He positioned the patients on hands and knees, used the "Bozeman speculum" identical to the Sims speculum, pared the edges of the fistula and then wire sutures 18 inches long were passed through the freshened edges of the fistula and the two ends brought together with a special instrument so bringing the fistula edges into apposition. The metal button was passed over the end of each double suture and a perforated shot fed along the wires to be pressed

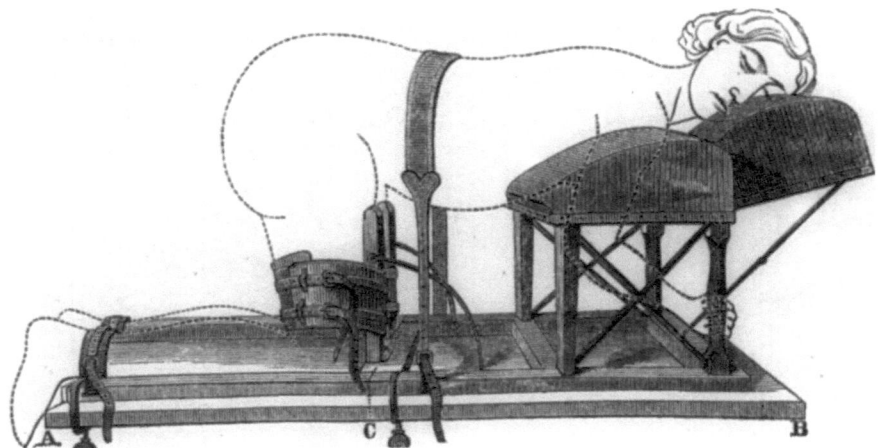

Figure 20. Bozeman's supporting and confining apparatus which allowed freedom of the abdomen from pressure, and did away with the need for assistants. (From Bozeman)

against the plate then squeezed tightly after which the redundant wires were removed. The difference from the Sims clamp method was in the use of one plate rather than two (Figs. 19 a, b). Baker-Brown (1861) who was greatly impressed by Bozeman further modified the technique by using fixed nipples on the plate with which to fix the sutures in preference to the perforated shot. In 1858 Bozeman demonstrated his techniques in Edinburgh, Scotland where success with fistula closure had been very rare. In 1861, when visiting Baker-Brown in London, Sims was pleased to hear that his vaginal speculum was now correctly named. Baker-Brown remarked, "I've been imposed upon and deceived, and so has the profession at large, not only here, but all over Europe, by your countryman who pretended to be the inventor of the speculum—I shall rectify the error and will hereafter do you the justice that is due you." In Paris where Bozeman had operated four years previously but unsuccessfully, Sims again paid him his due branding him as a plagiarist and liar. Bozeman (1869) further advertised his skills and inventions in the New York Medical Journal, in particular the apparatus to support a fistula patient in a "right angle position upon the knees and chest" (Fig. 20). Although originating with Roux and later modified by Wützer, Bozeman claimed that freeing the abdomen from pressure and effectively securing the patient witout the need for assistants, were distinct improvements. He described "our spring self-retaining speculum" further enabling examination to proceed without as-

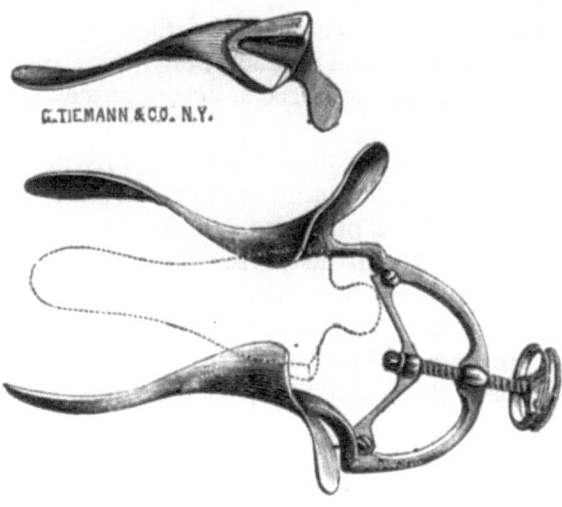

G.TIEMANN & CO. N.Y.

Figure 21. Bozeman's improved speculum—"the spring and self-retaining speculum". (From Bozeman)

sistance (Fig. 21). He noted several modifications to his speculum had been made, notably "by my friend Dr. J. C. Nott of New York who does not do me the justice to say his instrument is a modification of ours, it is nevertheless true". He laid claims of priority for his button suture devised and used for 14 years and composed of silver wire, a leaden plate and perforated shot, the advantages of which were a separate independent action of the sutures, and perfect coaption of fistula edges with perfect steadiness and support of these edges. Furthermore the grooved under surface applied to the healing fistula edges protected the area from vaginal and uterine discharge. He devoted several pages to denigration of the clamp suture which he claimed produced inaccurate wound apposition and consequently poor healing and then described a patient in whom Dr. Sims had failed repeatedly by using this technique which of course he was able to correct in eight days using the button suture—this is the only mention of Sims in the entire paper. Such claims and counter claims of priority in putting forward surgical techniques and designing surgical instruments are common in the literature of this period and frequently it is difficult to decide the rights and wrongs of some of these statements. It was quite acceptable in those times to begin a publication with a merciless attack upon contemporaries engaged in similar surgical activities. Ovariotomy, which carried a high mortality—1638 procedures of which 400 were performed by Spencer Wells, resulted in 504 deaths—still excited a fair controversy. Sims began his paper thus, "when Clay of Manchester and Peaslee and the brothers

Atlee of America began to perform ovariotomy, they met with nothing but rebuke from their brethren, who stood aghast and called them by the hardest of names. I was among the great herd that could scarely find terms strong enough to condemn what were then characterized as acts of butchery and murder".

After Sims' death in 1883, probably in expiation of his sins Bozeman wrote: "I do not wish to be understood as attempting to detract from the great credit due from the profession and the public to Dr. Sims for his untiring perseverence in bringing his method to its present high state of perfection. I consider that this gentleman is fully entitled to more than all the praise that has been bestowed upon him both in America and Europe. To the honor of his professional brothers in this country it may be stated no-one has been found who has not gladly accorded to him the high distinction that he at present occupies."

The idea that health problems peculiar to women deserved separate and distinct medical and surgical attention was not conceived before the middle of the 19th century. Some physicians even refused to examine or treat females because of their own clinical shortcomings and pseudo-modesty, so sick women suffered in silence and seclusion (Bender 1961).

Sims paid $15,000 for a home on Madison Avenue regarded as being on the outskirts of New York and discussed his plans for establishing a hospital in New York, for diseases of women, with John Wakefield Francis, the consulting physician to Bellevue Hospital and the best person to promote a new and worthwhile undertaking. He in turn sent him to Valentine Mott, Professor of Surgery at University Medical College and a variety of people including the Reverend Dr. William Muhlenberg who was about to build a new hospital in New York to be called St. Luke's. He recommended one of its wards should be reserved for diseases of women, and Sims should be made surgeon-in-charge, so with high hopes Sims waited for the hospital to be finished. In addition a call was issued for a public meeting to be addressed by Sims on the importance of organizing a Woman's Hospital and practically all New York papers on May 17th 1854 carried an appropriate announcement.

At about this time when New York doctors were acquiring Sims' techniques, many withdrew support for the proposed Woman's Hospital and Sims exclaimed: "As soon as the doctors learned what they wanted of me, they dropped me. As soon as they learned how to perform these operations successfully at the New York Hospital and elsewhere, they had no further use for me. My thunder had been stolen, and I was left without resources whatever." A typical critic was Dr. David M. Reese a prominent

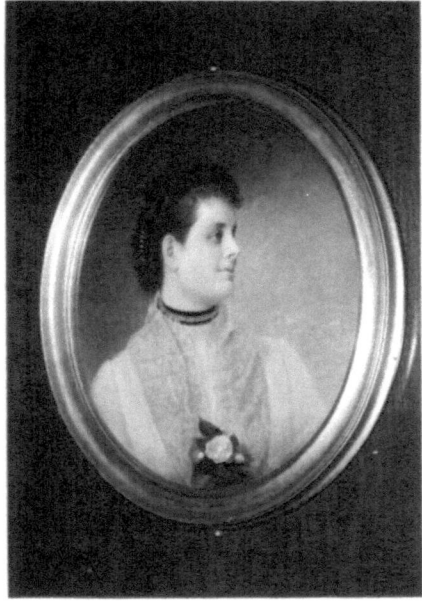

Figure 22. Sarah Platt Doremus

practitioner, who said it was easy enough "to apply silver of nitrate through a cylindrical speculum in any case of ulceration, and infusion of red-oak could be given for leukorrhea and anyone could insert Meigs ring or Physick's spherical pessary for a prolapse. It was ridiculous to speak of the necessity for a Woman's Hospital, and it would be impossible to find enough sick women to fill it". In desperation, Sims appealed to a group of intelligent New York women and on the 10th February 1855. 30 women held a meeting at 27, St. Marks Place. Mrs. Thomas C. Doremus, who was actively engaged in various community projects aiding worthy poor women, was instrumental in soliciting the help of wealthy women to start the Woman's Hospital in the state of New York (Fig. 22). New York City Council voted $2,500 for the project, and with this initial capital, a four-storey building at 83 Madison Avenue was rented for a period of three years for $1,500 a year. The rent was guaranteed by Mr. Doremus. The location was chosen because of its proximity to Sims' house since he preferred not to make to and from work because of his poor health (Fig. 23). When the Woman's Hospital opened its doors on May 4th 1855 with 30 beds, all were filled quickly ... so the first Fistula Hospital began. Sims performed one fistula operation each day and the publicity attracted more patients than he could handle alone, so it became necessary to find an

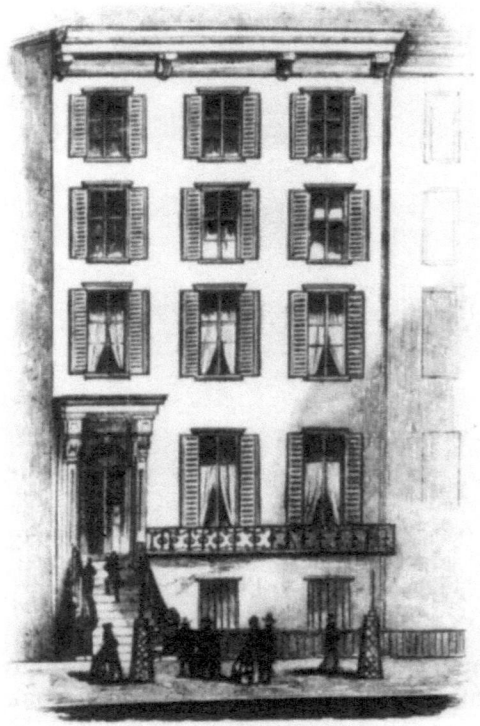

Figures 23. The Woman's Hospital 1855–83 Madison Avenue, New York

assistant and this golden opportunity fell to Thomas Addis Emmet, a promising young surgeon from the south land. Shortly after graduation, Emmet had been appointed resident physician to the newly opened Emigrant Refuge Hospital situated on Ward's Island, where patients were held in poorly built unplastered frame buildings. Most emigrants came from Ireland in the great exodus at the time of the potato famine, and on board the ships, the mortality from dysentery and typhus was appalling. In some instances half the passengers died and were buried at sea. During his three years as resident physician, he had 11,000 miscellaneous patients in his charge and in addition, performed 1,000 post-mortem examinations so becoming acquainted with a wide range of pathological conditions. In 1855 he met James Marion Sims, and there are two accounts of this meeting. Sims related that he had been acquainted with Miss Kate Duncan (recently married to Emmet) since her early childhood, adding, "so to the accident of good fortune in marrying a beautiful southern young woman, Dr. Emmet owes appointment to a position which he has long and honorably filled in the Woman's Hospital". Emmet's account however was as follows, "Late one night in March 1855 I was engaged working in my office having no idea of the hour, as a snow-storm had been raging all day and the general quiet was conducive to continued mental effort. Suddenly I was startled by a loud rap on my window and opening the door I admitted Dr. Sims whom I did not recognize. He asked some questions about the work spread out on the table before me but suddenly turned and said, 'You are just the man I am looking for. If you will come up to 83 Madison Avenue tomorrow morning 9 o'clock, I will show you something that you have never seen before.'" In fact Sims was very much in need of someone with Emmet's painstaking analytical methods for he had neither the time nor inclination to handle detail, and each day it became increasingly apparent that the Woman's Hospital needed someone to keep adequate records. His position did not become official until later in 1855 since at that time the by-laws called for a female assistant. The position of assistant surgeon to the Woman's Hospital carried a salary of $500 a year, which Emmet refused saying the hospital needed it more than he did. The primary motive in opening the Woman's Hospital was to devote it solely to the cure of vesico-vaginal fistula using Sims' technique, and Emmet assisted Sims daily, until fully acquainted with the procedure. Before long he was performing two thirds of the operations, besides keeping all the case histories and a record of each operation with hand-colored drawings showing the location of the fistula (Figs. 24 a, b). After becoming proficient in the Sims technique, Emmet suggested minor improvements to the method, and in fact did more than any other surgeon to spread what he had learned from his famous teacher, to the American profession. With Sims' departure to Europe in 1861, suddenly, at the age of 33, he found himself surgeon-in-chief, in complete charge of the Woman's Hospital; but when Sims returned in 1868, because of their former friendship and association, he offered to resign and yield the directorship to Sims or divide the service between them. Sims declined both suggestions, so eventually at Emmet's request the position of senior consulting surgeon was created for Sims together with election to the Board of Governors.

Early in Sims' career, between 1856 and 1861 he operated upon vesico-vaginal or urethro-vaginal fistulae once or twice each week and by 1867, could report details on 275 cases of injury to the vesico-vaginal septum.

Emmet's painstaking efforts took him further than the Sims' technique which he improved gradually, employing denudation well beyond the edge of the fistula using his own special angled scissors. Also he employed wide dissection of scar tissue, mobilization of bladder from vagina with liberal

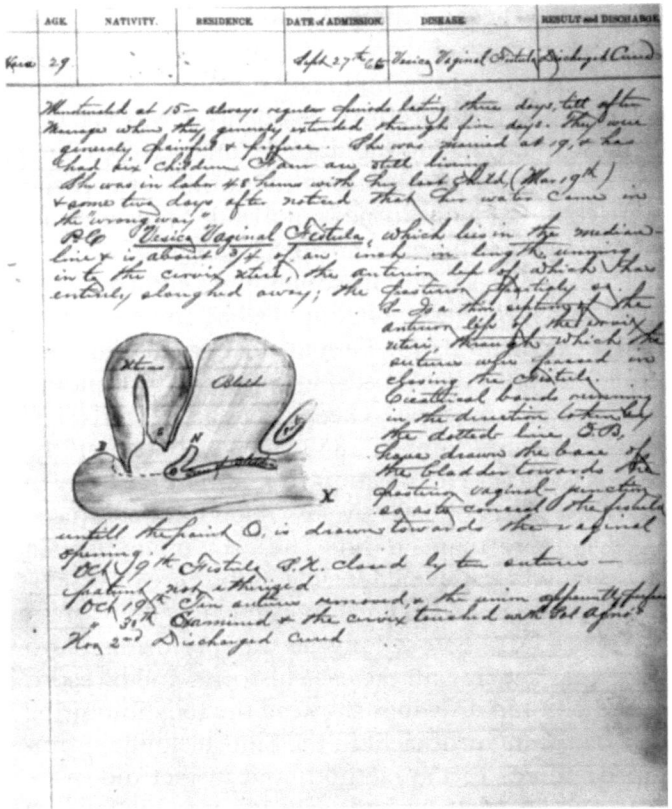

Figure 24 a

Figure 24 a, b. "Photographs of operation notes taken from the "case register" of the Woman's Hospital. There are three such volumes hand written by either Sims or Emmet—mostly Emmet—and include all cases admitted to the hospital between 1855 and 1871." (From the Archives of the Woman's Hospital, Bolling Medical Library, Archival and Historical Collection, St. Luke's/Roosevelt Hospital Center, NYC, NY)

use of sponges, and needles with silk threads to carry the silver wire sutures. In 1868 he published "Vesico-Vaginal Fistula From Parturition and Other Causes With Cases Of Recto-Vaginal Fistula". The book was dedicated "to James Marion Sims M.D. my instructor, and the lady managers of the New York State Woman's Hospital". In the preface he paid homage to Lamballe, Metzler, Sims and Bozeman. The 18 chapters dealt with all manner of fistulae, and early chapters discussed details of positioning and

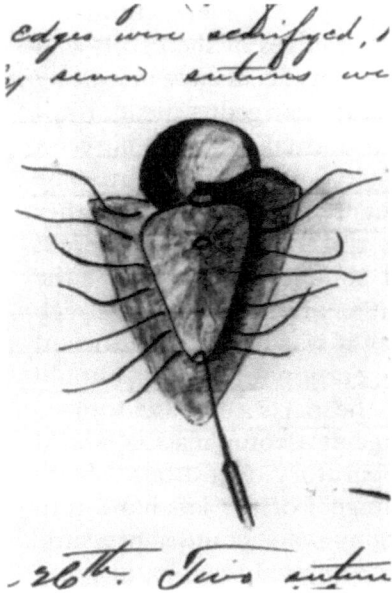

edges were rectified, 1
'y seven sutures we

26th. Two suture

Figure 24 b

necessary instruments. He introduced the subject stating that "prior to the application of the metallic suture by J. Marion Sims and a proper mode of explanation furnished by his speculum, any attempt for the relief of the injuries under consideration was uncertain in result, and the operation regarded as opprobrium by the profession".

Fistula patients attending the Woman's Hospital came in greater numbers than the available accommodation, and as a class belonged to the poorest, having not received proper attention during their confinement— the injury was exceedingly rare amongst the better class—or they came from the frontier and thinly settled sections of the country. Emmet states as a principle, that scarcely any case could be regarded as incurable in consequence of tissue loss alone. Prior to October 1867 he had 270 cases in his care of which 200 had been cured, five were incurable and the others returned home improved. The major problem of the incurable case was "excessive obesity which rendered it difficult to bring the parts into view, and others who were unable to bear a long operation on their knees". He commented that a small number of patients had been discharged for disorderly conduct! He described in great detail the use of silver nitrate on the raw surfaces and frequent sitz-baths to achieve cleanliness of recently sloughed tissues. Surgical correction was not to be considered until the vaginal wall and the hypertrophied and indurated edges of the fistula had attained a natural color and density, and the secret of success was in waiting until these tissue changes had occurred; but many surgeons did not appreciate this fact. After tissues had returned to normal, then the surgeon could decide upon a definite plan of procedure for fistula closure. The fistula edges should be seized at opposite points by a tenaculum in either hand and the degree of tension judged by an approximation in different directions. "If at any point the edges did not come together readily, the finger could detect the seed of resistance while the parts were kept on strech and when the bands were slight and superficial, it was generally sufficient to divide them with scissors at the time of the operation for closure. Should tension be due to more extensive sloughing, the parts could seldom be properly freed without more or less hemorrhage as a complication, and it was then necessary to make one or more preparatory operations." With the patient on her back, he introduced two fingers of the left hand into the rectum as a guide and the thumb in the vagina made counter-pressure, enabling him to snip freely with a pair of blunt-pointed scissors, at point after point, indicated by the thumb pressure. After opening the vagina as widely as deemed prudent, a glass vaginal plug devised by Sims, just long enough to stretch the canal without fear of producing sloughing or pelvic inflammation, was introduced and held in place with a T bandage. After the parts were healed properly, if necessary, the operation for enlarging the vagina could be repeated. He described a special self-retaining speculum with a large fenestrated blade attached, which clamped around the buttock and obviated the need for an assistant (Fig. 25 a). He re-described Sims position, scarification of the edges of the fistula with a pair of scissors, and removal of the inner edges in a continuous strip. Should the denuded portion be not of sufficient width, a further strip could be removed just beyond it. The scarification should be extended as near as possible to the bladder mucosa without actually involving it, then sutures were placed in deep bites, about four or five to the inch, avoiding the bladder surface. As each suture was introduced, it was followed at once with silver wire, for the silk trim became weakened after saturation with blood and urine. He emphasized the point, "that the sites of entrance and exit of the sutures should be at the same distance from the fistula edges, in order to avoid approximation of the scarified surface with an opposite portion which had not been denuded". After completing the surgery, the patient was placed on her back, a catheter introduced, and should the urine be discolored, tepid water was injected to wash out any blood clot. The catheter was

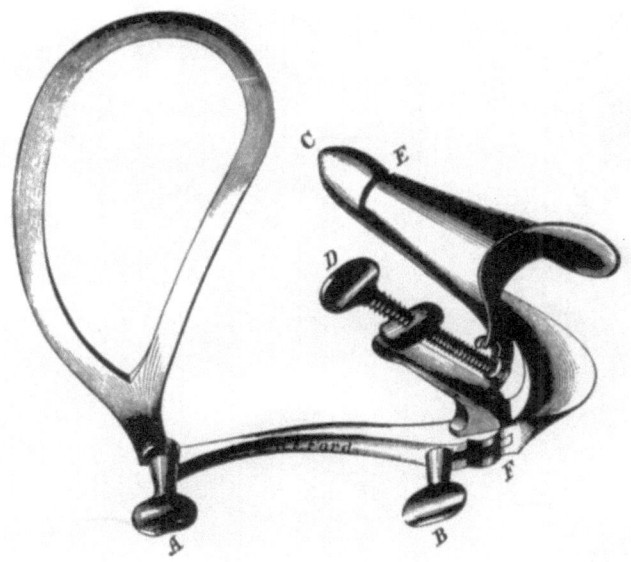

Figure 25 a. Emmet's self-retaining speculum. (From Emmet)

removed several times a day for cleaning and the patient instructed to notice carefully that urine had a free escape at all times, and it was well to have two catheters, so one could be introduced immediately after removal of the other. He advocated suture removal from the eighth to the tenth day with the catheter in continual use for a few days longer. He detailed some horrendous case histories and in particular, a female who had commenced labor on a Saturday in August 1864 then nothing further was done until Thursday night when a stillborn child weighing 14 pounds was delivered. The head had been impacted in the pelvis for 131 hours.

Bissell (1928) described the method of fistula closure taught by Emmet, and indicated many differences from the early Sims technique, in particular a change from the knee-chest position to the semi-prone Sims position, a much more extended denudation about the fistula in the general line of the vagina rather than transversely, and a change from the clamp or quill suture, to a simple twisting of the wires over the line of the approximated surface, the wire points being protected by perforated and crushed shot. Bissell believed several changes were due partly to Emmet's influence (Fig. 25 b).

Emmet first pointed out that methods of fistula prevention were entirely in the hands of obstetricians, and advocated forceps delivery after the foetal

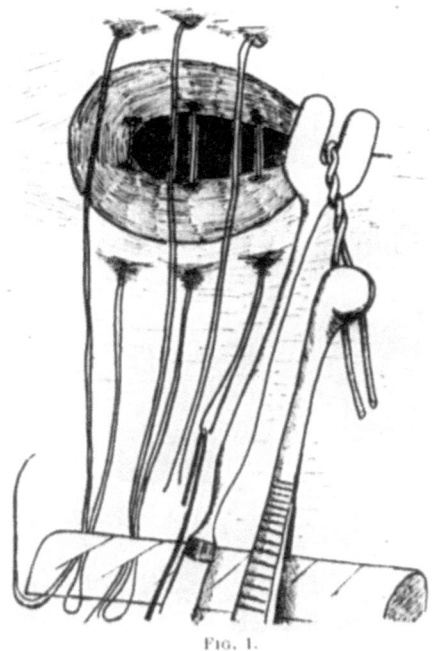

Fig. 1.

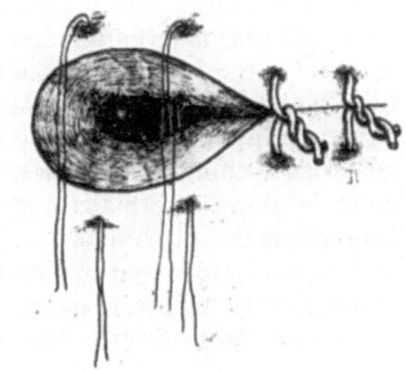

Figure 25 b. Changes in technique attributed to Emmet: *1* more extended denudation; *2* suture method changed to simple wire twisting. (From Bissell)

head had been visible for some time, frequent catheterization during labor, and he condemned the use of ergot to expedite delivery. In later years he wrote: "I did not realize that it was to be part of my life's mission to render this loathsome and almost incurable injury not only curable; but that I was able to be the means of restoring to perfect health nearly 600 women thus afflicted, and finally to discover the cause and thereby revolutionize

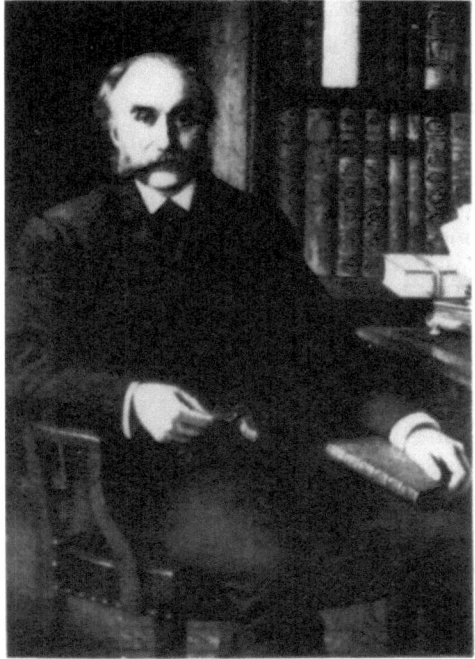

Figure 26. Thomas Addis Emmet

the obstetrical practice of the world, so that now the occurrence of this injury is almost unknown." In November 1900 Emmet resigned from the Woman's Hospital after 45 consecutive years of service and died at the age of 91 on the 1st March 1919 (Fig. 26).

The first patient at the Woman's Hospital in 1855 was Mary Smith, a recently arrived immigrant from Western Ireland "a pitiable, ill-smelling, repulsive creature with an extensively excoriated vulva, the result of constant escape of urine". A huge encrusted mass was discovered in her vagina about the size of a closed fist, thought to be a calculus; but after a great effort and much suffering by the patient, the object was dislodged. It was a wooden float of a kind used on fishing nets, inserted in an attempt to plug the fistula to stop the urine flow and prevent bladder inversion. Most of the bladder base and part of the urethra had been destroyed; but after more than 30 reparative operations performed in the knee-chest position without anesthesia over a period of five years, bladder function was restored partly and she became an assistant at the hospital, working there for many years. Nevertheless her tragic history continued with the development of a bladder calculus and against the advice of Emmet, the urethra was dilated to remove it and the bladder neck lacerated, returning the incontinence, "so that the hospital's first patient was still living in suffering, in poverty and incurable".

Soon the hospital became too small, new ground had to be secured and finally the site chosen was the burial place of victims from a cholera epidemic 25 years previously. The western half of the land was filled with coffins buried in tiers 18 deep, and during the summer of 1857, 47,000 bodies were removed, transferred to wooden boxes and reburied on Ward's Island. New York City owned this land at Park and Lexington Avenues 49th to 50th Streets, now occupied by the Waldorf Astoria Hotel, and the charter for the Woman's Hospital was granted in 1857.

With the approach of civil war, Sims' open display of southern sympathies made him extremely unpopular in New York where a majority of his patients came from below the Mason-Dixon line, so with their return home for financial and other reasons, the practice dwindled. In June 1861 he left for Europe to study hospital architecture, since he was dissatisfied with plans for the new Woman's Hospital, and following his return in 1862, he persuaded the Board of Governors to adopt the pavilion style. The 75 bed Wetmore pavilion was the beginning and in 1877 the addition of the Baldwin pavilion doubled the beds (Figs. 27 a, b). During his overseas tour he met Florence Nightingale, Sir James Young Simpson and Sir Thomas Spencer-Wells and demonstrated fistula surgery in London, Brussels, Paris and Dublin. Unfortunately in London, the fistula operation performed at Samaritan Hospital resulted in the patient's death, and autopsy revealed ligation of both ureters, but this was the only fatality that marred his European jaunt.

Until Sims, there had not been any consistently successful operation for fistula in France, and attempts at cure had produced many failures. Sims operated at the Charity Hospital on a suitable case giving first a graphic description, then performing the operation with his usual skill. The scene was described by Edmund Sauchon (1894). "On the day of the operation, the famous little operating theater in the old Charity Hospital was overcrowded with students, and the arena below filled with the most distinguished professors of surgery in the French capital—Velpeau, Nelaton, Ricord and Malgaigne but not Lamballe, who would not come. Before beginning the operation Dr. Sims proceeded to demonstrate graphically by using a piece of thick and hard cotton batting through which he cut a hole representing the fistula, then he pared the edges slantingly in one strip and next passed the silk thread and the wires. I was called to translate as he spoke. Following the demonstration, Sims proceeded with

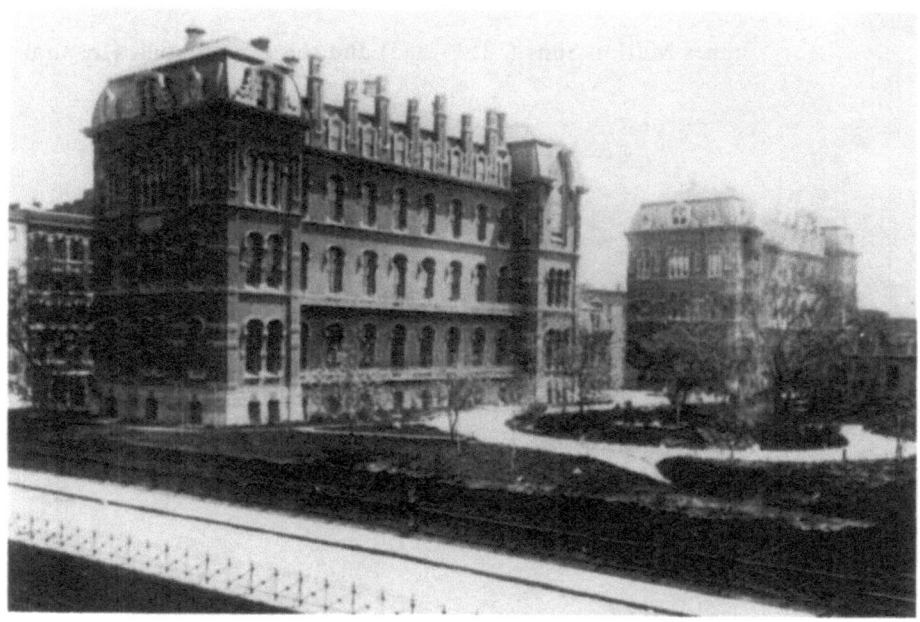

Figure 27 a. The Woman's Hospital in the state of New York, 1890 showing the Wetmore and Baldwin Pavilions. The present site of the Waldorf Astoria Hotel, Park Avenue, NYC

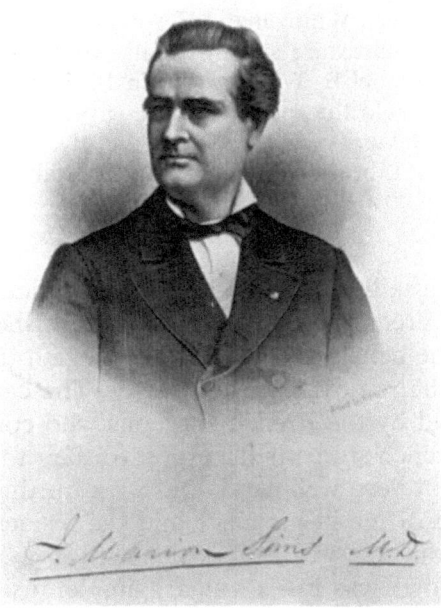

Figure 27 b. James Marion Sims circa 1862. (Courtesy James Ingram)

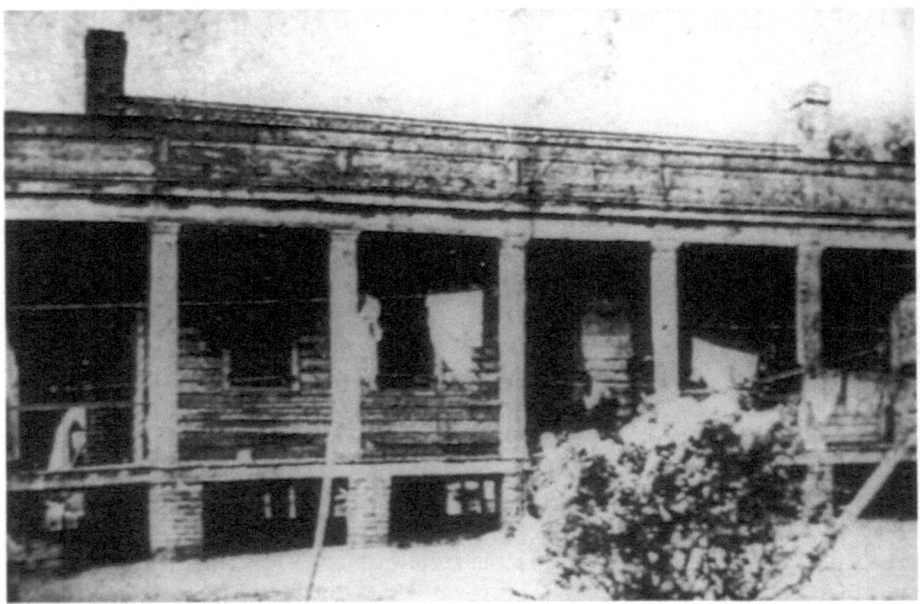

Figure 28 a

Figures 28 a–c. Photographs taken by Dr. Thigpen in Montgomery, Alabama circa 1890. *a* The house on Hammich Street, between Whitron and Heron occupied by the first patients; *b* building formerly the hardware store of Hall, Mores and Roberts; the building was identified by Colonel B. Wyman who in 1843, was a boy clerk in the store and perhaps himself sold the spoon; *c* building previously housed the jewelry store of Swan at 108 Dexter Avenue in which the silver wire was drawn. (From the Reynolds Historical Library—the University of Alabama at Birmingham)

the operation which he performed with skill and grace. It was done quickly and watched closely all the time by the French professors, and when finished a salvo of applause broke out from the benches. On the 9th day again the ampitheater was packed to witness the removal of the sutures. The case was pronounced cured, and confirmed by the French surgeons who congratulated him. Enthusiasm of the French students far exceeded their former outburst and since they could not very well carry Dr. Sims on their shoulders in triumph, they took hold of me in his place and the resident students carried me to their mess room for breakfast with them; a great unprecedented honor in those days for I was but a vulgar, simple, insignificant first year student."

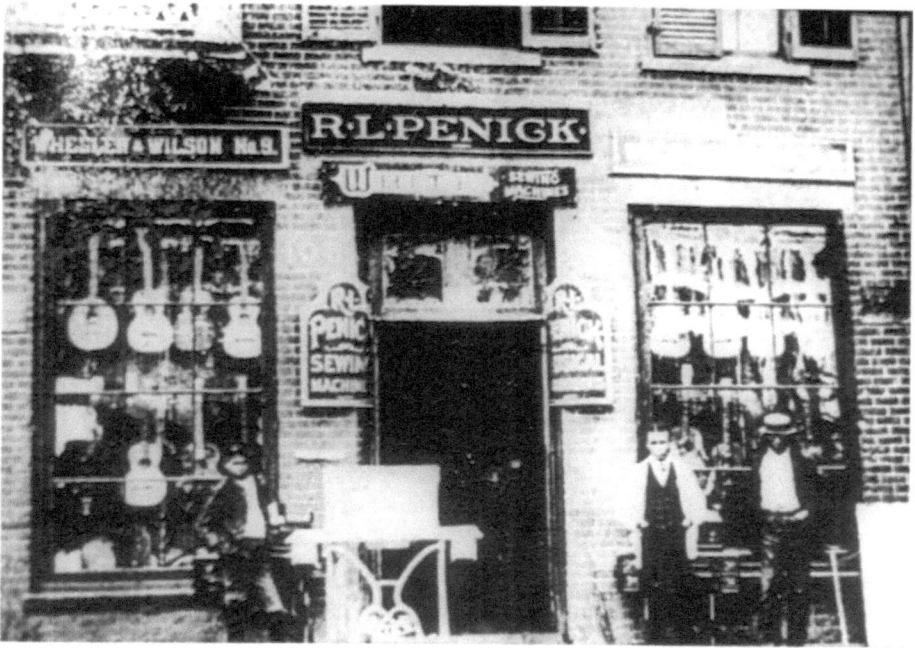

Figure 28 b

In 1895, en route to a meeting of the American Surgical Association in New York, Sauchon passed through Montgomery Alabama "to visit those places rendered famous by their connection with James Marion Sims". He commented with interest upon photographs taken by Dr. Thigpen to preserve for posterity the dilapidated house occupied by the first patient, the modest office in the rear yard of which was erected the forever famous hospital, the hardware store where Sims bought the legendary pewter spoon from which developed the great and celebrated duck-bill speculum, and the jeweller's store where the memorable silver wire for sutures was drawn. Edmund Sauchon, was Professor of Anatomy and Clinical Surgery at Tulane University, New Orleans (Figs. 28 a–c).

In Belgium, Sims was elected a Fellow of the Royal Academy of Medicine and after six months in Europe returned to New York on January 11th 1862; but with the Civil War in full progress and he still a pronounced southern sympathizer, the situation in New York was untenable, so immediately he returned to Europe remaining abroad for much longer than planned, and engaged in private practice both in France and England. He moved in high circles becoming physician to Eugenia, wife of Napoleon

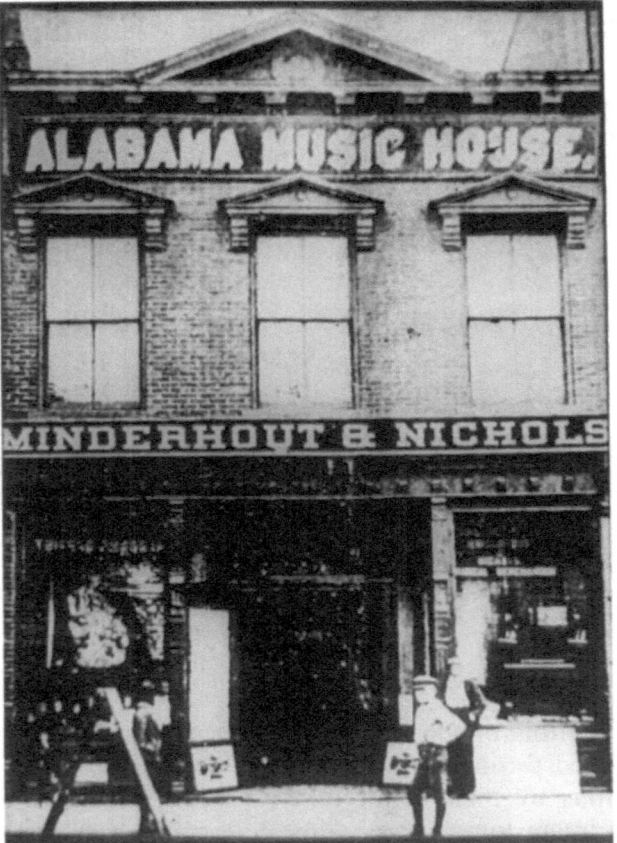

Figure 28 c

III., the Duchess of Hamilton, Winston Churchill's grandmother and ac-
coucher to the Empress of Austria. The French government bestowed the
Medal of the Legion of Honor.

In 1866 he published a text-book entitled "Clinical Notes on Uterine
Surgery" which was a sensation hailed as a valuable text by many, yet
sharply criticised by others. Filled with original concepts and inventions,
he was years ahead of his contemporaries advocating use of the microscope
in diagnosis and treatment of sterility, post-coital examination of sperm
and artifical insemination, so much so that the Medical Times and Gazette
of London expressed, "An unfeigned regret that Dr. Marion Sims had
thought proper to found an odious type of practice on such methods. Better

to let ancient families become extinct than keep up the succession by such means." Furthermore, also in 1866, a reader, H. L., who had followeed the vigorous criticism of his recently published work, offered the following verses:

> Say, what is man? An atom at the first,
>   Waiting its nuptial atom in the womb;
> Too oft, alas, by fate untimely curst,
>   In place of fostering home, to find a tomb.
> Grieved at the thought, a tear thine eye bedims,
> Great son of Aesculapius, Marion Sims.
>
> Swift to thine aid inventive genius brings
>   Persuasive tent or glistening hystrotome;
> With these the obstructed portal open flings,
>   And guides the struggling sperm'tozoon home.
> Thus may the wished-for union perfect be.
> The mystery no human eye can see.
>
> Sims, should these fail, thou still wilt cherish hope
>   To find some other cause that breeds the ill,
> With learned digit, searching microscope,
>   Or peering speculum, exploring still:—
> Nay, wizard-like, ethereal sleep wilt shed,
> To win thy point, e'en o'er the nuptial bed.

When he returned to New York in 1868 he was acknowledged internationally as the foremost gynecologist in the world and in 1870 became surgeon-in-chief, in active command of the Anglo-American Ambulance Corp in the Franco-Prussian War where his selfless devotion to wounded soldiers won for him the French Legion of Honor for the second time, together with the Iron Cross and other decorations from the German government.

In 1871, at a Board of Governors meeting at the Woman's Hospital, two decisions were made to which Sims allegedly acquiesced.

(i) No case of carcinoma uteri should be admitted to the hospital for it was believed such patients were contagious.

(ii) Not more than 15 spectators in addition to the hospital staff should be present at any vaginal operation, for reasons of modesty.

Later, following the annual meeting of the Board, Sims delivered a fiery speech reflecting severely upon the tyrannical course of the Board of

Governors in establishing these two rules, saying he would not submit to such treatment and threatened to resign unless they were rescinded at their next meeting. His resignation was accepted. In 1874, he published a long reply to a circular prepared by Drs. Peaslee, Emmet and Gaillard which supported the action of the Board and in which they registered astonishment at Sims' behavior since he had voted in favor of these rules at the initial Board meeting. In his reply Sims began, "Having been publicly assailed, I can no longer remain silent, I am now free to tell the story of my resignation (almost expulsion) from the Woman's Hospital. In this I shall do my duty to myself, to truth, to justice, to honor and to my profession. I shall use no disparaging epithets. I shall deal in no questionable innuendos nor in constructive interpretations of facts which may lead to wrong conclusions." Sims claimed in this publication that he had abstained from the vote at the Board of Governors meeting and prior to that had attempted to convince the other three doctors to stand up to the Board with him against these rules.

Shortly after this incident, Mrs. George W. Cullum was refused admission because of the diagnosis of uterine cancer and went to London for treatment. She was the cousin of John Jacob Astor's wife and Astor offered $150,000 to establish a cancer wing at the Woman's Hospital; but this was declined by the Board of Governors. Sims' last great contribution to medicine which commenced with these incidents, was not finalized until after his death. For years he had urged without success that several hospitals should be established for the treatment of cancer and just two weeks before his death Sims appealed once more to the lay press by letter, "a cancer hospital is one of the great needs of the day and it must be built". This letter received wide publicity and provided the necessary final impetus, for within a few months, a committee of prominent citizens including Astor, met to begin the establishment of such a hospital and in May 1884, just six months after Sims' death, Mrs. George Cullum laid the corner stone of the New York Skin And Cancer Hospital. It was completed in 1887 when the first building—the Astor pavilion for women was opened. So began the institution known world wide as the Memorial Hospital of New York.

Sims' unpopularity in New York went unnoticed by the American medical world at large for in 1875 he was elected President of the American Medical Association, and on the occasion delivered an address on "The prevention and regulation of syphilis in America". In 1878 he described his treatment for stenosis of the cervix, suggested cholecystostomy for acute gallbladder disease, and in 1879 wrote a paper on epithelioma of the cervix

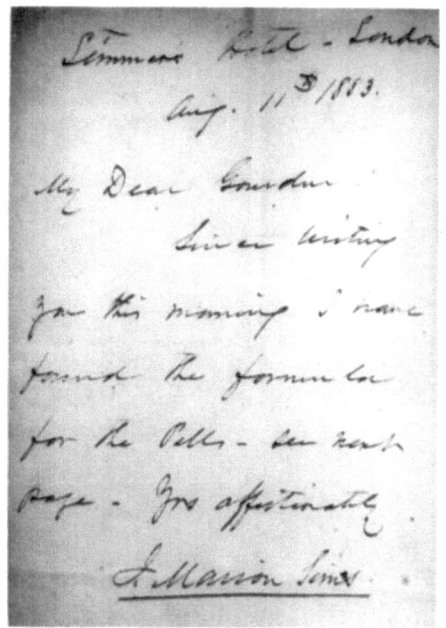

Figure 29 a. Letter written in London by Sims just prior to his death. (From the Alabama Department of Archives and History, Montgomery, Alabama)

in which local excision was the preferred surgical treatment. In 1880, he became President of the American Gynecological Society and was reinstated as consulting surgeon to the Woman's Hospital. He received considerable publicity in 1881, when he collaborated with three others writing an article entitled, "Surgical Treatment of President Garfield". The President had died of septicemia long after a gunshot wound and although Sims did not attend him, his experiences on the battlefields of France enabled him to contribute valuable information on management, recommending early exploration of the abdominal wounds and suture of bowel perforations before sepsis occurred.

On November 13th 1883, Sims was about to return to Rome, when apparently in robust health he was seized with dyspnea at 3 o'clock in the morning, while sitting in bed working on his autobiography. When his son Dr. Harry M. Sims reached him he had expired without a word. He was 71 years old (Fig. 29 a). An autopsy was performed by William H. Welch, then a new pathologist at Woman's Hospital and by Dr. Peabody. In addition to old pleural and pericardial adhesions he was found to have "obstruction of the circulation from atheromatous degeneration of the coronary arteries". Even in the manner of his death, he achieved medical

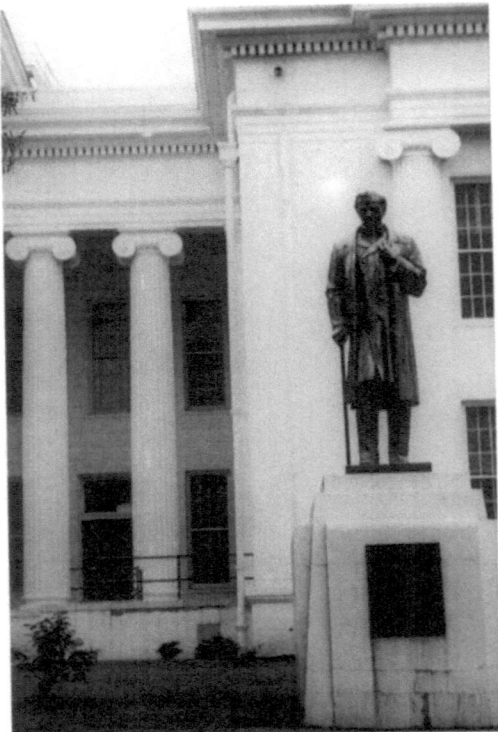

Figure 29 b. Sims' statue, Capitol Building, Montgomery, Alabama

distinction since he was only the second individual in the USA in whom a postmortem diagnosis of coronary occlusion had been recorded. He was buried in Greenwood Cemetery in Brooklyn, New York to be joined later by his wife Theresa, sons Willie and Harry, youngest daughter Florence and her famous surgeon husband John Wyeth.

In 1894 the Medical Records, a weekly journal of medicine and surgery made an appeal to the medical profession in the United States of America and other countries for funds with which to erect a monument to the memory of one of its acknowledged leaders. The subscriptions were limited to one dollar each and coming as they did from members of the profession in every part of the civilized world, attested, in an unmistakable manner the good name and fame of this American surgeon. The distinction came from his peers who were best able to judge his qualifications and who with one accord were delighted to honor him. The commission for the statue was awarded to Müller of Munich whose completed work was erected in

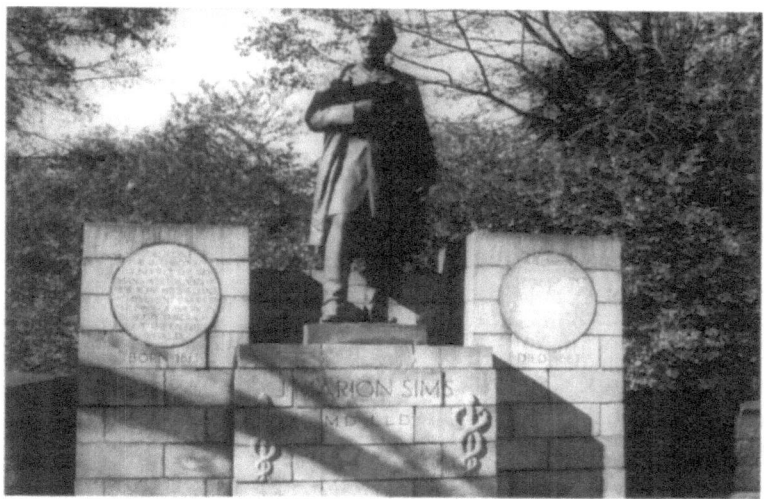

Figure 29 c. James Marion Sims' memorial at Central Park, New York

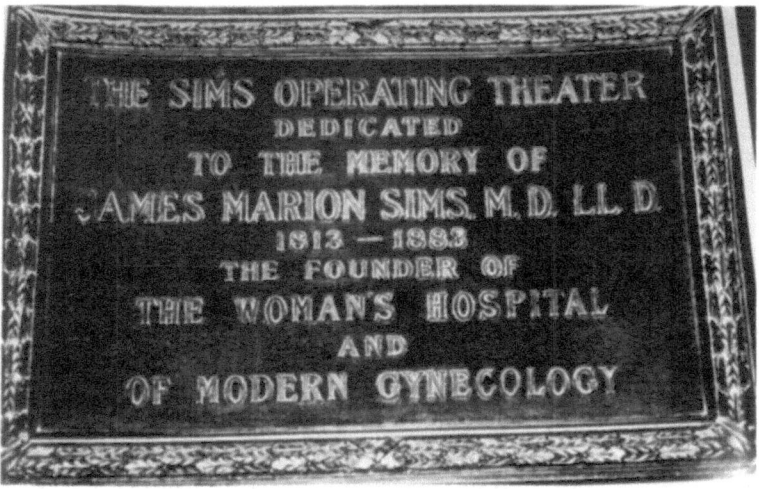

Figure 29 d. Memorial tablet at Woman's Hospital

Bryant Park, New York City and on October 20th 1894, George F. Shrady and Paul F. Munde delivered addresses. Shrady said that Sims' name was associated with more original operations and more new instruments for making such operations successful that that of any other American surgeon and Munde concluded that Marion Sims should with all propriety be called the father of modern gynecology, and it was to this universally admitted claim that he owed the distinction of being the first physician to whose memory a statue had been erected. Following the addresses, the concealing veil was drawn by a child, a grandson of Sims, and the statue formally presented to and accepted by the City of New York. On October 20th 1934 the statue was rededicated after being moved to a new site on the borders of Central Park on 5th Avenue and 103rd Street, where it was erected on a more beautiful pedestal opposite the Academy of Medicine. At this time Dr. Sach the President of the Academy presided. In the grounds of the capitol of both Columbia, South Carolina and Montgomery, Alabama, two other statues of Sims have been erected. Finally on March 14th 1922 a newly constructed operating theater in the present Woman's Hospital was opened and on that occasion a bronze memorial tablet unveiled and dedicated to the memory of J. Marion Sims, the founder of the Woman's Hospital (Figs. 29 b–d).

During his lifetime Sims published more than 60 papers and articles covering a wide range of medical and surgical problems. Emmet wrote, "he had heard Sims remark that he would have accomplished nothing without the aid and advice of his wife who devoted her life to him, and he had never seen a person more dependent on another than Sims upon her. She watched over him with a singleness of purpose equalled only in the care of a mother for her offspring".

In 1906, the present main Woman's Hospital was opened on Morningside Heights at 110th Street and Amsterdam Avenue, and in 1953 the consolidation with St. Luke's Hospital, a general hospital with all medical specialties except obstetrics, was effected. A stained glass window based on gynecology as discussed in the bible, had been placed in the chapel at Woman's Hospital in memory of Sims. With the closure of Woman's Hospital in 1964, the window could not be housed in the new location and was accepted by the University of Alabama at Birmingham to be placed in the J. Marion Sims room at the Medical Center library.

Howard Kelly (1928) commented upon Sims' technique thus: "Our forefathers especially Sims and Emmet succeeded under conditions of extreme awkwardness, where we today, with less of their special skills wrought out of an abundant experience would fail lamentably. Like the bow of Ulysses, there is scarcely one today who can handle these tools, or use their legerdemain in this field." James Marion Sims founder of the Woman's Hospital in the state of New York—the first fistula hospital—and one of the founders of modern gynecology, by force of his genius will and energy, invaded the unexplored field of surgical instruments and covered a wide

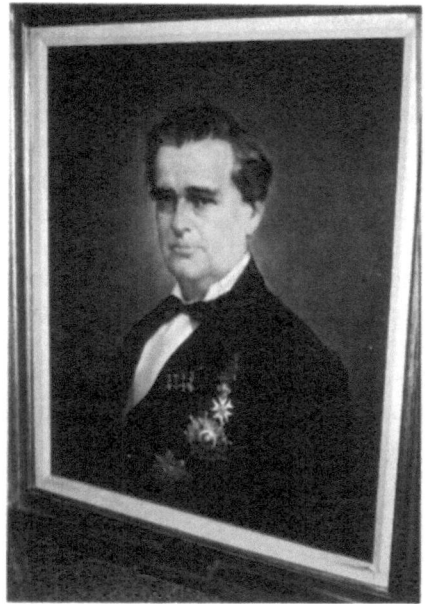

Figure 30. James Marion Sims M.D.—about 1874

range of surgery in the pre- and post-antiseptic era. Handicapped for most of his professional life by the dangers and difficulties associated with surgical intervention prior to general anesthesia and asepsis, his surgical feats, to this day, remain outstanding. In 1976, Barker-Benfield published "The Honors of the Half-Known Life" depicting Sims as racist and male chauvinist, and archetype of evil masquerading as good saying, "Sims garnered diseased black women into his back yard—to provide guinea pigs for his self-education, before he and others could convincingly offer care to the wives of the wealthy who were originally Sims' backers for the hospital". Also he cited Sims' refusal to appoint a female assistant despite article XVI of the hospital constitution which stated: "The surgeon's assistant must be a woman." Kaiser (1978) presented this material to the American Gynecological Society annual meeting and concluded, "it is not easy to decide whether Sims acted out of callousness or compassion. Sims' attitudes towards women were those of an ante-bellum southern gentleman." In the heated discussion which followed, such notions were vigorously refuted especially by Dennis Cavanagh.

Professor Chassar Moir (1940) wrote: "The treatment of vesico-vaginal fistula has a fascination of its own. No branch of surgery calls for greater resource, never is patience so sorely tried, never is success more dependant on the exercise of constant care both during operation and even more perhaps during the anxious days of convalescence. But never is reward greater. Nothing could equal the gratitude of the woman who wearied from constant pain, depressed by an ever-growing sense of the humiliating nature of her infirmity, and desperate with the realization that her very presence is an offense to others, finds suddenly that she is restored to full health and able to resume her rightful place in the family—who finds as it were that life has been given anew and she has again become a citizen of the world. To J. Marion Sims, more than to any man, is due the honor for this transformation. And if in these days a moment can be spared for sentimental reverie, look again, I beg, at the curious speculum and, gazing through the confused reflections from its bright curves, catch a fleeting glimpse of an old hut in Alabama and seven negro women who suffered, and endured, and had rich reward (Fig. 30)."

3

The Post-Sims Era

The Professor of Midwifery at Heidelberg, Germany, Gustave Simon, had visited Paris, earlier in his career, as a pupil of Jobert de Lamballe and whilst appreciating fully the merits of Lamballe's procedure, in 1854 made his own modifications to the technique of fistula closure by doing away with lateral relieving incisions except in special circumstances, substituting two rows of sutures—one to approximate the edges and the other to relieve tension of the primary closure. Using an exaggerated lithotomy position, the hips were raised high with the legs strongly flexed on the body, and the uterus drawn down and held by sutures passed through the cervix, so pulling the anterior vaginal wall out between the labia. The Simon speculum was a retracting speculum with long handles, and also he used lateral retractors. A steeply precipitous funnel-shaped denudation was prepared, and the first row of sutures united the wound edges accurately and without tension. Simon was not concerned whether or not the suture passed through the vesical mucosa. The second row of sutures entered and emerged at a greater distance from the wound edges than the first line, so removing all tension. He reported 35 cures in 40 cases (Kelly. 1912) Novel elements in this approach were relaxation sutures, and a more vertical incision which were important advances in the evolution of fistula surgery technique (Fig. 31 a, b). Between 1856 and 1868 he published several papers on the place of colpocleisis in the management of vesico-vaginal fistula, stressing the necessity for applying the transverse vaginal closure immediately beneath the defect. Circular denudation of the vagina was effected adjacent to the fistula, and the wound surfaces opposed with sagittally applied sutures, but inevitably a small diverticulum formed. In most cases, the normal lower vagina was adequate for cohabitation. Technically the method was simple and very successful since the anterior and posterior vaginal walls normally were in contact so tension was avoided (Fig. 31 c). In 42 vesico-vaginal fistulae he performed "occlusio vaginae" 12 times with 12 cures, nevertheless the excellent results reported by Sims and Bozeman made colpocleisis unnecessary and technically wrong, for even when the

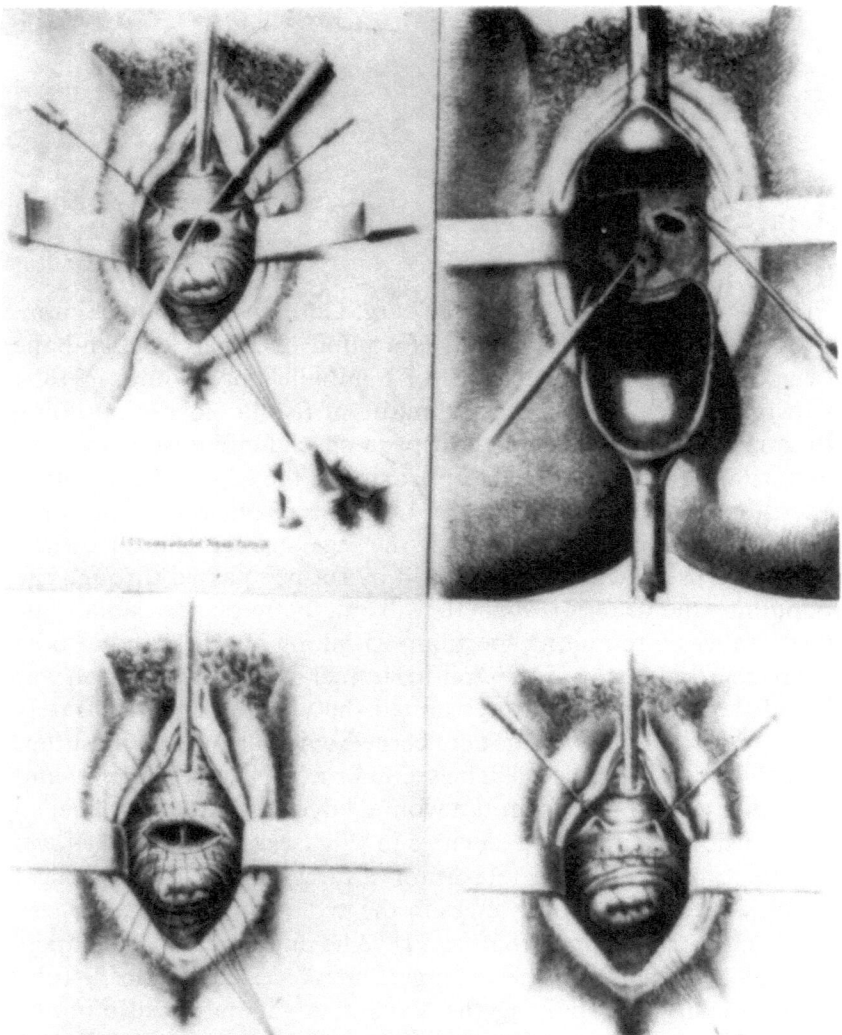

Figure 31 a. Gustave Simon's technique for fistula closure

diverticulum was very small, still, menstrual discharge with cervical and uterine secretions, commonly caused severe cystitis and calculi. Emmet (1879) stated that, "There was no greater blunder in surgery than the Simon operation, and in recent years all modern authors have regarded the procedure as obsolete and removed it from the list of fistula operations". More recently however, colpocleisis following total hysterectomy has been re-

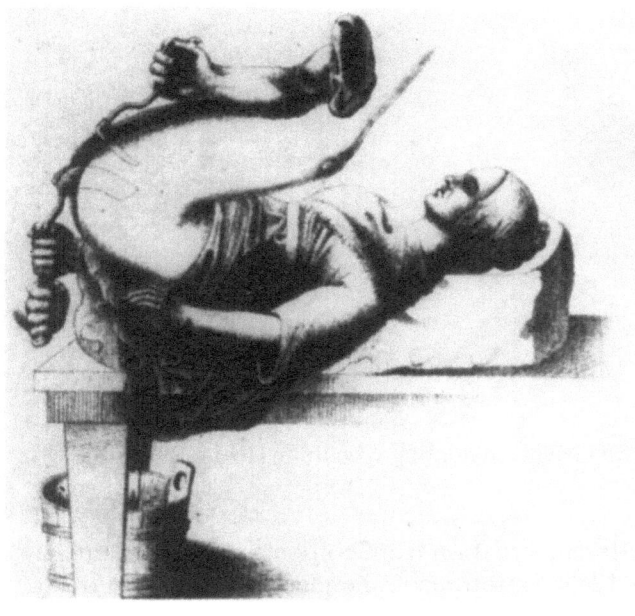

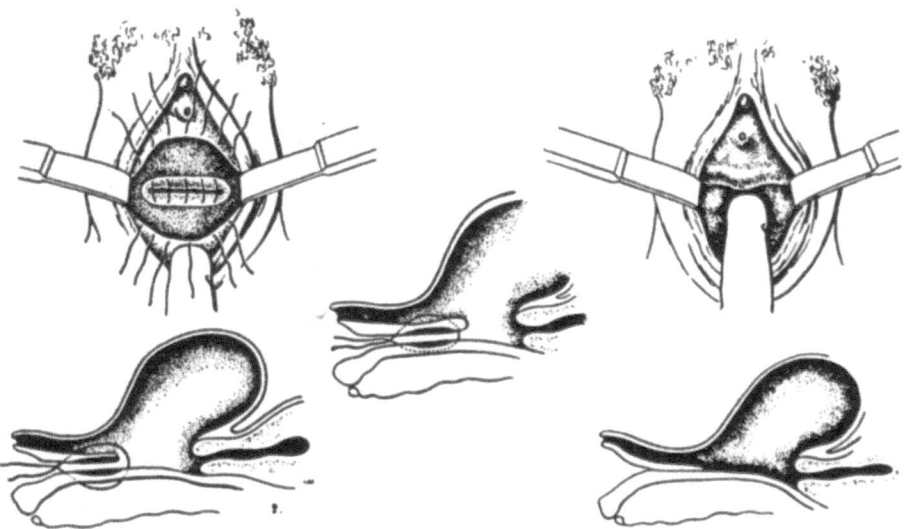

Figure 31 c. Colpocleisis after Maisoneuve, as performed by Simon. (From Miller)

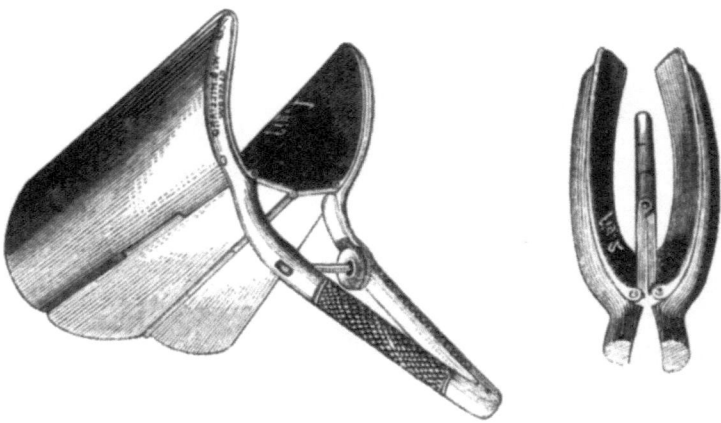

Figure 32. The self-retaining quadrivalved dilating speculum. (From Baker-Brown)

evaluated as an entirely different situation from colpocleisis with the uterus
present (Latzko 1942). In 1867, Simon recommended transposition of the
ureteric openings from the edge of a vesico-vaginal fistula into the bladder
interior by splitting the anterior wall of the ureter (Latzko 1942).

Baker-Brown of London (1859) gave an historical survey of the fistula
scene together with an enthusiastic description of the Bozeman method of
fistula closure, and even earlier, in 1856 recommended the use of episiotomy
to aid fistula exposure. He described a self-retaining quadrivalved dilating
speculum made by Mr. Hilliard, a surgical instrument maker from Glasgow,
designed to dilate the vaginal introitus and vaginal interior (Fig. 32). Prior
to surgery when there had been gross vaginal scarring, he advocated preliminary vaginal dilatation to improve subsequent exposure. Dividing all
strictures with a bistoury and cutting towards the sides of the vagina to
avoid the rectum, bleeding was staunched by plugging the vagina for 48
hours with strips of lint dipped in oil. This vaginal plug was replaced by
a tent of oiled silk, stitched like the thumb of a glove and well-filled with
small pieces of sponge. The tent was removed daily, the vagina syringed
clean, and progressively, a larger tent inserted. "When the whole vaginal
surface is again covered by mucus membrane, the operation to close the
fistula may be proceeded with." Surgical correction began by removing a
ring of mucus membrane around the fistula opening, paring the fistula
edges and then introducing sutures which were passed through the eyelet
hole of a simple bar clamp (Fig. 33) or in some cases, Bozeman's button—
"which has a superiority over clamps when the vagina is very large and

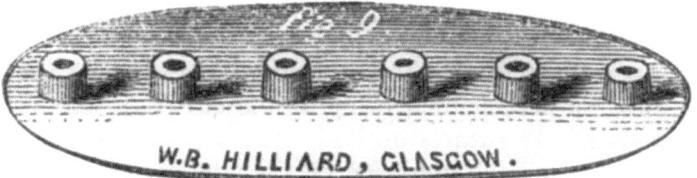

Figure 33. Baker-Brown bar clamp with nipples to replace loose perforated shot. (From Baker-Brown)

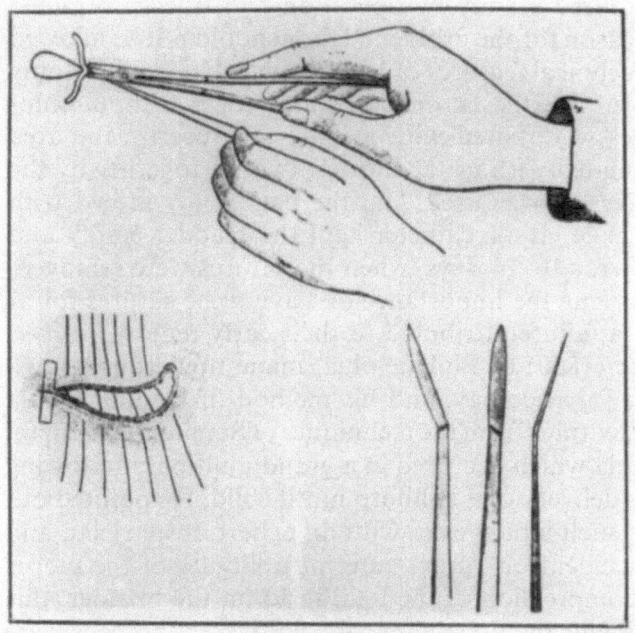

Figure 34. Baker-Brown's technique using single curved lead clamps which were straightened by forceps to oppose the fistula margins. The instruments shown were devised by Baker-Brown. (From Baker-Brown)

lax, or where there is an unhealthy condition of the fistula edges". Left undisturbed for ten days, the sutures were then removed. In later cases, Baker-Brown substituted a single lead clamp for each suture, each clamp having a nipple pierced to receive the wire suture. Drawing the suture tight, the clamp was nipped by special forceps to fix the suture (Fig. 34).

However, eventually he discarded both clamps and buttons favoring Sims' method of merely twisting the wire sutures together.

Should the fistula open through the cervix, he suggested splitting the cervix to lay it open into the fistula, then bringing the cut edges of the uterine walls into apposition with sutures in the ordinary way, but when the fistula was high and involved the uterine neck, he advocated closing the os itself, and diverting the menstrual discharge into the bladder. He claimed no ill consequences followed this maneuver.

Baker Brown (1864) reported 43 successful closures in a series of 55 vesico-vaginal fistulae, some of which were large. He stated that vesico-vaginal fistula could be cured readily by operation and since protracted labor generally was the reason for the problem, labor should not be allowed to become protracted. Technical features of his surgery included lithotomy position under chloroform anesthesia, or hands and knees without chloroform. The fistula edges were pared with a knife to saucerize the area which then was approximated with metal sutures, twisted together by the surgeon's fingers. No dressing was used, and the patient lay in bed with her knees drawn up. A male elastic catheter kept the bladder empty and the patient stayed quietly for 10–14 days, when the sutures were removed. He concluded by emphasizing the importance of leaving the sutures for at least nine days, quoting a failure attributed to their early removal.

Washington L. Atlee (1860) of Philadelphia, made numerous contributions to the advance of gynecology, and his method of bladder fistula repair combined the best features from the techniques of Sims and Bozeman. He described a large fistula which occurred in a grand multipara following the very difficult forceps delivery of a stillborn ninth child. He pointed out that fistula can occur in such labors even with an expert obstetrician and blamed this particular accident on "great anterior obliquity of the uterus together with constant compression of the fetal head on the bladder, this force constantly increasing as the pregnancy advanced". The forceps were exonerated since the incontinence occurred during the prolonged labor, and on several occasions the bladder was proven empty prior to delivery. Two months later, Atlee confirmed the large fistula; but declined surgery until after the approaching menstrual period. The fistula was $1^1/_4$ inch in diameter, almost a perfect circle, with most of the trigone destroyed and red bladder mucosa protruding through the opening. Surgery was performed in the knee-elbow position without general anesthesia, but nearly 30 drops of elixir of opium, were taken orally. "The rectum was elevated with a Sims speculum, the fistula was brought into good view and the whole vagina completely illuminated by sunlight."

Transfixing the fistula edge by bistoury, a complete circle of tissue was removed from the fistula opening with one swoop of the knife. At the completion of this dissection the patient was allowed to rest on her side. The second step was the passage of six blue wire sutures, using the alternates for fistula closure and the others passed through a Bozeman type lead plate to relieve tension on the wound. Some catheter drainage was used initially but later the patient voided without help and three weeks after surgery, "my patient walked downstairs with very little assistance, got into her carriage and rode home, a distance of several miles".

Maurice Collis of Dublin (1861) suggested splitting the fistula margin all round in order to separate bladder and vagina widely, one half consisting of vaginal mucus membrane and submucus tissue and the other, vesical mucus membrane and submucus tissues. The extent of separation was decided by fistula size, position, and the condition of its margins. Near the cervix, dissection was unnecessary to a great depth since a better blood supply in the area ensured ready union, but if situated on the bladder floor, dissection should be more extensive because tissues were thinner and a wider extent of raw surface was necessary to secure proper union. Separation should be proportionately extensive whenever fistula margins were unhealthy. Preferring wire or thread sutures to silk, he declared that the raw surfaces should not be drawn together too tightly, otherwise edges may slough since inevitably much swelling would arise during the first 24 hours. The effect of confining flaps tightly between two vaginal bars was interference with nutrition resulting in their death. When the raw edges were drawn together by quilled suture, he believed a ridge arose on the vaginal surface between the quills, and that a similar but larger ridge was thrown up towards the bladder which acted as a valve. In several instances, he succeeded in reducing a large fistula aperture to moderate dimensions after a succession of procedures, finally closing it completely. He attributed failure to overmuch haste in repeating operations before the fistula edges were restored to a healthy condition.

Schuppert of New Orleans, a great operator and critic, published "Treatise on Vesico-Vaginal Fistula" in 1866 which contained surgical pearls as well as well as spicy criticisms of his contemporaries. He believed that whether or not the vesical mucosa was perforated with the sutures did not matter, declaring that "fear of wounding mucous membrane of the bladder is a spectre not founded on reality". He advocated early ambulation saying the operation could be done without anesthesia; but used it to spare patient's feelings and gave an account of 17 patients, and of one he cured he remarked: "The patient did not long endure her happiness, for about 3 months later she died of yellow fever, a disease in which silver sutures are unavailing." He attempted to close one tiny fistula with silver nitrate and remarked, "Has the opening closed? I doubt the affirmative from the experience I have had with nitrate of silver, which seems to favor only French surgeons." In 1859 he attempted to close a large adherent fistula first by uniting the middle portion, and then at two subsequent operations, the small openings left at the sides. To counter-balance Diffenbach's classic but depressing and pessimistic description, Schuppert enthusiastically exclaimed: "The joy of the poor woman after 4 years of suffering, being besides previously told by several physicians that her case was a hopeless one, is beyond description in seeing herself freed from a loathsome disease. (Kelly 1912)."

Pawlik (1882) was first to advocate preliminary catheterization of ureters to avoid damage during fistula repair (Latzko 1942).

Milton (1887) in the St. Thomas' Hospital reports, gave details of 60 fistulae treated in Cairo, 50 of which were vesico-vaginal and 10 recto-vaginal. He took great pains before surgery to improve the patient's general health with good food and tonics, and "to bring the mucus membrane of the vagina and bladder and the integument of the external genital organs into the best possible condition by frequent emollient irrigations". Like Atlee, he emphasized that surgery should be performed one week after the menstrual period, although in most of his patients, the menses were suppressed. Cicatiricial contractions in the vagina should be divided 10 days previously, and the vagina dilated as far as possible to normal dimensions. He used both lithotomy and prone positions for surgery, and regarded silver wire as the best suture. Adequate exposure was emphasized, and to this end he employed the Sims speculum with a variety of techniques to bring the fistula well into view. He put thread through the cervix for traction or used a vulsellum, and in two patients with particular difficulty in exposure, dilated the urethra, introduced a finger into the bladder and prolapsed the fistula to the vulva. He believed it immaterial if wound closure was transverse to the long axis of the vagina, and practised wide mobilization of bladder from vagina so producing a funnel-shaped wound surface. The blunt apex of the funnel corresponded to the vesical edges of the fistula, and its base to the original incision. Generally irrigation was sufficient to check bleeding—he used weak sublimate solution—and sutures were passed by inserting the needle between bladder and vagina, to exit as far laterally as the dissection permitted. The wires were pulled through, both ends grasped with a pair of forceps, then handed to an assistant. A second stitch was introduced half an inch from the first, carefully avoiding bladder, and similarly further stitches were introduced at half inch intervals until the last, buried like the first was inserted. Then the stitches were tightened consecutively with a wire twister so they were neither too tight nor too loose. Tension on sutures was not uncommon and easily remedied by relieving incisions in the vaginal mucosa parallel to the wound. Finally, catgut sutures were introduced between the wires to ensure complete wound closure. Four hours after surgery, patients were encouraged to void spontaneously in the knee-elbow position, and if unsuccessful, he allowed periods as long as 10 hours to elapse, before catheterization.

Howard Kelly (1906) gave an excellent historical survey of the surgical events which led to the adoption of the suprapubic route in an endeavor to correct vesico-vaginal fistulae. The surgical victory of Lamballe, Sims, Emmet and Simon, with vaginal closure of vesico-vaginal fistula created such an impression upon contemporary thought that it seemed as though complete mastery over this difficult problem had been secured. However, succeeding decades revealed many cases in which the fistula was either so large or fixed in scar tissue and adherent to the pubic rami, that denudation and approximation by suture were insufficient to cope with the problem. Accordingly colpocleisis was used to close off the vagina, and Rose in order to obviate the risk of urine stagnation in the vaginal pocket formed by the colpolcleisis, effected a recto-vaginal fistula through which the urine drained into the rectum. It was with a view to avoiding such mutilating procedures that numerous ingenious methods were devised, and in fact almost every possible conceivable avenue was employed by which a fistula could be approached and dealt with to better advantage, to avoid difficulties which appeared to the operator as insurmountable by the usual vaginal route. In reality, the evolution of these new methods was a campaign conducted against colpocleisis. With large fistulae attached to bone Samter (1896) recommended removal of a pubic ramus by carrying the resection into the obturator foramen to gain adequate exposure, and von Bramann advised temporary resection of the pubic symphysis to give a wider abdominal wound without detaching the rectus muscles. Trendelenburg made two unsuccessful attempts to close a fistula by the suprapubic route in 1881 and 1884 (Fig. 35) and the procedure was suggested for fistulae lying high in the vagina and close to the peritoneum, or those in which a vaginal procedure had been tried and failed. The abdomen was opened through a transverse suprapubic incision dividing the rectus muscles at their insertion, entering the bladder extraperitoneally. Bladder mucosa denudation was made in the shape of a funnel, and if the fistula lay too close to the ureteric orifice, this was protected by introducing a sound. The fistula was closed

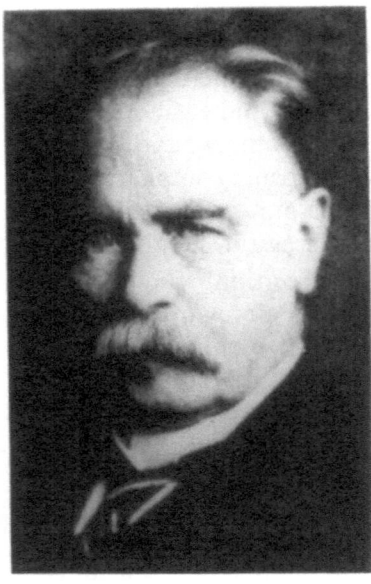

Figure 35. Friedrich Trendelenburg

with six silkworm gut sutures, and postoperatively the patient made to lie constantly upon one side or the other to assist bladder drainage. The patient, although successful had to return because of calculi which formed on the silkworm gut sutures, and these sutures were removed by dilating the urethra so a finger could be inserted into the bladder to remove both sutures and concretions. Following this misfortune, Trendelenburg advised closing the vesical wound with catgut. Kelly commented that perusal of the descriptions of Trendelenburg's interesting first case, suggested to him that a deft gynecologist experienced in vaginal surgery might well have succeeded in effecting a cure without the necessity for the suprapubic approach. Similar to and inspired by Trendelenburg was the work of McGill (1890) who reported two cases, the first a urethral epithelioma extending onto the base of the bladder which he removed by transvesical approach then closed the resulting defect, and so successful was this procedure that he used the same approach to close a large vesico-vaginal fistula. In 1893 Leopold von Dittel of Vienna, after two unsuccessful vaginal procedures to close a large vesico-vaginal fistula associated with destruction of the anterior uterine lip, attempted to close the fistula by an abdominal tran-speritoneal procedure. Drawing the uterus out through the abdominal incision, the vesico-uterine peritoneum was divided and the bladder freed from the uterus and vagina to expose the fistulous opening which was

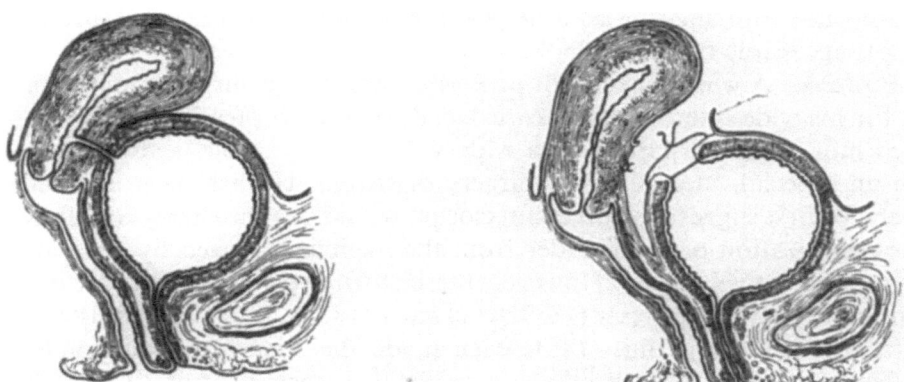

Figure 36. Von Dittel's procedure. (From Latzko)

denuded and closed. Unfortunately the operation failed because of the patient's interference with the wound. Subsequent writers suggested its use in management of the high postoperative vesico-vaginal fistula, and individual authors have achieved excellent results with this procedure (Fig. 36). Bardenhaeuer (1891) and Frank (1894) suggested bladder mobilization to enhance the ease of fistula closure. In two cases reported by Bardenhaeuer, the closure was effected abdominally, whereas in Frank's case, freeing the bladder enabled an artificial descensus of bladder and uterus to be secured so the fistula could easily be attacked from the vagina.

Schuchardt (1893) introduced the parasacral incision used successfully by him in 1896, to facilitate repair of a high vesico-vaginal fistula. The Schuchardt incision of that time, differed from Duhrssen's deep incision only in the fact that it was carried up into the vault and then down and out nearly to the tip of the coccyx thereby encircling the anus. Schuchardt wrote that, "For comfortable accessibility the levator need not be cut through. The incision leaves the levator tunnel entirely untouched." The Schuchardt incision now in general use and named by him the paravaginal incision, was proposed in 1901 as an introductory step in the radical vaginal operation for cervical carcinoma, and the principal difference from the original Schuchardt incision lay in cutting through the levator and coccygeus muscles, to open up the ischiorectal fossa. This incision opens the ischiorectal fossa widely, so that when the rectum has been forced back, the operative field in the upper vagina becomes superficial and no longer lies in the depths of a funnel. Many authors since that description have recommended the incision as a helpful preliminary to surgical closure of the less accessible fistula.

Professor Alwin Mackenrodt of Berlin, famed as a surgical innovator and for his wide interest and knowledge, during his professional life published more than 70 papers on a wide variety of gynecological subjects, with an especial interest in the surgery of fistula. He has been credited widely for first suggesting successful closure would be more likely to follow wide mobilization of the bladder from the vagina, followed by separate closure of the two defects. However, the historical record is clear on this point and shows Dupuytren (1829), Hayward (1839), Maisoneuve (1848): (Latzko 1942), and Collis (1861) each made the same suggestion independently. In 1894, Mackenrodt wrote: "Fistula surgery has not yet reached a point of technical perfection that would guarantee the complete cure of this unpleasant disorder. The small not too deeply situated fistula can be easily and perfectly closed using Simon's technique for angular trimming of the fistula edges, then simple suture. However when the vaginal wall is very scarred, the sutures cut through readily and the adaption of the edges soon is gone after the operation, and perhaps new small fistulae will develop through the suture holes." He pointed out the increasing problem with larger fistulas particularly those difficult of access, and cited Martin (1891) who loosened vaginal flaps next to the fistula edges, inverted them into the bladder and having plugged the bladder defect, endeavored to close the vaginal wall. He cured two patients by this technique; but clearly the method was applicable only with adequate vaginal tissues. Also in 1888, H. Fritsch had suggested flap-splitting the fistula edges to provide a larger wound surface than the Simon procedure, but useful only with smaller fistulae. Larger defects made closure without tension impossible.

Mackenrodt considered colpocleisis as "only excusable by the truly desperate state of women suffering from incurable vesico-vaginal fistula and in such cases, one must weigh sympathy for the patient against disapproval for an operation that cannot be justified scientifically". He believed von Dittel's transperitoneal approach was dangerous, "there is no doubt this intervention puts the patient between life and death", and regarded the suprapubic extraperitoneal approach as "less dangerous but more difficult". To avoid dangers of the abdominal approach to a large fistula, Mackenrodt proposed wide bladder and vaginal separation, for then no matter the size of the defect, "the bladder detached from the vagina does not resist primary union and the vaginal defect may be left open". The fistula was exposed using a large episiotomy if necessary, the upper and lower edges of the fistula were caught with a tenaculum, and the

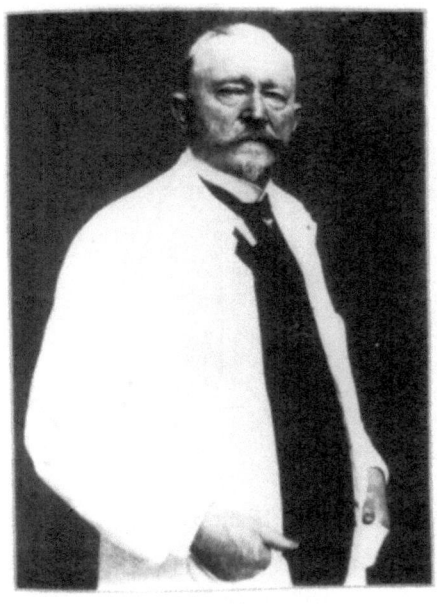
Alwin Mackenrodt †

Figure 37. Alwin Mackenrodt

anterior vaginal wall made tense by traction. An incision extended through the vaginal wall in the median line across the fistula, and then the fistula margins were split so as to detach the bladder completely from the vaginal wall on all sides. The mobile bladder was closed after denuding its edge then opposing them with fine silkworm gut sutures, followed by a second and even third layer of sutures, and finally closure of the vaginal wound. Following bladder closure, the vaginal wall was sutured to the uterus—vaginofixation—and the vaginal flaps closed across the midline if feasible; but if not, each flap was stitched separately to the uterus, leaving a central defect. Postoperative treatment was simple, "the patient must urinate frequently or a catheter must be applied", and twice daily the vagina was douched with mild antiseptic. Usually the bladder sutures caused little reaction, and their discharge spontaneously through the urethra was to be anticipated. Although this paper was based only on two successful cases—one a 3 cm defect and the other, after 4 previous failures by 3 different surgeons, nevertheless both were cured after 14 days, and Mackenrodt believed the benefit of this method to be so great, that he no longer regarded any vesico-vaginal fistula as incurable. He considered neither colpocleisis nor laparotomy necessary, for this vaginal technique was the natural way to operate on such large fistulas combining successful outcome with minimal risk (Fig. 37).

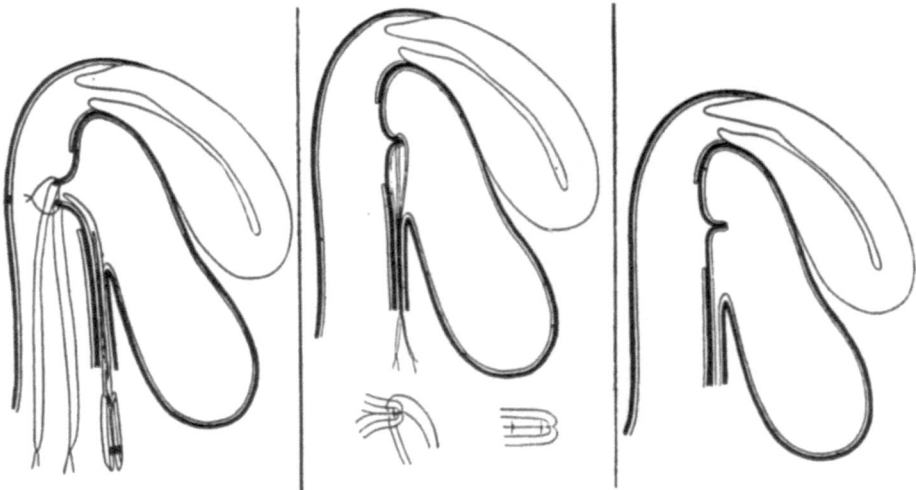

Figure 38. Stanmore Bishop's technique. (From Stanmore Bishop)

Stanmore Bishop (1897) describing a new method of operating upon
vesico-vaginal fistula commented, "that operations for the cure of vesico-
vaginal fistula are even now futile will, I believe, be admitted. Even in the
latest list of any importance, that of Milton of Cairo, out of 79 operations,
41 were useless." He believed "any union depending on primary adhesion
for success, if exposed to the action of urine, will be extremely likely to
break down and allow percolation through into the track of sutures, with
consequent failure". He claimed the past 50 years had seen little alteration
in the mode of attack, for in all, the fistula edges were the parts attacked,
the principle being to obtain a large raw surface, whether by paring or
varying degrees of splitting. Colpocleisis had been the only procedure
avoiding the fistula edge and he quoted a pregnancy which had occurred
after successful colpocleisis, doubtless due to urethral insemination! Accordingly he suggested mobilizing the fistulous tube as a whole, including
an annulus of vaginal wall attached to the fistula edge, the width of this
annulus depending upon the size of the fistula. "When mobilized the vaginal
mucosa lies like a truncated glove finger attached solely at the edge and
continuous with the mucus wall of the bladder." At four equidistant points
on this frill, sutures were passed, but not knotted and the frill was inverted
into the bladder by pulling the sutures through the urethra. So the mucus
membrane faced the bladder and the raw connective tissue faced the vagina
and came into apposition with ease. A purse string of silk was placed at

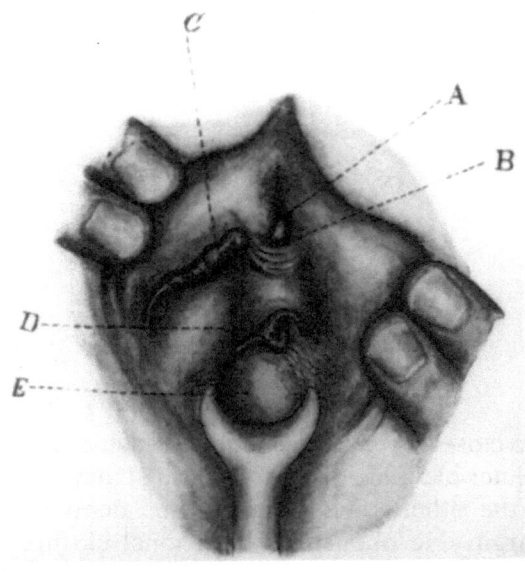

Figure 39. Noble's labium minor flap. *A* Clitoris; *B* artificial urethral orifice; *C* right labium; *D* left labium minus; *E* anterior vaginal wall. (From Noble)

this site and tightened as the inversion was effected then further sutures were placed burying deeper sutures as further inversion occurred and finally the guiding threads were removed. The raw vaginal surfaces were closed without tension (Fig. 38).

Charles Noble (1901) made an historic contribution to the problem of reconstructing an entirely destroyed urethra. Few experiences had been reported prior to this time, the most important being that of Emmet (1868) when he described six or seven cases all of which had failed. Noble offered two important contributions, the first a wide mobilization of the bladder fistula, followed by deep incisions parallel to the long axis of the vagina on either side of the proposed urethra, in order to raise flaps with which to form a new urethra. He emphasized the importance of detaching the soft parts from the pubic bone to overcome tension, then the tissues were sutured around a small catheter to form a new urethra. His second contribution was the idea that a flap was better than using local tissues when tension was unavoidable along the line of union, so he selected the left labium minor as tissue for the flap, since this could be detached easily from subjacent structures. The tissues were very elastic, and the mobilized labium could be drawn easily over the raw suture, then back into the vagina (Fig. 39).

Howard Kelly (1896) reviewing management of large vesico-vaginal fistula, mentioned especially the Mackenrodt mobilization and the work

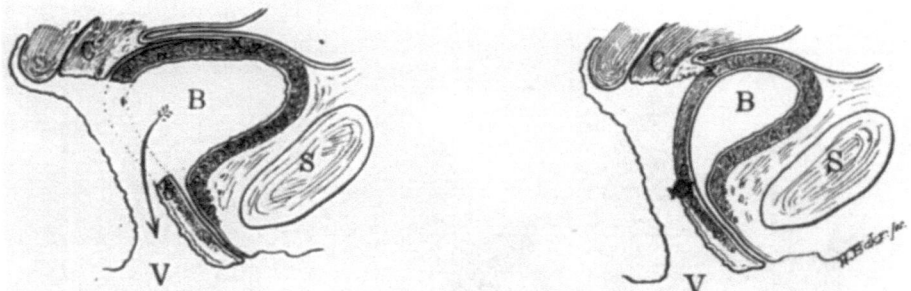

Figure 40. Kelly technique for dealing with a large vesico-vaginal fistula. (From Kelly)

of E. C. Dudley from Chicago, who closed a very large fistula by fashioning a semicircular denudation on the inner bladder surface extending from one margin of the fistula around to the other, then attaching the denuded surface to the anterior fistula margin. He obtained a functional closure despite the exclusion of a portion of the posterior part of the bladder. Kelly's patient presented with the bladder mucosa everted through a large defect, both ureteric orifices opened onto the fistula edge, and after five previous attempts at closure, several centimeters of each ureter had been sacrificed. The fistula margins were densely fibrotic with no possibility of bringing these tissues together by any known means of denudation or suture, so he devised the following procedure: the ureters were catheterized, and making a crescentic incision around the posterior two thirds of the fistula, the bladder and vagina were separated widely with the bladder freed to the peritoneum. Then a strip was removed from the anterior one third of the fistula, and the mobilized bladder accurately applied to this fixed, denuded anterior area, so bladder mucosa and ureteric orifices were inverted (Fig. 40). In 1902, Kelly contributed to the surgery of difficult high vesico-vaginal and recto-vaginal fistula following hysterectomy, when he suggested opening the peritoneal cavity widely from side to side, so freeing the bladder from its fixation to the vault, and rendering it more mobile. This step enabled the entire area to be moved so the fistula could be closed more easily and without tension. Separating the rectum on all sides to mobilize it and make it more accessible could be applied with even greater satisfaction to the surgical closure of the high recto-vaginal fistula. Here previous hysterectomy was not required to facilitate exposure, it was necessary only to open the cul-de-sac behind the cervix, then from side to side and down the sides of the rectum to gain great advantage from the

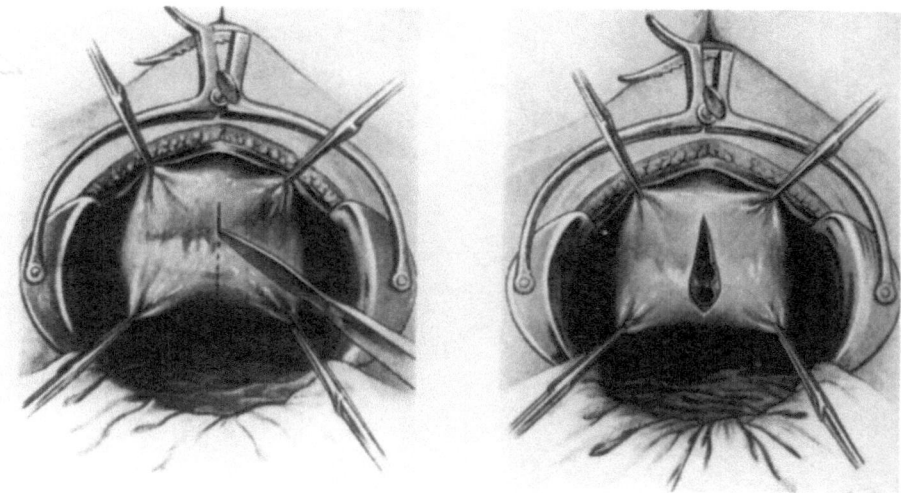

Figure 41. Midline incision into the bladder and vaginal vault exposing the fistula orifices

increased bowel mobility. In 1912 Kelly chose as his title for the Presidential address to the American Gynecological Society, "The History of Vesico-Vaginal Fistula". This detailed paper with an excellent bibliography covered the field of fistula surgery in detail up to that time. He invited the audience to contemplate efforts which had been made to cure fistula before Sims' time, the work of Sims and his contemporaries, and finally what had been done since Sims' death 27 years before to perfect this operation.

Felix Legueu of Paris (1914) suggested yet another suprapubic fistula operation namely a transvesical-transperitoneal method, a combination of the Trendelenburg and von Dittel procedures, in which the bladder was opened by a sagittal incision via the peritoneal cavity, and the incision extended to the fistula (Fig. 41). Following this, the vagina was separated from the bladder and individual closure effected (Figs. 42 and 43). Although ingenious and effective, in those days the problem with such surgery was fatal peritonitis, so the relatively high mortality from the procedure as well as its technical difficulty, argued in favor of the vaginal approach since vaginal fistula operations really had no primary mortality (Bandl 1878).

Charles Dowman of Atlanta, Georgia (1920) reported an unusual method for dealing with a large vesico-vaginal fistula. His young patient suffered an extensive fistula following difficult delivery after a six day labor. The defect involved the anterior portion of the cervix together with the

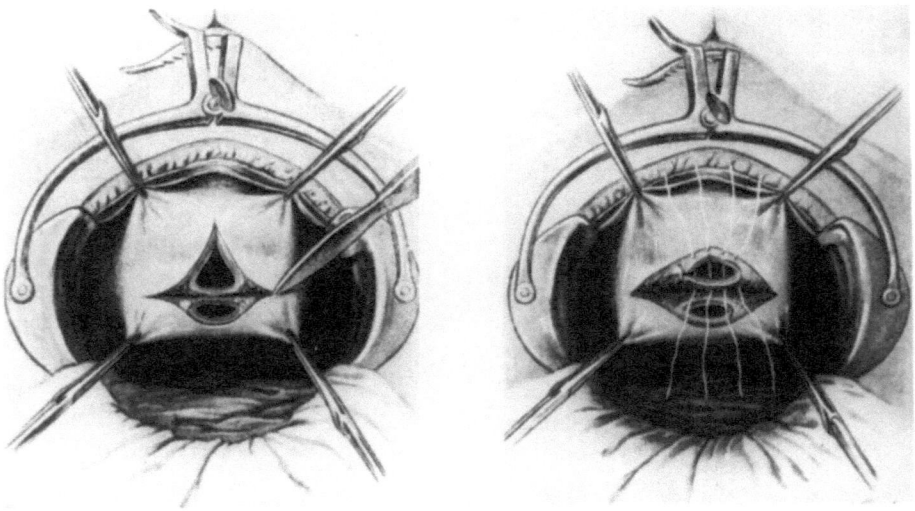

Figure 42. Complete separation of fistula orifices and sutures placed in bladder defect

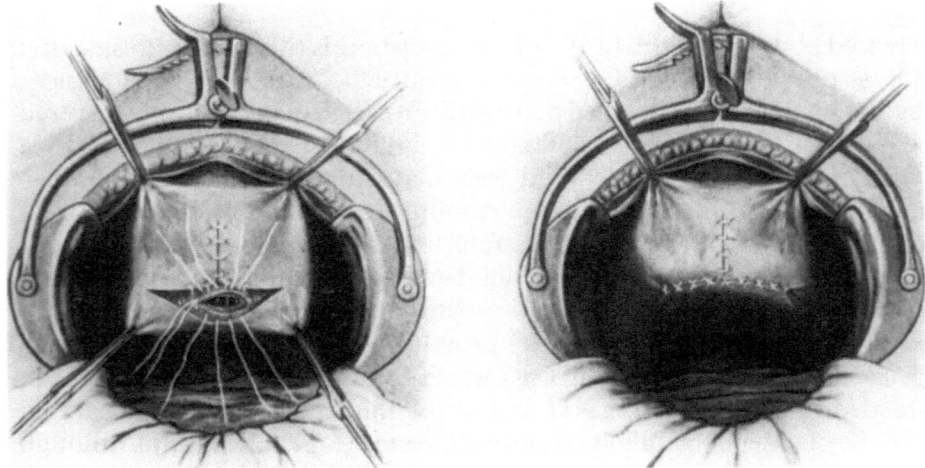

Figure 43. Closure of vault defect, then peritoneum. (From Legueu)

anterior vaginal wall, and complete destruction of almost the entire posterior wall of the bladder, excluding ureters. A combined vaginal and abdominal approach was employed with the patient in lithotomy position, and the vaginal surgeon commenced the procedure with an incision made at the junction of bladder and vaginal mucus membrane, freeing the bladder

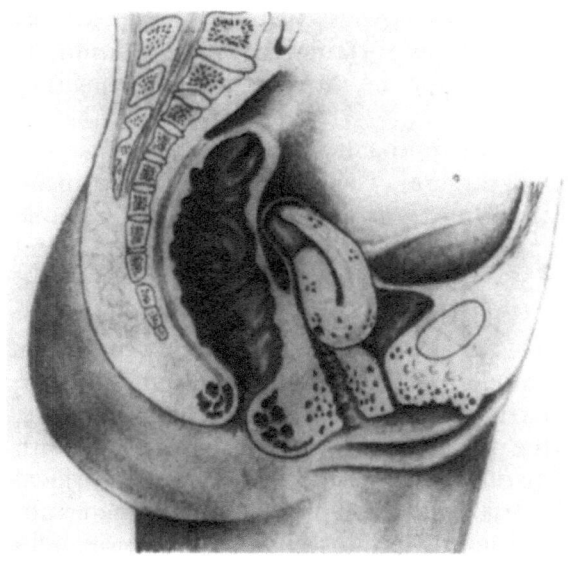

Figure 44. Edges of bladder defect sutured to the posterior uterine wall. (From Dowman)

wall extensively from the anterior vaginal wall on all sides. With the abdomen open, the Fallopian tubes, round and broad ligaments were divided and the bladder opened at its attachment to the anterior uterine wall. This dissection continued until the bladder was freed completely from all uterine attachment and the uterus placed in an extreme anteverted position, so the posterior wall of the fundus could be utilized as the posterior wall of a reconstructed bladder. That part of the bladder wall accessible through the abdominal opening was sutured to the posterior surface of the uterus, so bladder mucus membrane was in contact with and approximated to the peritoneal surface of the uterus. The second line of sutures reinforced the first. Returning to the vagina, the operation was completed by continuing approximation of bladder wall to the peritoneal surface of the uterus, then a rentention catheter was placed in the urethra (Fig. 44). Three months later, cystoscopy showed that normal bladder and the part of the uterus forming its posterior wall scarcely could be differentiated. Six years afterwards the patient was healthy with a bladder functioning normally. There is nothing really new under the sun, for in 1895, Freund had succeeded in closing two large fistulae by utilizing the body of the inverted uterus brought through the posterior fornix into the vagina, then sewn to the anterior vaginal wall.

Herbert Spencer of London (1925) described his experiences with a variety of unusual genital fistulae in which he claimed success by using a hollow needle, designed by him in 1916, to pass the silver wire sutures. Like so many unaware of the contributions of Henry Levert and Montague Gosset, he gave full acknowledgement for the introduction of this suture material to Sims.

In 1906, Kelly reported a variety of approaches for correction of vesico-vaginal fistula which included parasacral, ischiorectal, transperitoneal, paravaginal, transvulval, transurethral, transpubic by removing a pubic ramus, trans-symphysial, suprapubic extraperitoneal and transperitoneal transvesical. Many approaches were destined to be short-lived or reserved for selected cases and today only vaginal, transvesical and combined are accepted as sound and practicable. The gradual favoring of the suprapubic route was attributed to the fact modern fistulas more commonly were the result of surgical trauma than parturition, frequently much less accessible, and urologists more often were the primary consultant than formerly. With the historical development of fistula surgery, the principles of surgical correction, developed largely by trial and error, gradually became established until 1852 when Sims, clarified uncertainties and stated principles categorically, which are just as valid today. More recently the principle of interposing healthy tissues as a plug between vagina and bladder or between rectum and vagina has been added to the armamentarium.

The Grafters

The concept of a graft to lie between bladder and vagina originated with Heinrich Martius of Göttingen, Germany and John Garlock of New York, USA in 1928. Martius, Professor of Obstetrics and Gynecology in the University of Göttingen, had a major interest in gynecological radiology and radiotherapy, and also gynecological surgery. His textbooks on obstetrics and gynecology were translated into several languages; but it is for the bulbocavernosus graft, which carries his name, that he is remembered throughout the gynecological world (Fig. 45). Initially (1928) he described a grafting technique using pelvic floor muscles in an endeavor to reinforce a urethra, reconstituted following a large urethro-vaginal fistula after forceps delivery. The muscle transfer was made also with the hope that it would function as a sphincter and help continence control. In the past, similar procedures had been proposed using the body of the uterus; but there were obvious technical difficulties and later problems with uterine disease. Martius dissected the ischiocavernosus and bulbocavernosus mus-

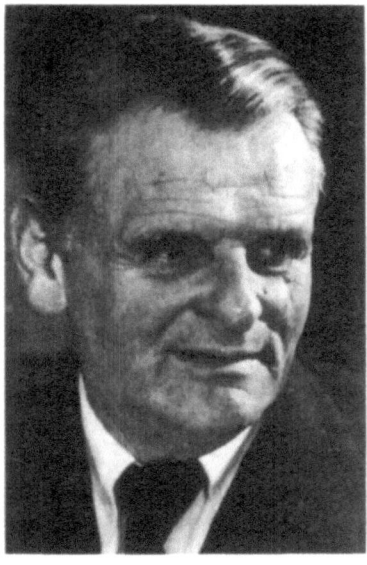

Figure 45. Heinrich Martius

cles subcutaneously until he obtained a flap "as thick as a finger and as long as a small finger" attached at the point of origin, and this flap was placed across the bladder neck to act as a sphincter, then fixed to the pubic ramus on the opposite side (Figs. 46 and 47). The skin was closed over the graft. Writing again in 1942 he stated that the "bulbocavernosus supplement was used only when special reasons seemed to make it necessary". For simple fistulae, it was used only when there was difficulty closing the vaginal skin without tension. He believed the graft assisted sphincter fuction by muscular activity, and by the pad acting as a valve on the bladder neck area. With large fistulae, the graft was used more and more as a tissue substitute, to protect fistula closure and he believed the technique was simple, without risk and guaranteed in high degree to cure the fistula. "The risk is low, the gain is high and the flap can always be enlarged to meet the need with sufficient material in the labia majora and mons pubis, and can conventiently be pulled through the undermined labia minora and used for the simple coverage of all cavities and corners." The flap also had a place covering a closed recto-vaginal fistula especially those which followed radiation. A further benefit claimed was in provision of adequate soft tissue in the area making any further fistula surgery for a small recurrence, so much easier. Initially, Martius described the graft as bulbocavernosus; but in later reports used the term bulbocavernosus fatty flap and commonly today the graft is known as the Martius fat graft (Figs. 48 and 49). Professor

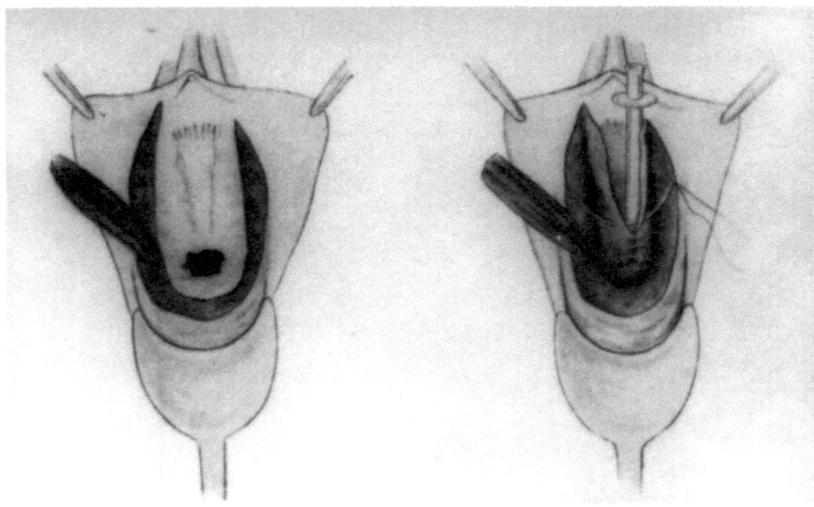

Figure 46. Mobilization of ischiocavernosus and bulbocavernosus and commencing urethral reconstruction

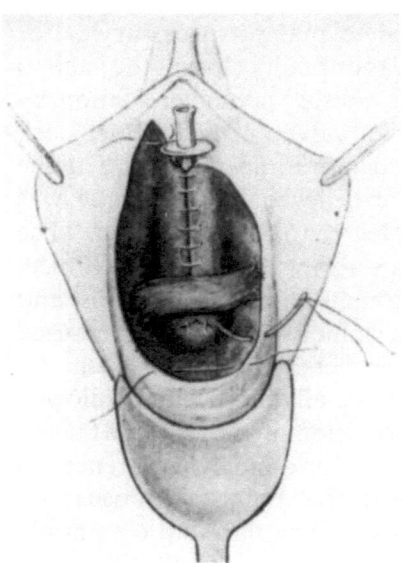

Figure 47. The ischiocavernosus and bulbocavernosus graft in place

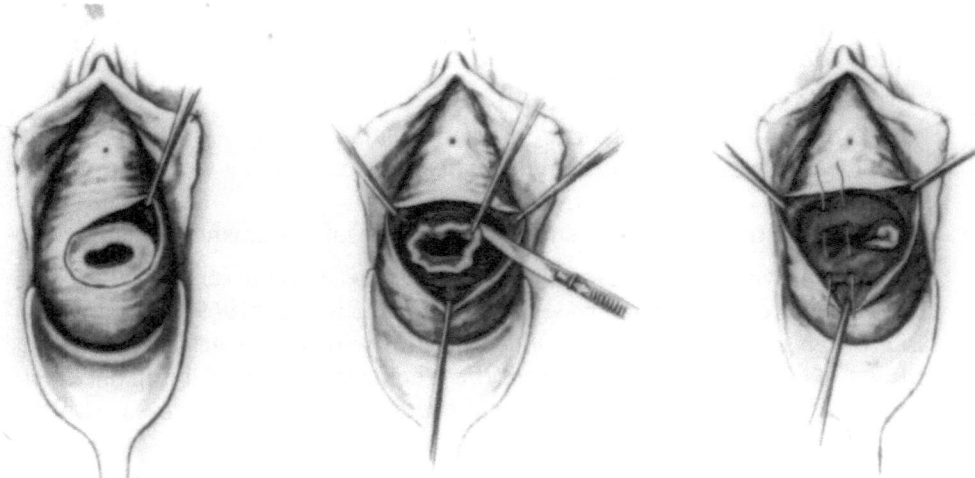

Figure 48. Martius technique of fistula closure

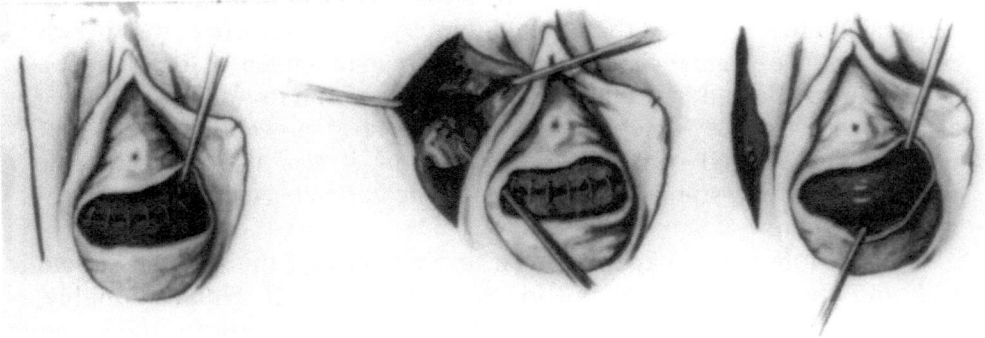

Figure 49. Fashioning and placement of the Martius fat graft. (From Martius)

Martius died in 1965 a few weeks after his 80th birthday and having perhaps a premonition of impending death, invited a large circle of relatives, friends and students on that occasion. Since initial publications, the Martius graft gained immediate and wide acceptance amongst fistula surgeons and its place as one of the important principles of surgical correction of fistula is secure. Shaw (1949) used the graft in repair of urethro-vaginal fistula and vesico-vaginal fistula, and regarded it highly. "The results have been so good that I have thought fit to draw attention to what I regard as the extraordinary value of the method in vaginal surgery." Betson (1961) attributed four functions to the graft:

1. Adds support to the urethral neck.
2. Adds bulk to the bladder neck and bladder base.
3. Decreases and/or obliterates the dead space between vaginal mucosa and bladder.
4. Brings in a new blood supply to an area of diminished vascularity.

He employed the technique with both large or recurrent fistulae and with severe stress incontinence. Hamlin and Nicholson (1969) used a Martius graft in all but the smallest fistulae, and with the largest defects, the graft was used selectively to reinforce the gracilis muscle graft, lying between the muscle and the vaginal skin, "to make security, doubly secure". Birkhoff et al. (1977) used the graft with success in 10 fistula patients, many having repeat surgery, and believed the fat pad a significant factor in successful closure with alleviation of stress incontinence. They recommended the procedure should be used in repair of all fistulae. Clegg (1979) expressed similar views. Webster et al. (1984) reviewing surgical managment of urethro-vaginal fistula stated that labial fat interposition improves the success rate of urethro-vaginal fistula repair, and recommended it for all cases. The pad provided additional blood supply and lymph drainage to the area as well as a surface for epithelization, while also preventing overlap of urethral and vaginal suture lines. In addition, it was also suggested the pad facilitated re-establishment of continence after correcting a urethro-vaginal fistula.

Some more recent papers give an impression that the surgeon should pick and choose whether or not to use a Martius graft. Unquestionably, the graft enhances the chance of surgical success, and except for the tiniest defects, there can be no good reason for not using the graft in every case whether the bladder, urethra or rectum is involved. To repeat Martius' words: "The risk is low, the gain is high."

John Garlock (1928) New York, USA reported cure of an intractable vesico-vaginal fistula using a pedicled muscle flap. He reviewed the development and refining of the principles of fistula surgery, whilst appreciating that each operative attempt at cure caused more tissue slough, establishing a vicious circle. Such a dilemma formerly had spawned a variety of heroic measures, including suprapubic cystotomy, colpocleisis and ureteric transplantation. In 1927, a patient aged 44, in whom three well-planned, well-executed procedures had failed, came under his care. Following the third failure, the fistula was $^3/_4$ inch in diameter and involved

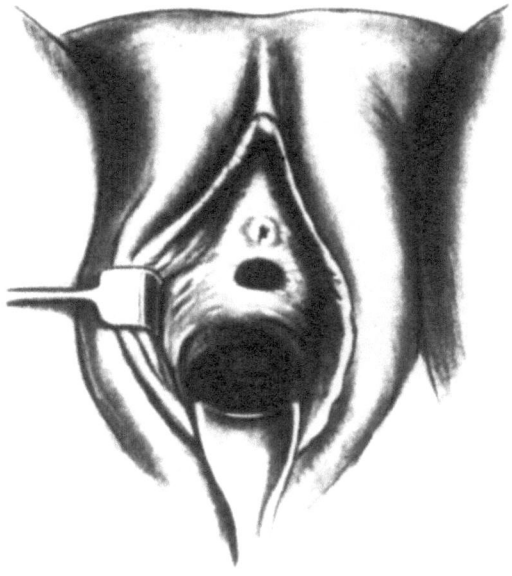

Figure 50. Garlock's patient with a large bladder fistula involving the urethra

part of the urethra (Fig. 50). The bladder was markedly contracted and its base a mass of dense scar tissue. The vaginal mucosa was atrophic and encrusted with urinary salts. Evidently something different was required for success, and three factors were judged to be of vital importance.

1. An atraumatic technique.

2. A layer of normal tissue should be interposed between bladder and vagina—a tissue with good blood supply and known resistance to infection.

3. The bladder should be kept dry at all times using continuous intravesical suction through a retention catheter. With this particular patient, it was necessary to close the defect and attempt repair of the divided sphincter. Two weeks' preoperative local cleansing preceded the surgery which followed standard techniques of flap-splitting and bladder closure, but performed through transverse anterior vaginal wall incisions. A longitudinal incision on the medial aspect of the right thigh exposed the gracilis muscle (Fig. 51). The lower nerve supply was divided and the muscle cut across at its insertion and turned back upon itself, dividing the upper nerve supply; but the upper blood supply remained intact. The lower thigh incision was closed, and the upper extension of the thigh incision made continuous with the vaginal wall incision by dividing the vulva transversely. The gracilis was placed across the bladder base and repaired fistula, then

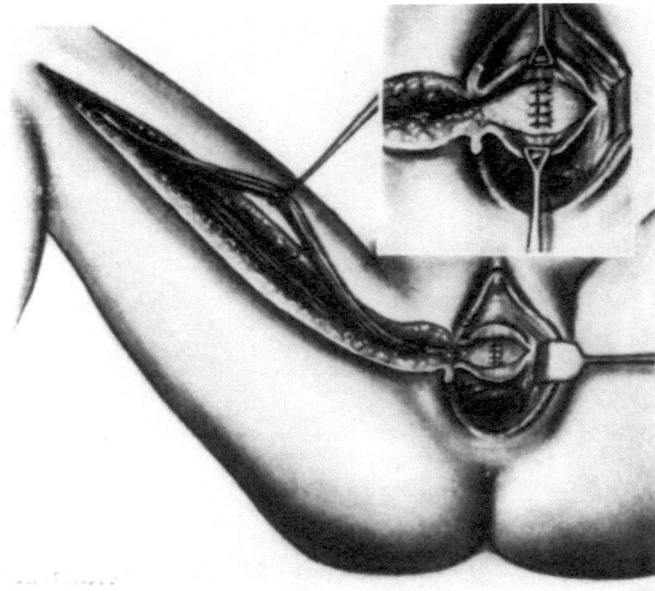

Figure 51. After raising anterior and posterior vaginal flaps, the fistula was closed in two layers. Medial thigh incision extended through the vulva and the gracilis muscle was isolated and retracted

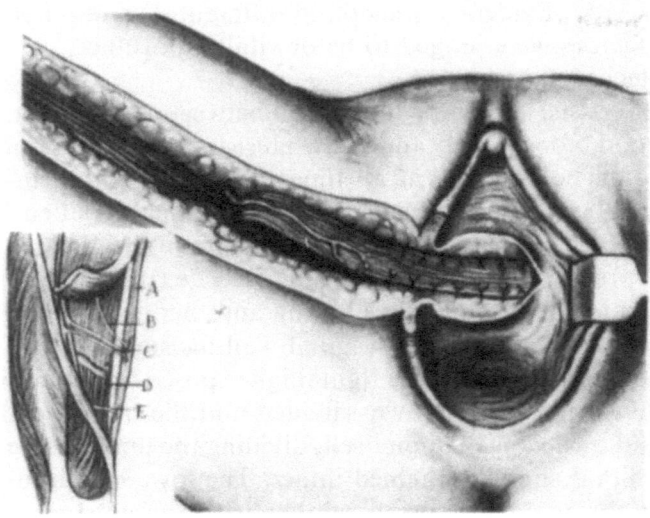

Figure 52. The gracilis muscle turned upon itself and anchored over the closed fistula

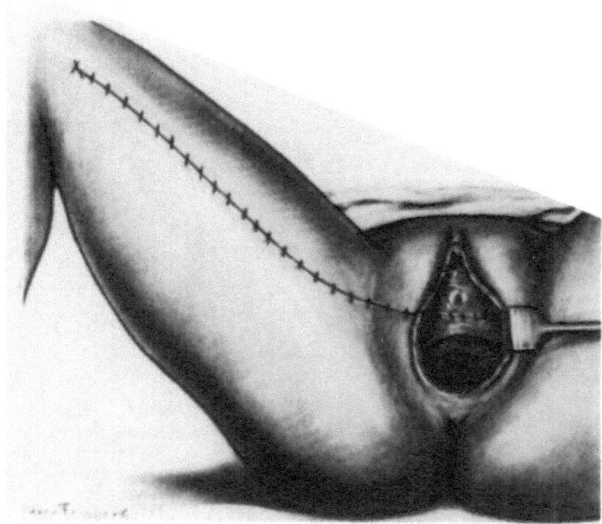

Figure 53. Closure of incisions in thigh, vulva and vagina. (From Garlock)

held in position by fine chromic catgut anchor sutures (Fig. 52). The vaginal mucosa was closed over the muscle, and the remaining thigh wound repaired (Fig. 53). After a bladder wash-out, an indwelling catheter was passed and a tight vaginal pack inserted. The thighs were immobilized with a moulded plaster splint of triangular shape placed to separate the knees. Intravesical suction was maintained for 24 days, and the catheter changed each 48 hours to maintain adequate suction. The pack was removed on the fourth day and although the anterior vaginal flap was sloughing, the muscle was intact and united to the bladder. There was no leakage. The fistula healed well; but continence control was imperfect. Ingelman-Sundberg (1960) discussed a variety of grafting techniques for use with fistula surgery including the pubococcygeal flap and bulbocavernosus fat graft of Martius, the rectus abdominus and gracilis muscle grafts. An innovative change in the technique of gracilis muscle grafting came by taking the muscle through a new canal in the obturator foramen rather than via the transvulval incision of Garlock, however other details were unchanged. The canal through the obturator foramen was made by index finger palpation on either side of the obturator membrane—between the gracilis and adductor magnus on one side, and between bladder and vaginal wall on the other. Care was necessary to avoid injury to the obturator nerve, and a long Kelly clamp guided by the fingers made a track, two fingers in

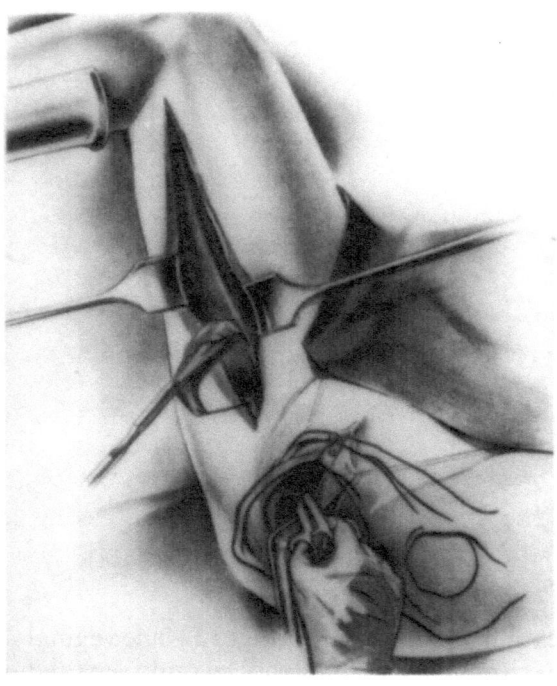

Figure 54. A suture through the gracilis tendon employed to draw the muscle graft through the canal in the obturator foramen. (From Ingelman-Sundberg)

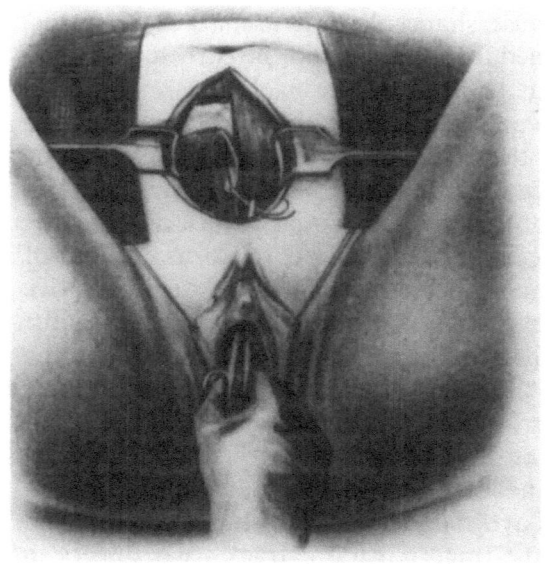

Figure 55. Flap of distal rectus muscle and inferior epigastric vessels drawn extraperitoneally into the vagina. (From Ingelman-Sundberg)

diameter to minimize muscle compression (Fig. 54). Similarly, the rectus abdominus muscle could be used as a pedicle flap graft, one rectus being divided at the umbilicus taking care not to damage the blood supply. An extraperitoneal canal was fashioned by the finger through the paravesical space down to the site of fistula closure, and the mobilized muscle drawn down to the vagina where it was anchored (Fig. 55) (Ingelman-Sundberg 1948). Banerji (1966) described a variant of the Ingelman-Sundberg procedure using a $^1/_2$ inch strip of rectus muscle and rectus sheath as a pedicle graft passed through the paravesical space to the vagina. Graham (1965) revived the principle of the Garlock procedure by suggesting the gracilis muscle could be brought into the upper vagina through a deep Schuchardt incision. However such an incision could endanger the pudendal nerve branch to the anal sphincter, and produce fecal incontinence. An important and much simpler technique of gracilis muscle grafting was introduced by Hamlin and Nicholson (1969) when they took the mobilized muscle through a subcutaneous tunnel into the vagina. The tunnel was made from thigh to introitus, deep to the skin and superficial fascia of the upper thigh and labium, using the handle of a large scalpel as a director. They emphasized "the tunnel should cross the ischiopubic ramus almost as high as the level at which the destroyed urethral meatus formerly emerged". The gracilis tendon was guided through the sublabial tunnel and under the pubic symphysis to be fixed to the anterior lip of the cervix. Patil et al. (1980) gained excellent results in the correction of 18 difficult urinary fistulae using both gracilis and Martius fat grafts. Chassar Moir (1965) wrote: "The methods used by Ingelman-Sundberg and Hamlin and Nicholson are essentially different. In the former, the gracilis muscle is brought by a deep route to the upper vagina where it provides a new blood supply and serves as a plug for the fistula; in the latter, the muscle is brought by a superficial route to the lower vagina where it provides a direct support to the bladder and urethral wall." In addition to muscle and fat interposition between bladder and vagina, other structures—peritoneum, homograft of placenta or fetal bladder, omentum and myocutaneous flaps—have all been employed with varying degrees of success and acceptance. Peritoneal flap interposition described first by Bardescu (1900) and modified by Solms (1920) has enjoyed an upsurge in popularity since the 1960's. Eisen et al. (1974) proposed the following indications for the use of such a flap:

1. Vesico-vaginal fistula involving ureters.
2. Failed previous attempts at closure.
3. Post-irradiation fistula.
4. High fistulae, especially vesico-cervico-vaginal.

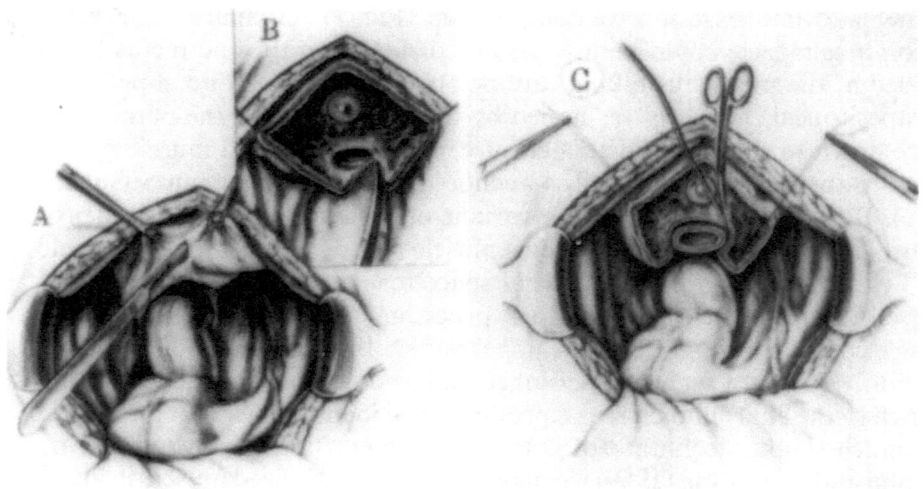

Figure 56. The bladder incised posteriorly to and through the posterior fistula margin, then bladder and vagina detached

Using a transperitoneal approach, the bladder was split, the fistula circumcised then freed from the vaginal wall, which was closed and re-inforced with a paravesical peritoneal flap cut from the lateral pelvic wall. The bladder was closed and drained by both suprapubic and Foley catheters, and both intraperitoneal and prevesical extraperitoneal drains were employed. The peritoneal flap offers enhanced success with closure, since the flap sticks quickly to the vaginal wall minimizing urinary leak. It is applicable to vesico-vaginal fistula at any location or of any size, and useful with a vesico-cervico-vaginal fistula.

Laffont (1946) introduced the placental graft in the repair of vesico-vaginal fistula because of the high regenerative capacity of embryonic tissue, and this early report prompted Tozum et al. (1975) to suggest and use fetal bladder as a homograft for such a repair. They reported two cases, both successful. The bladder was obtained from a five to six month stillborn fetus, removed en block within one hour of death and placed in saline. Routine vaginal surgery was employed with wide bladder and vaginal separation, then the fetal bladder was sutured to the bladder defect, both mucosal surfaces lying in apposition. The vaginal wall was closed and bladder drainage effected by urethral catheter for 12 days. Because of the difficulty having both patient and fetal bladder available simultaneously, they suggested establishment of a fetal bladder bank.

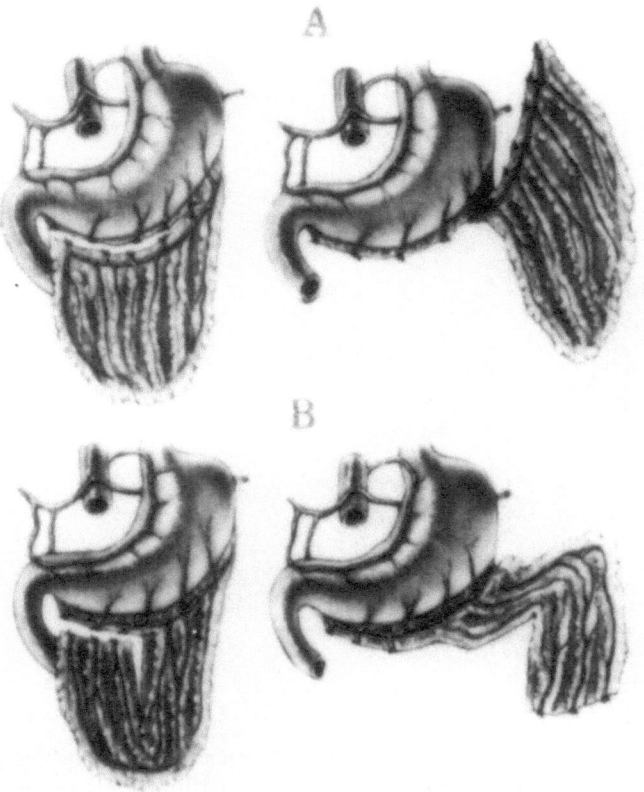

Figure 57. Mobilization of entire omentum (*A*) or omental flap (*B*)

Kiricuta and Goldstein (1972) first described the use of pedicled omentum in the repair of extensive vesico-vaginal fistula in 1955. The procedure included extensive median cystotomy with separation of the fistula from the vagina (Fig. 56). The bladder wall and ureters were mobilized from surroundihg tissues and the vaginal defect closed if feasible; but if not, it was left open to be occluded and healed over by the omental flap. Fashioning the omental pedicle depended upon vascularization of the omentum—if poorly developed, the whole omentum was mobilized based on the gastroepiploic artery; but when well-developed, the flap could be fashioned without including this artery (Fig. 57). Mobilization was from left to right or from right to left depending on the size of blood vessels; but should the omentum be very long and the free end easily brought to the

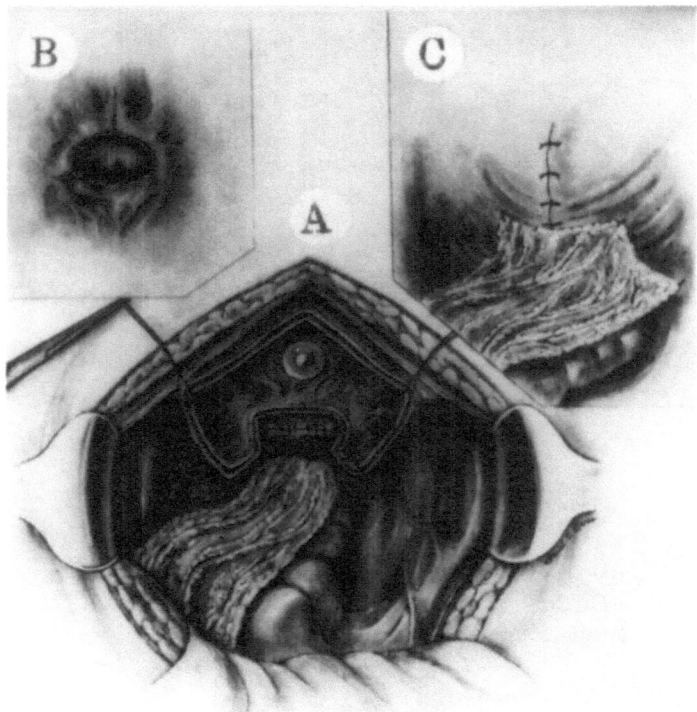

Figure 58. Vaginal defect closed with omental attachment to anterior lip of bladder defect (*A*). (*B*) represents the "curtain appearance" seen from within the bladder (*C*) following closure of the cystotomy incision, the omental pedicle was attached to the outer bladder surface, 2–3 cm away from the former defect. (From Kiricuta and Goldstein)

pelvis, no preparation was required. The pedicle was fixed to the right or left paracolic gutter or anterior abdominal wall lateral to the laparotomy incision to minimize small bowel obstruction. The cystotomy incision was closed, leaving the former defect open, the omentum covered the vesical defect from behind "such as an open window is covered by a curtain" and soon adhered to the posterior bladder wall (Fig. 58). Such a technique obviated the need to close the bladder or reimplant ureters, for the patch soon was covered by transitional epithelium and eventually contained smooth muscle fibers. Goldstein and Dearden (1966) experimented on rabbits with bladder defects occluded by pedicled omental grafts. Removing a circular segment of posterior bladder wall 12 mm in diameter, a collar of mucosa was stripped from the lumenal surface of the bladder around the margin of the defect, and an omental flap sutured to the bladder to cover the hole. Most critical histological change occurred in the first 15 days, and 24 hours following surgery, the lumenal surface of the omentum was covered by a thick layer of exudate. Vasodilatation was pronounced in the omentum attached to the bladder near the defect, and by the third and fourth days the margin of the bladder wall defect was covered in part by islets of epithelium from one to three layers thick. Tracing these epithelial islets by serial section showed they were not continuous with transitional epithelium of the bladder, and on the lumenal surface of the graft, groups of large epithelial-like cells formed a discontinuous layer of flattened cells between exudate and the newly formed connective tissue layer. By the 10th postoperative day a large portion of the omentum as well as most of the posterior bladder wall was covered with epithelium, and smooth muscle bundles were present in the newly formed connective tissue covering the lumenal surface of the omental patch. These bundles appeared to extend from the muscular layer of the bladder. By day 15, the omentum over the bladder wall defect was covered by transitional epithelium, and at 44 days mucosa covered the defect. Transitional epithelium covering the graft was continuous with that of bladder epithelium in the periphery of the defect; but also it seemed some originated from multipotential mesenchymal cells in the omentum.

Most of 27 patients reported by Kiricuta and Goldstein had developed a large fistula following irradiation and radical pelvic surgery, where healing and surgical problems were accentuated, and omental grafting prevented a diversionary procedure or reimplantation of ureters in these difficult cases. In the present context dealing with obstetric fistula, there is an important place for such a graft when abdominal closure of the fistula is contemplated, especially the vesico-cervico-vaginal fistula.

Baines et al. (1976) treated 19 large obstetric fistulae using "omental grafts and slings" in a combined abdomino-perineal technique. Beginning with wide vaginal mobilization of the fistula the bladder was opened extraperitoneally, vagina and bladder separated, and the fistula closed by sutures passed through one fistula edge from below to the abdominal surgeon, who returned the suture through the other edge. No effort was made to achieve water-tight closure, the mobilized omentum was fed into the vagina and fixed by anchor sutures to the site of fistula closure, and the procedure completed by closing both vaginal and suprapubic bladder incisions. With selected urethro-vesical fistulae, the omental graft was used also as a sling, passing it beneath the urethra to be tethered to the pubic

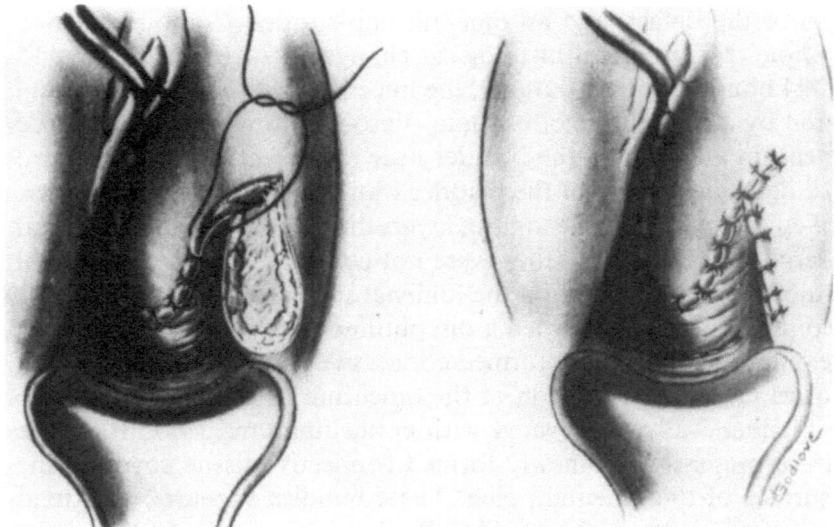

Figure 59 a. Symmonds' myocutaneous labial flap

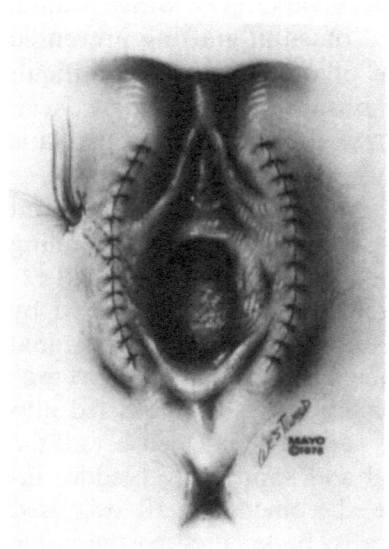

Figures 59 b, c. Symmonds' myocutaneous patch graft. (From Symmonds)

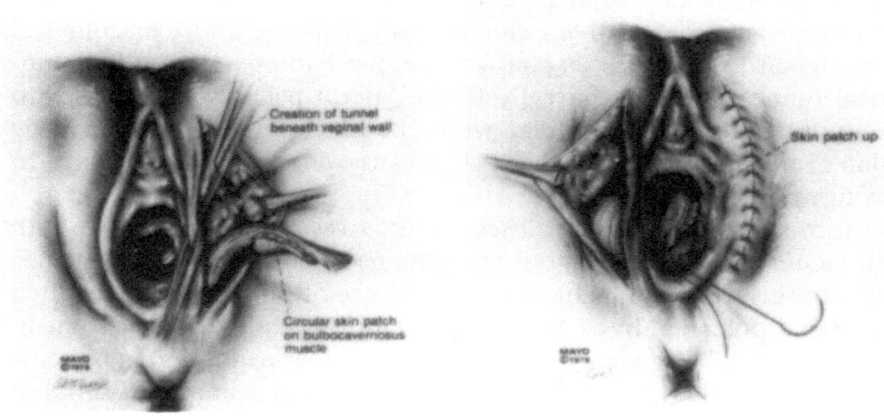

Fig. 59 b

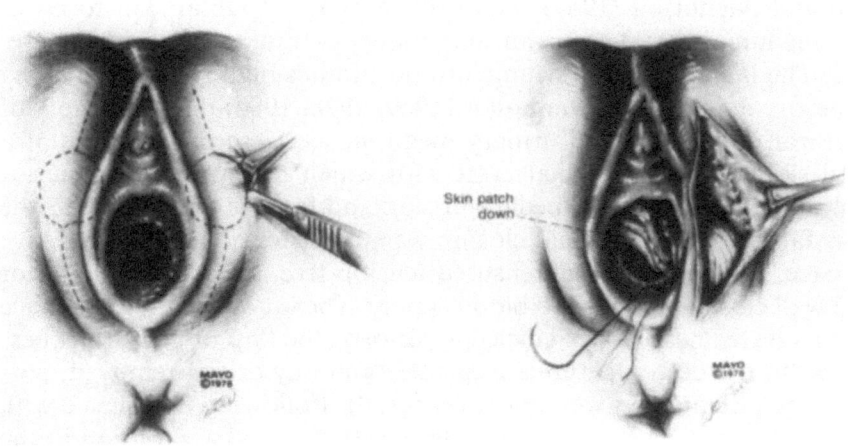

Fig. 59 c

symphysis by the abdominal surgeon in the hope that stress incontinence would be reduced.

Turner-Warwick (1976) agreed the interposition of an omental pedicle graft often ensured a reliable outcome with obstetric and gynecological vesico-vaginal fistulae. He emphasized the need to create an abdomino-perineal tunnel extending laterally to the lateral pelvic wall in order to ensure unsuspected lateral fistulae would be free, and also to allow wide overlap of the graft. The tunnel should be large enough to accept three to four fingers.

Orford and Theron (1985) closed 52 of 59 vesico-vaginal fistulae with the aid of an omental pedicle graft and obtained a cure rate of 93%. Major benefits of the graft were reduction of incidence of pin-hole fistulae, often a distressing postoperative complication, and the ability of omentum to form new tissue. They concluded an abdomino-perineal approach incorporating an omental graft was the treatment of choice in all but simplest fistulae.

Attempts to use labial skin as a graft to plug a fistula began in 1834 when Jobert de Lamballe of Paris, tried the technique; but with few successes. Similarly, in Germany, Döderlein suggested a flap of vaginal epithelium, rolled into a tube to plug the fistula and buried beneath vaginal mucosa. Charles Noble (1901) of Philadelphia reported a patient with entire destruction of the urethra and after repeat reconstruction, the left labium minus was used to form a flap graft. Noble's suggestion was used with success by Gray Ward (1923) to cover the raw area after reconstruction of a large vesico-vaginal fistula complicated by complete loss of the urethra. Hamlin and Nicholson (1969) used pedicle grafts of labial skin to cover the gracilis muscle graft, since in most patients little vaginal mucosa remained. The labial flap was swung into position as high as possible along the anterior vaginal wall. Symmonds (1969, 1978, 1984) discussing loss of the urethral floor with total urinary incontinence, described the use of a pedicled skin—fibrofatty labial graft with which to replace the anterior vaginal wall. This combined pedicle of skin and fat was preferrable to the Martius fat graft when vaginal closure was under tension, or might leave dead space, for the labial flap ensured tension-free, suburethral, anterior vaginal wall closure and a good blood supply. The fat pad filled dead space and kept suture lines apart. Pedicled anteriorly, the flap of good thickness was fitted to the defect, sutured accurately and any excess removed, particularly the potentially avascular tip (Fig. 59). Following experience with myocutaneous pedicle flaps Symmonds (1984) reported a variation in the Martius graft technique adding an attached skin patch for use as an onlay graft in either bladder or rectum. Taken from the medial nonhair-bearing area of the labium, the skin patch passed through an adequate sublabial tunnel, positioned to lie so the skin surface faced bladder or anal canal, and used to close the defect. A second patch could be taken from the other side and placed with the skin surface out, to close the vaginal wall defect and offer additional support to the repair (Figs. 59 b, c). Davis et al. (1980) reported favourably on both the Martius and labial flap grafts in dealing with urethro-vaginal fistulae. Hoskins et al. (1984) used the Symmonds bulbocavernosus myocutaneous flap technique to repair difficult urethro-vaginal fistulae successfully, and believed the graft paticularly suitable because of its excellent blood supply.

4

Fistula Surgeons in the Modern Era

From May 4th 1855 when the first fistula hospital in the world began in New York until the opening of the second fistula hospital in Addis Ababa, Ethiopia on the 24th May 1975, there has been an overwhelming number of publications dealing with the problem of genital fistula due to both obstetric and surgical causes. Many publications dealt with relatively small numbers of patients, but certain authors have had a vast experience and international recognition for their expertise with the problem, beginning with Naguib Mahfouz of Cairo, Chassar Moir of Oxford, a group of surgeons in West Africa headed by John Lawson, surgeons in South Africa and India, and the Hamlins of Addis Ababa, Ethiopia.

Naguib Mahfouz, Professor of Obstetrics and Gynecology at University Hospital, and gynecological surgeon to Kasr el Aini and Coptic Hospitals in Cairo, was born in 1882 in the village of Mansoura about 60 kilometers from Alexandria (Fig. 60). He began medicine in 1898, when for the first time the medical course was conducted in English because of the appointment of foreign professors. Later, as Professor of Obstetrics and Gynecology, he was the only Egyptian professor; but in fact, there was no department of obstetrics and gynecology. He had great problems establishing himself as a gynaecologist with few beds and all under the direction of British surgeons, yet gained extensive experience from liason with pubic health department medical officers, who called him to difficult domiciliary confinements. (2,000 in 15 years). The turning point in his life occurred with the appointment of Dr. Roy Dobbin, assistant master of the Rotunda Hospital, Dublin, as Professor of Obstetrics and Gynecology in the University of Cairo. Mahfouz his protegee, learned the techniques of obstetrics and gynecology from this master, then proceeded to Europe to be influenced greatly by Bland-Sutton, Wertheim and Schauta and although unimpressed with Wertheim's manners or surgery, he found Schauta quite different.

During the 1914–1918 war he was consultant in obstetrics and gynecology to wives of British officers in Cairo and established lasting friendships with leading United Kingdom surgeons.

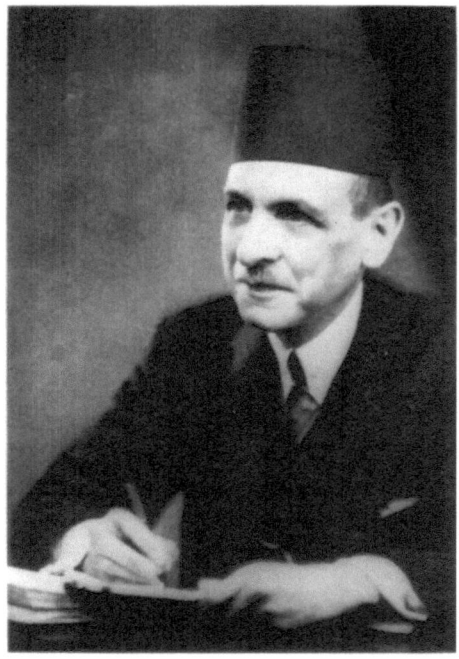

Figure 60. Pasha Naguib Mahfouz

Early in his professional life and largely self-taught, he dealt with obstetric fistulae following Mackenrodt's layered closure technique. Lady Cromer, wife of the British Ambassador, had created the Lady Cromer refuge for abandoned children, and in 1919, by his own efforts, this was converted to a maternity center where women could be delivered in relative safety, minimizing the great problem of obstetric fistula. So successful was this scheme that the department of health, formerly antagonistic, opened many similar centers and eventually antenatal clinics were set up at these centers.

Although the famed Mahfouz Obstetric and Gynecological Museum commenced with his own specimens and it was necessary for him to import jars and chemicals, nevertheless some years later a special room at the hospital was provided and the museum began with 300 specimens. Later there were 1,500 in sinks, all with descriptions, microscopic sections and microphotographs together with a printed guide to the museum. The museum was divided into three sections, obstetrics, gynecology and fetal abnormalities and in 1945 Sir Eardley Holland the President of the Royal College of Obstetrics and Gynecologists who was visiting Cairo at the request of the Egyptian government to report on the state of the depart-

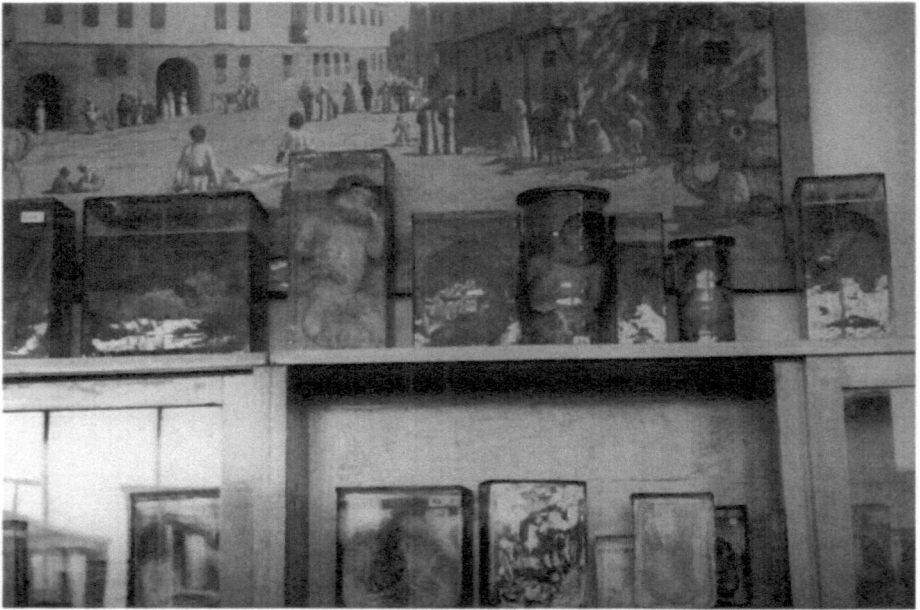

Figure 61. Part of the Mahfouz Obstetrical and Gynaecological Museum, Cairo

ments of gynecology at Cairo and Alexandria Universities, was quite over-whelmed by the museum. He regarded it as being more complete and better catalogued than any collection anywhere (Fig. 61).

Another saga in Mahfouz' life was the preparation of the atlas depicting all the specimens in the museum. Due to poor communications during the war, the manuscript, photographs and diagrams were taken to the United Kingdom in a diplomatic bag by the wife of the British Ambassador. Sir Comyns Berkely undertook the United Kingdom arrangements, which included solving the problem of partial destruction of the manuscript and photographs by a mad employee at the printing works and ultimately the intervention of Mr. Attlee the British Prime Minister was required to obtain special paper for the book. The first of three volumes was completed in 1949. He was made a Fellow of the Royal College of Obstetricians and Gynecologists, the Royal College of Physicians and the Royal College of Surgeons of England. He died on 25th July 1974 at the age of 92 and during his lifetime he published many papers on "Urinary and Recto-Vaginal Fistulae in Women". The first (1929) gave a brief historical in-troduction to the problem then details of 234 operations performed on 276 fistulae under his care between 1907 and 1928. He succeeded in 86.5% of these women, 259 patients having developed the fistula due to pressure necrosis from obstructed labor. He noted that while most urinary fistulae in men were due to bilharzia it was uncommon in the female and responsible for the problem in only two of his patients. The site of the fistula depended upon the level of obstruction and in about two thirds of his patients a contracted pelvis of the flat type was the responsible factor. He followed closely the principles enunciated by Sims, emphasizing good exposure, wide mobilization, not sacrificing any tissue, and accurate approximation of the bladder with mucosal inversion, the sutures not being tied too tightly. Before closing the vagina, the integrity of the bladder repair was tested. A self-retaining catheter was inserted for ten days postoperatively and the sutures removed at two weeks with the patient instructed not to have intercourse for a further two months. Of all cases, only in five was the abdominal route chosen to correct the defect and he suggested this route was applicable to an inaccessible vault fistula caused by narrowness of the vagina due to dense scar tissue; but emphasized that the abdominal route under such circumstances still would offer considerable technical difficulties. In a further publication on urinary fistulae (1930) he cleverly divided their history into four distinct periods and discussed the ancient period which included Queen Henhenit and the period of discovery to which Avicenna, Mercado and Felix Platter all contributed. The third period characterized by the despair of many surgeons attempting without success to close a fistula concluded with a fourth period or period of victory when Sims and Emmet in the United States and Simon in Germany put the surgical situation onto a proper footing. Because of continuing problems with fistula closure, abdominal correction was attempted in 1890 by Trendelenburg and in 1893 by von Dittel, and Mackenrodt (1894) developed a layered operation in which he practised wide separation of bladder from the vaginal walls on all sides, suturing each layer independently. All later techniques he believed were merely modifications of the Mackenrodt operation. The paper published in 1934 dealt with superior recto-vaginal fistulae and in 1938 in a lecture delivered at Hammersmith Postgraduate School, London again he covered fistula history in great detail together with a discussion on etiology, diagnosis and a detailed description of surgical methods of closure including the suprapubic route. In London (1957) he gave the William Flechter Shaw memorial lecture at the Royal College of Obstetricians and Gynecologists. This great man reiterated the principles of fistula closure with such clarity and wrote so eloquently of the problem based on a unique experience, that he stimulated all the surgeons who

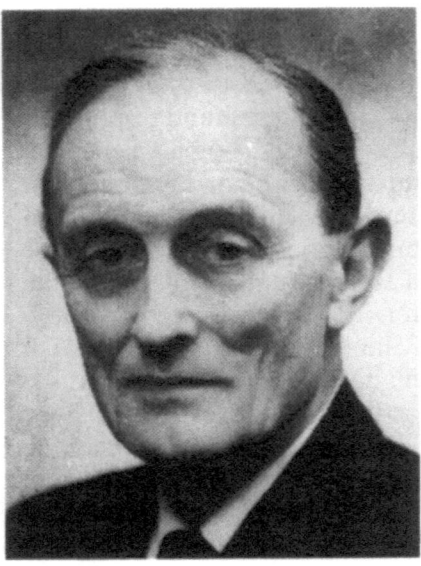

Figure 62. Professor Chassar Moir

came after him in north, west and east Africa to continue in this great
tradition.

Professor Chassar Moir was appointed Nuffield Professor of Obstetrics
and Gynecology at Oxford, England at the age of 37 years and occupied
the position for 30 years (Fig. 62). Graduating in Edinburgh in 1922, he
began his medical career as a general practitioner but in 1930 gained an
M.D. by thesis on the subject of internal rotation. Early studies of muscular
activity of the pregnant and nonpregnant human uterus led to the discovery
of an active principle in ergot and in collaboration with Dr. H. W. Dudley
F.R.S. he isolated ergometrine from a liquid extract of ergot, described as
a major contribution to safer obstetrics comparable only to Domagk's
discovery of sulphanilamide. At Oxford he became interested in the application of diagnostic radiology to obstetrics becoming expert at pelvi-
metry then in its infancy. Following the death of Munro Kerr, he assumed
the authorship of "Operative Obstetrics". His was a meticulous approach
to the surgery of vesico-vaginal fistula and it was his scrupulous attention
to detail which produced results both the envy and admiration of his
colleagues. He was a perfectionist, and it was not unknown for him after
a long surgical procedure to correct a fistula, to appraise the result and
then decide to remove the sutures and begin again. "Vesico-Vaginal Fistula", published in 1961 was the standard book on the topic and ran to
two editions, also he contributed many papers and lectures on various

aspects of both vesico-vaginal and recto-vaginal fistulae. A great protagonist of James Marion Sims, he emphasized Sims' principles in all his writings. In praising the excellent results achieved by Sims and Emmet, he believed that the older technique of saucerization, rather than the more modern layered repair, still merited attention and could be used with great advantage in many cases. Although he used the "flap-splitting method" when it seemed specially indicated—urethral fistula or vesico-vaginal fistula adherent to the pubic ramus—generally he preferred the simple saucerizing procedure which was not to be termed "edge-paring operation" for this gave a totally inadequate idea of both its form and extent. He admitted that closure under tension was more likely with this technique but this could be overcome readily by relieving incisions. He advocated silver wire sutures for 20 days, bladder washout following fistula closure to remove clot, and the avoidance of a self-retaining catheter "since the mushroom head may press harmfully on the repair". Finally, he preferred vaginal cystotomy rather than a urethral catheter should the urethra be extensively involved. Professor Moir died on 24th November 1977 at the age of 77 years (Fig. 63).

From the early sixties until the late seventies, many important contributions were published by surgeons from Africa, the Middle East and India which dealt with many facets of the fistula problem and common to each country were three important features—first the social circumstances which led to a high incidence of obstetric fistula and the social upheavals which followed, second the very large number of patients presenting for help and third the difficult technical problems produced by the large tissue deficit, together with gross scarring and bony adhesion, which tested the ingenuity of each surgeon, many contributing new, unusual and exceedingly clever techniques to overcome their difficulties. John Lawson, formerly Professor of Obstetrics and Gynecology at the University of Ibadan, Nigeria has written extensively on the surgery of vesico-vaginal fistula based on his own wide experience. A major contribution by him to the art of fistula surgery was the organization of a highly specialized fistula unit in that university, and the teaching of reparative surgery. His many papers and text-books cover etiology, classification and surgical technique, and the influence of his teaching methods has extended widely into other areas of West Africa. In 1970, John Lawson became consultant to the Newcastle General and Princess Mary Maternity Hospital, Newcastle upon Tyne in the United Kingdom and also, the Director of Postgraduate Studies at the Royal College of Obstetricians and Gynecologists, London. He has maintained his interest in fistula surgery although the incidence of obstetric

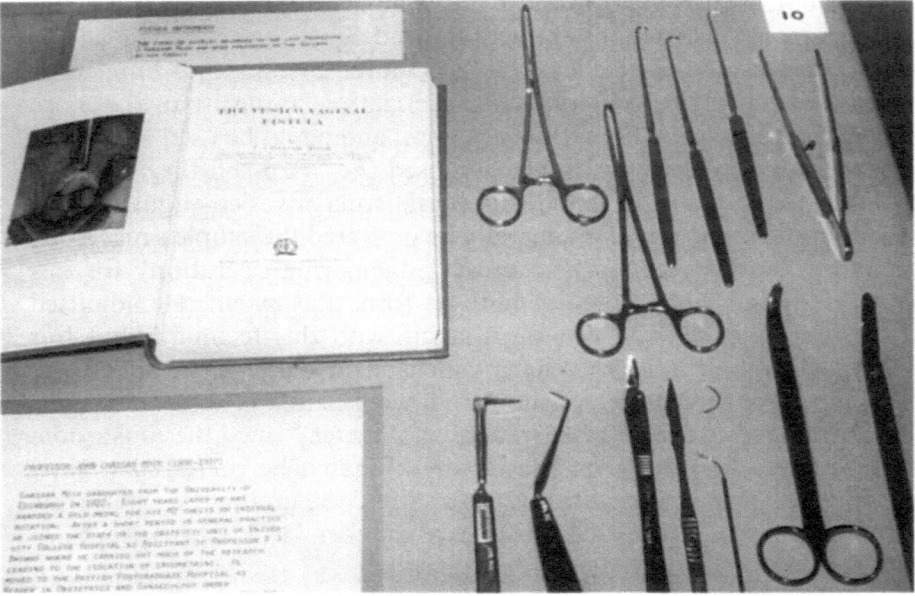

Figure 63. Chassar Moir's famous text. "The Vesico-Vaginal Fistula" and his special fistula instruments

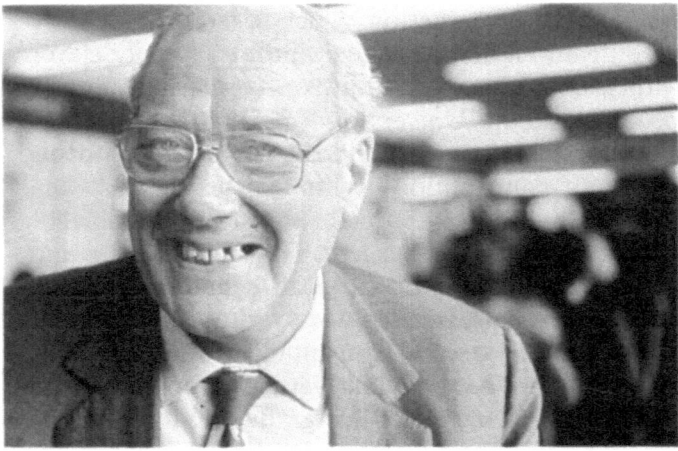

Figure 64. John Lawson

fistula in the western world has fallen dramatically, replaced by fistula due to surgery and radiotherapy. In the J. Y. Simpson oration delivered in 1985, he indicated that of the 377 fistulae treated in Ibadan, 369 were obstetric, whereas of the 135 since his return to the United Kingdom, only 16 were due to obstetric causes (Fig. 64). Two other surgeons with an extensive experience of fistula surgery in Nigeria are Professor Una Lister and Sister Ann Ward. Professor Una Lister, recently retired from the Ahmadu Bello University Hospital, Zaria, Nigeria. Each year nearly 250 patients were admitted for operation to that hospital with vesico-vaginal or recto-vaginal fistula, and that figure constituted almost 50% of all admissions for major gynecological conditions, making fistula by far the commonest single major condition seen in that area. Sister Anne Ward, presently in charge of the Mission Hospital of St. Luke's at Anua, Nigeria reported 1,789 cases of genito-urinary fistula in an 11-year period and of these, 1,445 were vesico-vaginal (Ward 1980).

5

The Hamlins of Ethiopia and the Second Fistula Hospital

Reginald Hamlin was born in Napier, New Zealand and graduated from medical school at the University of Dunedin. He gained a University of Otago and University of New Zealand government travelling scholarship, which after war service with the Royal New Zealand Navy, took him to Crown Street Women's Hospital in Sydney, Australia, where eventually he became medical superintendent of the busiest maternity hospital in New South Wales. The assistant superintendent was Catherine Nicholson, a graduate of Syndney University, and following their hospital term they married and moved to London. After working in the United Kingdom for a time, they spent six months at Queen Mary Hospital in Hong Kong, returning to Australia for Reg to become superintendent at the Queen Victoria Maternity Hospital in Adelaide, South Australia and Catherine an obstetrician on the staff. For quite a time both had felt their medical skills would be more usefully employed in countries with poor health services rather than in their own privileged countries, so in 1959 they accepted a challenging position in Addis Ababa, Ethiopia, setting up a midwifery training school at the Princess Tsahai Hospital, a hospital commemorating a daughter of Haile Selassie, the Emperor, who died in childbirth in the United Kingdom following a severe postpartum hemorrhage. They travelled by ship to Aden and then by air to Addis Ababa.

Addis Ababa, which means new flower, owes its existence to the Tasmanian Blue Gum. The nomadic Ethiopians cut existing flora to build houses and cook food, so gradually the upper Ethiopian plateau became denuded and the tribes moved on repeating the process. Emperor Menelik— Haile Selasie's uncle—founded Addis Ababa and in 1895 introduced these rapidly growing eucalypts from France, aided by Mondon-Vidaillet, the French engineer supervising the building of the railway from Djibouti in French Somalia to Addis Ababa. These most typical of all Australian trees arrived in France in 1803 brought there by two famous botanists, Leschenault and Guichenot, who accompanied the scientific and cartographic

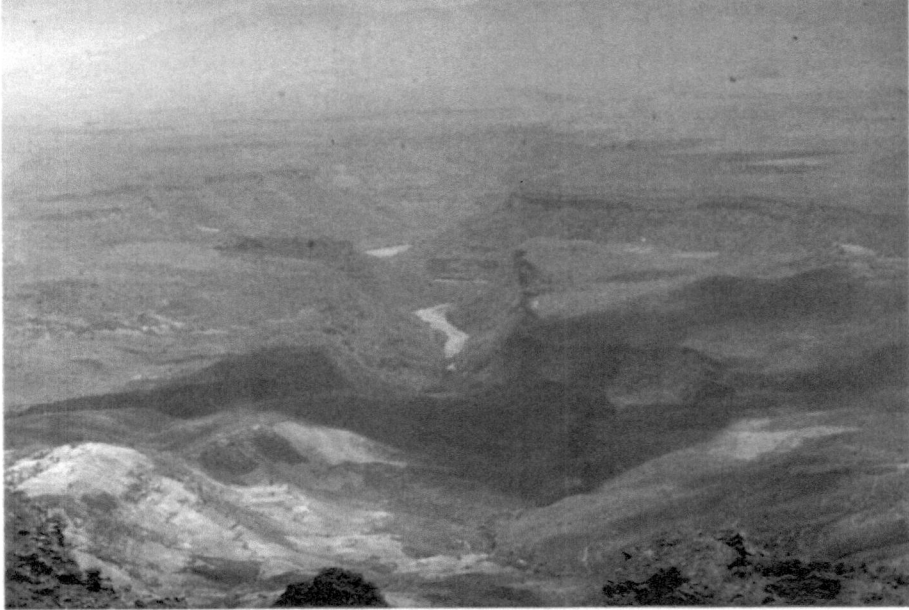

Figure 65. The gorge of the Blue Nile

voyage of Nicolas Baudin to Australia. The trees grew at the Jardin des Plantes in Paris and at Empress Josephine's summer palace, Malmaison. The particular characteristic of eucalypts which appealed to Menelik was that when lopped, they did not die like native flora; but new shoots appeared rapidly replacing the old, and this feature allowed Addis Ababa to become the stable capital of Ethiopia, a capital city which owes its existence to this tree (Zacharin 1978).

Although the Hamlins' early days were successful and four midwives graduated from the first school, with the passage of time they restricted their activities to the Princess Tsahai obstetrical and gynecological wards where they saw the first fistulae and were appalled at the surgical problems involved. They wrote: "The high Ethiopian mountains with innumerable canyons, escarpments and gorges, filled in the rainy season with rushing tributaries of the Blue Nile make it one of the most spectacularly beautiful countries in the world; but mothers who live in such remote areas, cut off by these physical barriers from rapid access to medical help, must, when childbirth becomes difficult, endure the torture of unrelieved obstructed labor (Fig. 65). Those who survive find themselves afflicted with the most

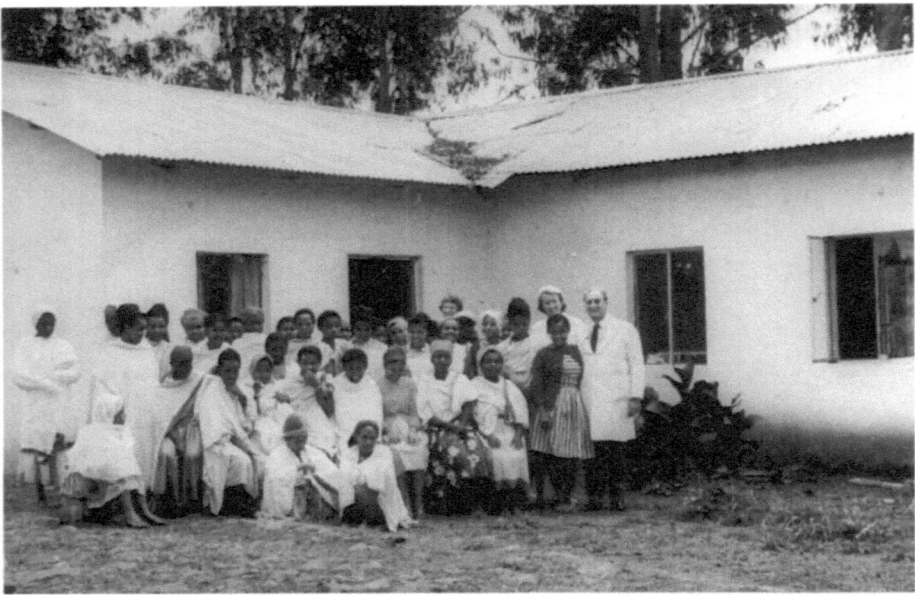

Figure 66. The annexe "Fistula House" in the grounds of Princess Tsahai Hospital. The Hamlins with fistula patients awaiting surgery. Note the Australian eucalypts behind the building

appalling damage, and mourning the still-birth of their only child, incontinent of urine, ashamed of their offensiveness, spurned hy husband and families, homeless, unemployable except in the fields, they endure, they exist from early womanhood throughout life without friends and without hope. They walk with downcast eyes as if ashamed, as indeed they are, ashamed of a tragic injury suffered in their first, their only experience of childbearing." These women travel incredible distances to seek help from any hospital which offers hope a cure and their gratitude when cured is overwhelming.

Many colleagues had tried unsuccessfully to manage these difficult cases and so the Hamlins read widely—Sims, Mahfouz, Ingelman-Sundberg and Chassar Moir—then began tackling the problems gradually improving and refining their techniques, and as their skills developed they became convinced about the necessity to employ a graft. Nothing succeeds like success, and since such afflicted females had none to whom they might turn for help, a multitude appeared creating enormous problems.

Restricted to six beds for patients in those early days, the Hamlins

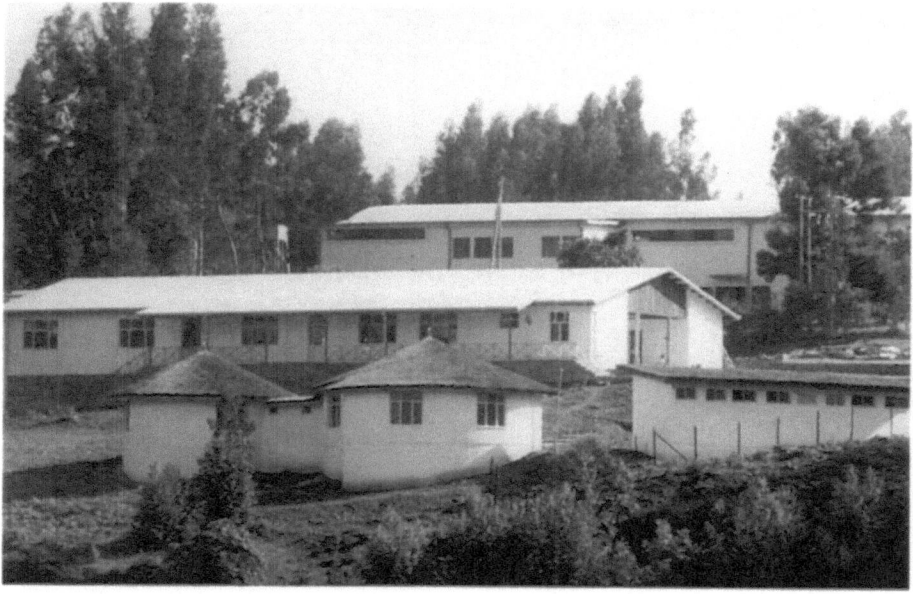

Figure 67. The Second Fistula Hospital, Addis Ababa, Ethiopia, surrounded by eucalypts

kept new arrivals in the hospital grounds, in hospital corridors, even under other patients' beds. They built four large hostels in the hospital grounds, and each morning at 6 a.m., Reg, Catherine and Mamite would collect their charges and feed them (Fig. 66). Eventually 68 women stayed in these hostels, for delays were great with only two operating theaters in the general hospital and greatly restricted operating time. At one time Reg and Catherine were even paying for extra hospital beds for these unfortunates from their own meagre salaries, so obviously this state of affairs could not continue and they decided a special hospital was needed. Such a prospect would have daunted lesser mortals; but not the Hamlins.

Really it is remarkable how the fortunes and fate of the Hamlins paralleled that of their eminent predecessor and founder of the first fistula hospital, James Marion Sims, nearly a hundred years before the Hamlins faced up to the same problems in Addis Ababa. Sims learned humility and pangs of failure when dealing with these dreadful problems, and developed tenacity and persistence necessary for success. Such characteristics still are displayed admirably by the Hamlins.

The proposed new hospital had to be close by Princess Tsahai so the Hamlins could fulfill their salaried duties for the Ethiopian government.

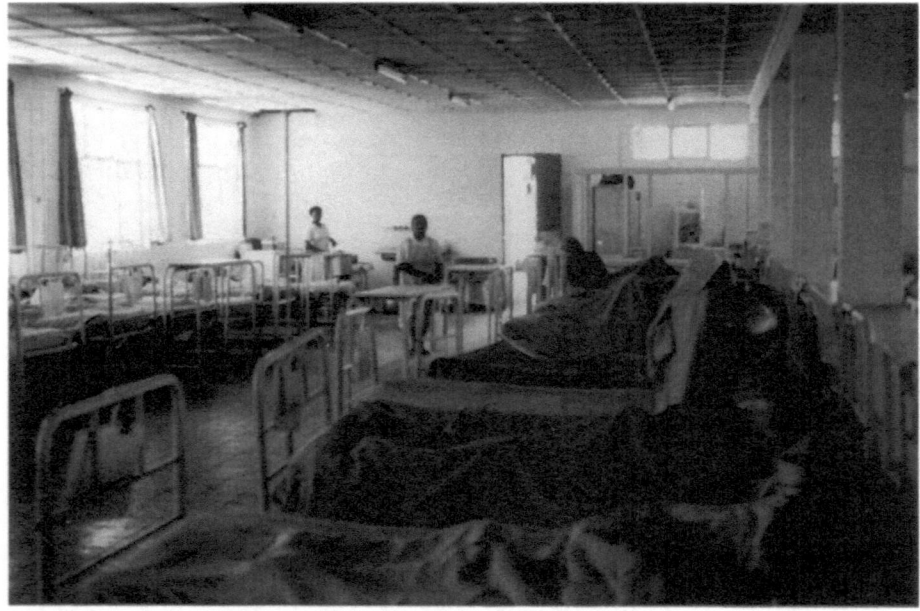

Figure 68. Portion of the main ward and the sisters' desk at the Fistula Hospital

Accordingly, suitable land was found near the old airport which belonged to the Armenian community, a group granted Ethiopian citizenship when they needed refuge from Turkish oppression. The land was promised, and a tour of the United States of America to raise funds, culminated in financial help arranged by the Bishop of Connecticut—so the land was purchased. The building of the second fistula hospital began financed by C.O.R.S.O., New Zealand and the outbuildings from an appeal held in Victoria, Australia following a visit to Ethiopia by the then premier, Sir Henry Bolte. The first fistula hospital, the Woman's Hospital, New York, opened its doors on 4th May 1855 and the second, in Addis Ababa on 24th May 1975 (Figs. 67 and 68) and on 19th October 1971, the James Marion Sims Chapter at the Woman's Hospital, New York, presented $1000, a brick from the wall of the first fistula hospital, and a commemorative wall plaque to the second fistula hospital in Addis Ababa. These actions were appreciated greatly by the Hamlins, and the brick is a cherished possession (Fig. 69).

When completed it had been planned to equip the hospital slowly and move patients in gradually, but the revolution, and then the death of Emperor Haile Selassie changed the situation rapidly. Princess Tsahai hos-

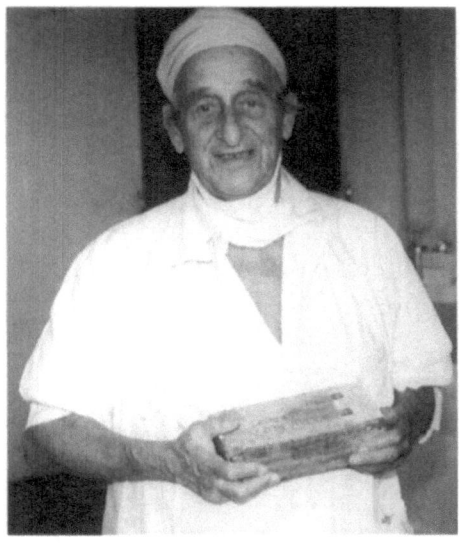

Figure 69. Reg Hamlin with the brick from the First Fistula Hospital

pital was taken over by the Ethiopian army, and the Hamlins moved into the fistula hospital, incompletely finished and unfurnished, to begin work. Subsequently the Ethiopian government gave a substantial grant of land, doubling the size of the hospital grounds. Total running costs of about U.S. $90,000 are met by voluntary donations from many countries around the world and also various Ethiopian charities, and this money runs the hospital for one year, providing nursing salaries, maintainance, drugs, surgical equipment, food etc., the Hamlins surviving only on their Ethiopian government salaries. They established a blood bank, now supported by the Ethiopian Red Cross, and ask relatives to supply blood prior to correction of a large fistula (Fig. 70). Most theatre and nursing staff are former patients who have elected to stay and help their less fortunate sisters. This dedicated band of women have a unique knowledge of the techniques of fistula surgery, and so skilled are they that they manage much of the day to day routine work and in fact Mamite is quite capable of closing a difficult fistula, and the skill of these nurses in detecting aberrant ureteric orifices at the fistula edge, needs to be witnessed. Mamite has been with the Hamlins during their entire stay and well she remembers laboring for many days in her first and only pregnancy in a remote village, then the horrendous journey over mountain tracks carried on a goat-skin stretcher by four male relatives to the nearest road. Eventually she arrived at Princess Tsahai, and after successful fistula surgery elected to remain and help, to become the Ethiopian equivalent of Sims' Mary Smith (Fig. 71).

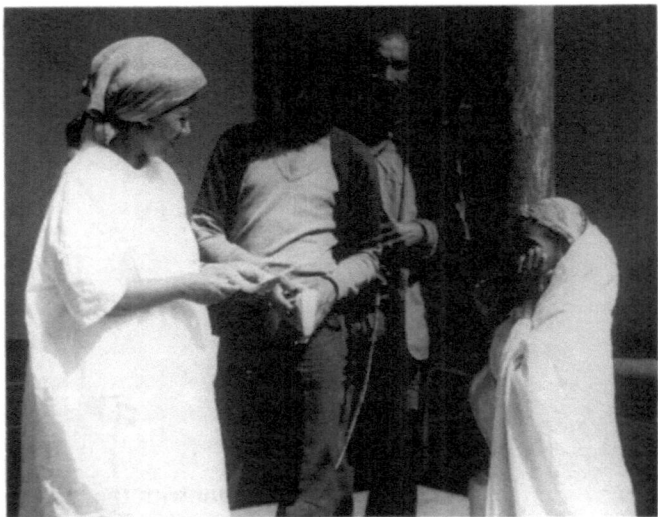

Figure 70. Matron arranging admission of a fistula patient and discussing the necessary blood donation with her husband and father

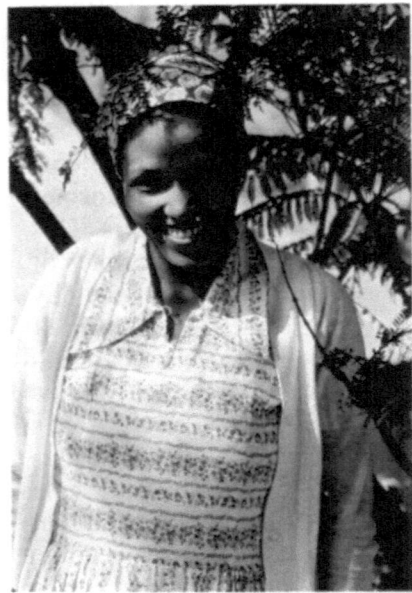

Figure 71. Mamite

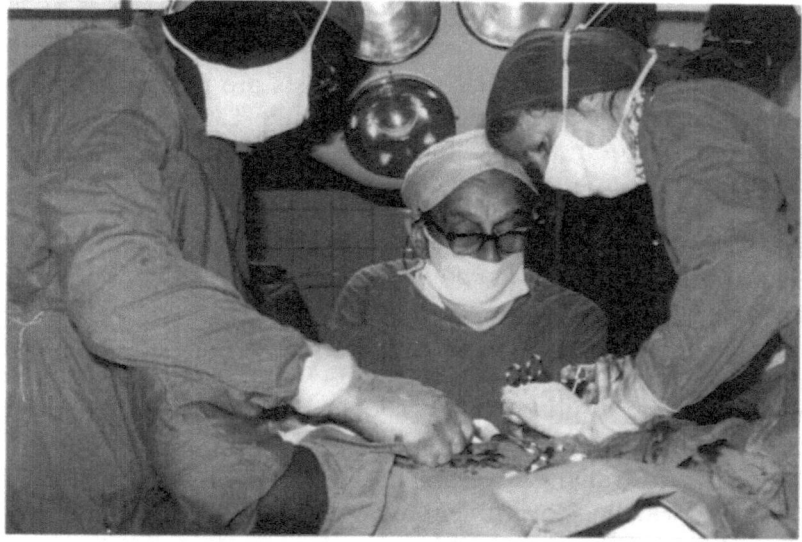

Figure 72. Teaching fistula surgery to a surgeon from Khartoum

With an annual admission rate of approximately 700 patients, the closure cost of $130 per fistula is excellent value for money. One must remember most patients have very large defects with great tissue loss and extensive scarring, so a primary success rate exceeding 90%, truly is remarkable. During their time in Ethiopia the Hamlins have dealt with over 10,000 patients. Gynecologists from Europe, United Kingdom, United States of America, many African states and Australia have visited them to assist and learn their techniques, and it is of particular importance for the future that surgeons from many African countries—Sudan, Malawi, Nigeria, Ivory Coast, Cameroon and Zaire—have visited the hospital for periods of instruction (Fig. 72). Regularly Reg gives illustrated lectures to social workers, medical students, nurses and other interested parties emphasizing that fistula is not peculiar to Ethiopians, but is due to a combination of obstructed labor and obstructed transport and he pleads, "For understanding, charity and compassion for these innocent fistula pilgrims who appear with only faith, hope and urine-soaked clothes." Several young Ethiopian gynecologists now are competent fistula surgeons capable of training others so these skills will be passed on. Medical supplies arrive regularly from Ethiopian government medical stores and donors in the western world, and many local expatriate women have formed auxiliary groups to help with bed linen, sewing etc. Originally the enormous daily load of linen was washed by hand; but thanks to the present Australian High Commissioner in Nairobi, Geoffrey White, they have a commercial-size washing machine. Half the annual running costs are met by World Vision of Canada, part of the remainder by the Hamlin-Churchill Fistula Trust in the United Kingdom, by aid for International Medicine in the United States of America, and various charities in New Zealand. All New Zealand donations are trebled by the New Zealand Government; but still a deficit remains, met by private donations from interested people in many countries. Finance and management really is the big headache, and possibly the easiest part of their lives is the surgery.

The Hamlins have had many honors bestowed by various bodies and governments. In 1972 they were awarded jointly the prestigious Haile Selassie humanitarian prize and Catherine has been elected a Fellow ad Eundem of the Royal College of Obstetricians and Gynecologists, a signal honor, and also the Australian Government awarded her the Order of Australia. The New Zealand Government awarded Reginald Hamlin the O.B.E. and more recently the Returned Services League of Australia bestowed the 1984 Peace Prize for meritorious service. Although such honours are wonderful and much appreciated, regrettably they do not finance hospitals, so still a large part of their time is devoted to fund-raising. Luxuries are few, and they return to Australia only every three years when he Ethiopian government pays their fare together with one month's salary. Reg drives his 1959 Volkswagen and Catherine has a nearly worn-out Peugeot, since new cars attract a high tax. Recently they said: "What we always think of in our mind is what we can give to these women who have lost their husband, homes, babies, self respect and hope, and who have come all the way from their villages out in the countryside on foot, by camel, donkey, horse and mule, looking for help. We give them love, welcome and the necessary medical care, and our reward is seeing them cured, their lives, bodies, minds and hope revived. We love the work, and it is our joy to do it." The Hamlins will remain in Ethiopia forever, so attached are they to this unfortunate band of women for whom they care. One has only to listen to Reg when a new fistula patient arrives after a long and difficult journey as he promises a new life, a new dress and a new husband and baby. Following cure the revolting urine-stained clothes are burnt, and phoenix-like the arisen patient departs in bright new clothes with her fares paid. She is warned to return when she achieves another pregnancy and over 3,000 women have done so. It is their wish for the future, that like the first fistula hospital in New York, the second in Addis Ababa should continue to function until no longer required, and it is their

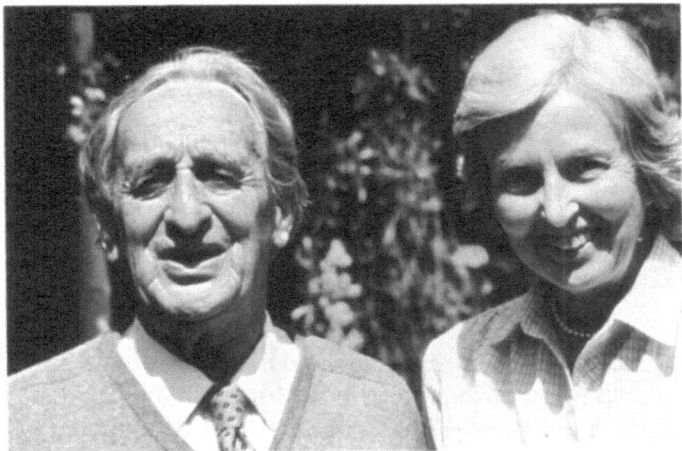

Figure 73. Reg and Catherine Hamlin

hope that Ethiopian fistula surgeons will care for the patients until that time arrives and obstetric fistula has vanished as it did, a hundred years ago in the United States of America (Fig. 73).

6

The Incidence, Etiology and Pathology of Obstetric Fistula

"Kaltume Bakar had been married seven years and menstruation began two years after marriage. No preparations were made for the baby because nobody knew if it would be a live birth. During labor an old woman came and stayed with her. She was not a midwife but there was nobody in the village with any knowledge of midwifery. She was three days in labor and the old woman just sat in the room, asking now and then if she wanted help. The husband sat outside doing nothing either. It was the rainy season with a river between them and a motorable road.

After three days kneeling most of the time and lying when tired, she delivered about midnight. She had not passed urine for three days but it gushed out after delivery and one month later she became incontinent of stool also. Following delivery she had the usual hot baths—continued usually for 40 days— and pap with potash.

She remained in the room for six months, for she was unable to walk. Her husband divorced her and she lived with an aunt, continuing the baths for a further 18 months and still unable to walk properly.

Later, when able to walk, some Shua Arab cattle traders who had travelled widely in Nigeria told her that fistula could be repaired in Zaria, so she travelled from town to town asking of Zaria and finally arrived."

Una Lister
Zaria, Nigeria.

Incidence

The clear-cut relationship between obstetric fistula and poor or absent medical care associated with a wide range of contributing social conditions, is shown by the large number of papers published in the last 30 years, originating from a variety of countries around the world. An important feature of these publications is the large number of patients reported. Yenen et al. (1965) reported 197 fistulae from Istanbul of which 65 were obstetric. Mustafa (1971) dealt with 121 fistulae at the University Hospital of Khartoum, Sudan, all due to obstructed labor, and a visit to Khartoum in 1985 showed the situation unchanged, the major hospital dealing with more than 200 new fistulae each year, with a majority in the difficult category, and referred from smaller hospitals. In addition, these more peripheral hospitals managed a further 200 fistulae annually, so the total number of new fistulae occurring each year in the Sudan averages 500, most coming from the western and south-western regions where the population is mobile. Massoudnia (1973) Iran, reported 420 fistulae seen between 1966–1970. There have been many reports from Africa over the years particularly East, West and South Africa. Abbott (1950) Kenya, reviewed the literature, adding 40 difficult fistulae together with detailed results of treatment, and from Johannesburg, Lavery (1955) described 157 large fistulae with an average diameter of one inch many of which were multiple, and Coetzee et al. (1966) reported 309 cases, 248 following complicated labor with 185 vesico-vaginal. Bird (1967) described 69 fistulae from Kenya, 65 following obstructed labor and other reports were published by Linke et al. (1971) Rhodesia, Quartey (1972) Ghana, Kelly (1979) Ethiopia and Clegg (1979) Rhodesia. In India and Pakistan, many large series have been reported since the paper of Das (1928) and include Benion Thomas (1945) Madras, Hayes (1945) Lahore, Naidu (1962) and Aziz (1965) Hyderabad, Dass et al. (1969) Assam, Ingle et al. (1969) and Vaidya et al. (1915) Bombay. Already mentioned are the big series of fistulae recorded by Mahfouz; but a visit to Cairo in 1985 indicated the situation virtually had been reversed. Discussion with Professors Mahran and Sherbani and other gynecologists of that city, indicated obstetric fistula almost to be a problem of the past, following improvements in antenatal and general midwifery services. In Jordan, the story was similar with obstetric fistula now almost unknown. (Akasheh and Batayneh 1985) In Ethiopia and the Sudan the problem remains as it has always been and in West Africa, Nigeria in particular, recent communications with Lawson, Ward and Lister (1986) indicate the position has not altered.

Etiology

(i) Spontaneous Development

Most obstetric fistulae follow pressure necrosis caused by impaction of the presenting part during difficult labor, and it is the length of impaction

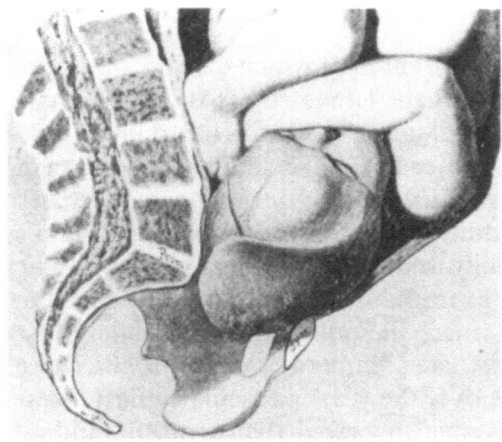
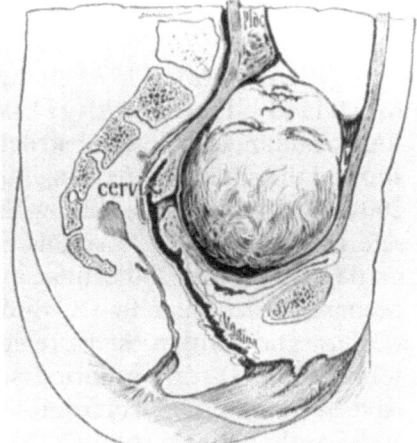

Figure 74 a   Figure 74 b

Fig. 74 a, b

a Brim obstruction with marked moulding and caput formation

b Brim obstruction with pressure on cervix, bladder, ureters and rectum

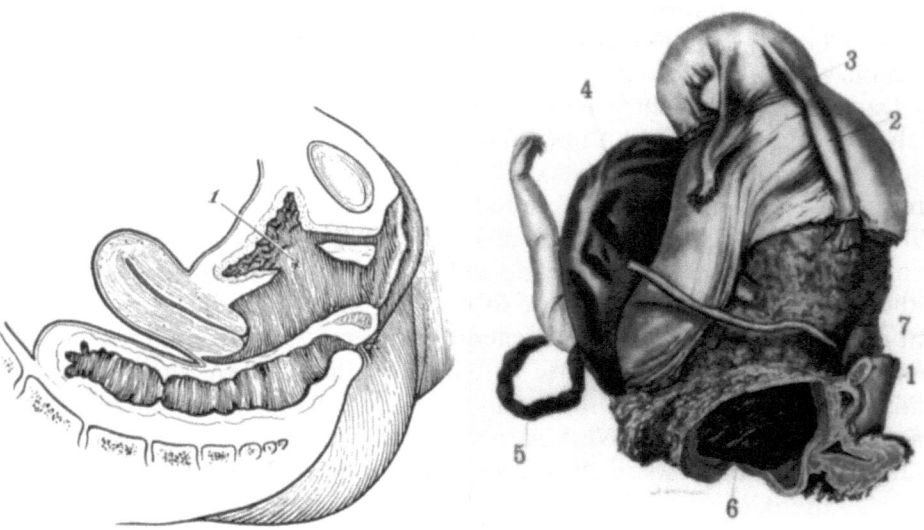

Figure 74 c   **Figure 74 d**

Figure 74 c, d

c The large urinary fistula which results from brim obstruction

d Mahfouz museum specimen of uterine rupture following brim obstruction—bladder and ureter (*7*), compressed against the pubis (*1*), by the fetal head (*6*). (*3*) is the retraction ring above the greatly distended lower uterine segment. (From Mahfouz)

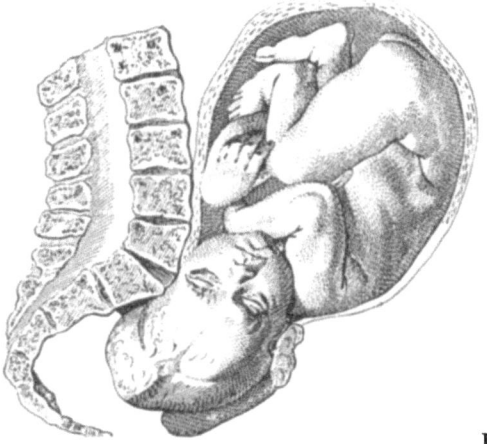

Figure 75 a. Midpelvic obstruction

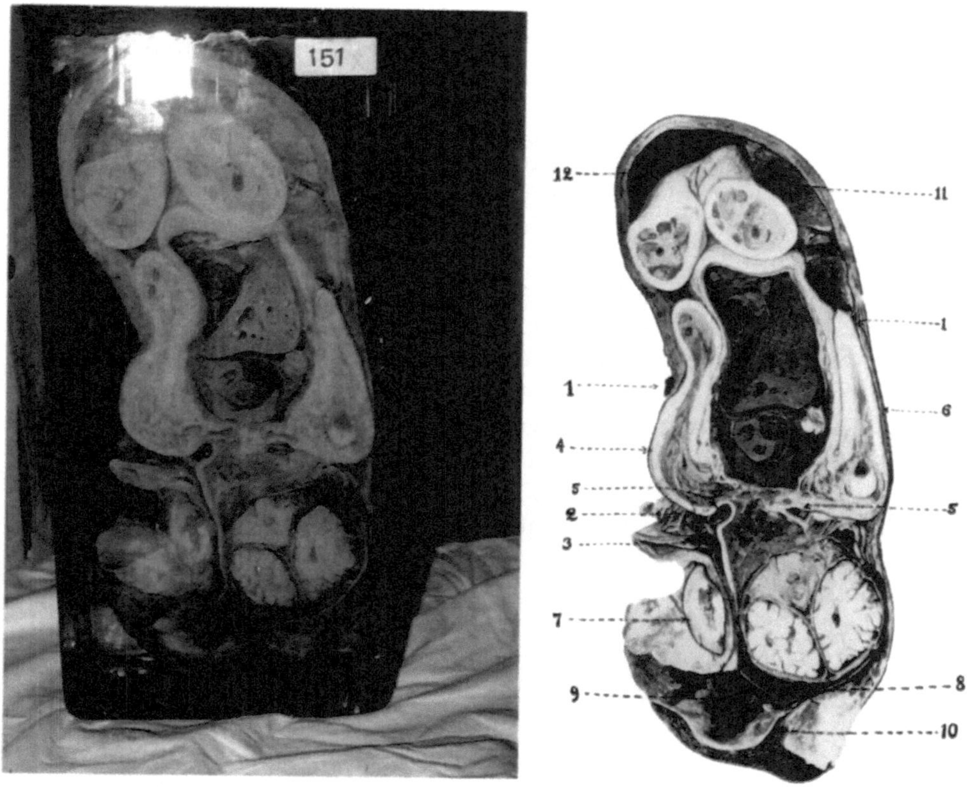

151

12 ---- ---- 11

---- 1

1 ---- ---- 6

4 ----

5 ----

2 ---- ---- 5

3 ----

7 ----

9 ---- ---- 8

---- 10

Figure 75 b. Specimen from Mahfouz museum showing a sagittal section through a ruptured uterus. (*1*) and (*2*) show the upper and lower edges of the lower uterine segment tear. (*3*) bladder elevated above the symphysis pubis (*7*), against which the trigone and upper urethra are compressed by the fetal head

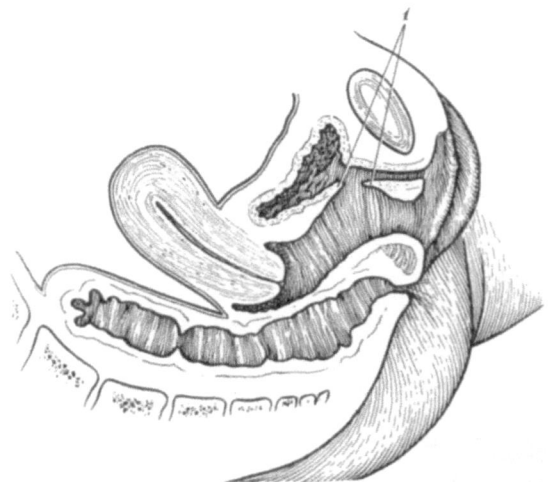

Figure 75 c. Fistula following midpelvic obstruction involves bladder floor, bladder neck and urethra. (From Mahfouz)

without relief rather than the magnitude of pressure, which determines the degree of tissue necrosis. The fistula site depends greatly upon the degree of cervical effacement and dilatation, and level at which the presenting part impacts. Should impaction occur at the brim before complete cervical dilatation, continued pressure on the insufficiently effaced and undilated cervix as well as on the vaginal vault, bladder and rectum, eventually will produce necrosis, and tissues slough to form a fistula which can involve, cervix, bladder, ureter and rectum (Figs. 14 a–d). Should impaction occur in the pelvic cavity or outlet, urethra, bladder base and trigone lie in the direct plane of compression, so vesico-vaginal and/or urethro-vaginal fistula may occur (Figs. 75 a–c). When compression occurs at the outlet and persists for a prolonged period, with grossly neglected cases, the entire urethra, vagina and rectum might slough to be replaced by a narrow slit, surrounded by scar tissue with numerous fistulous tracts (Figs. 76 a–c). The duration of compression in such cases usually is long but Mahfouz (1938) reported a fistula which developed after three hours of compression.

Many factors contribute to the development of spontaneous genital fistula following obstructed labor, including abnormalities of the bony or soft genital passages, large babies, and circumstances delaying the diagnosis allowing obstruction to persist. Mahfouz (1929) noted two thirds of fistulae caused by difficult labor, were due to contracted pelvis of the flat type and the other third included malposition—expecially neglected shoulder presentation—and hydrocephalus as chief causes. Poor nutrition, with frequent childhood and adolescent infections leads to growth stunting and poor

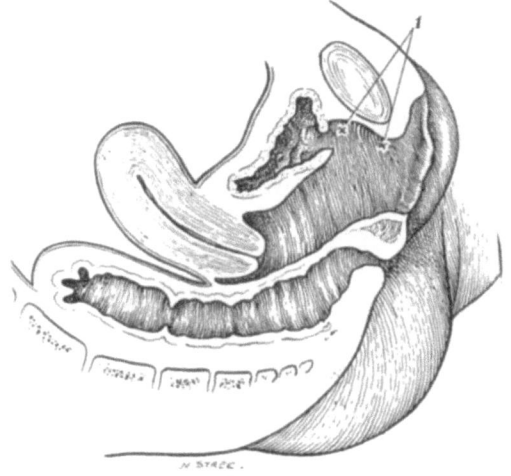

Figure 76 a. Diagram of the fistula which follows prolonged outlet obstruction involving trigone, bladder neck and all the urethra. (From Mahfouz)

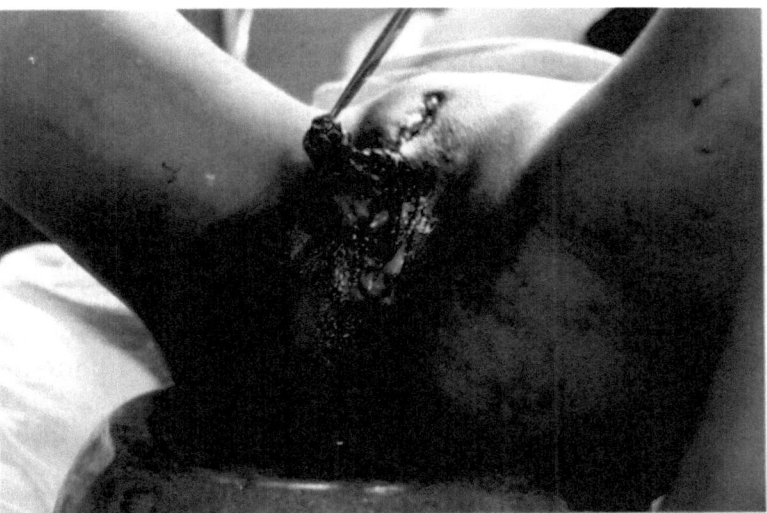

Figure 76 b. Necrotic tissues discharged through the vulva some weeks following obstructed labor

pelvic development. The pelvis does not reach mature size until two to three years after height ceases to change, and Moerman (1982) stated the pelvic basin followed a different pattern of growth from the more familiar adolescent growth curve for stature and maturation of the reproductive system, so attainment of adult size and stature did not indicate pelvic birth canal growth was complete. Accordingly, immaturity of the pelvic basin

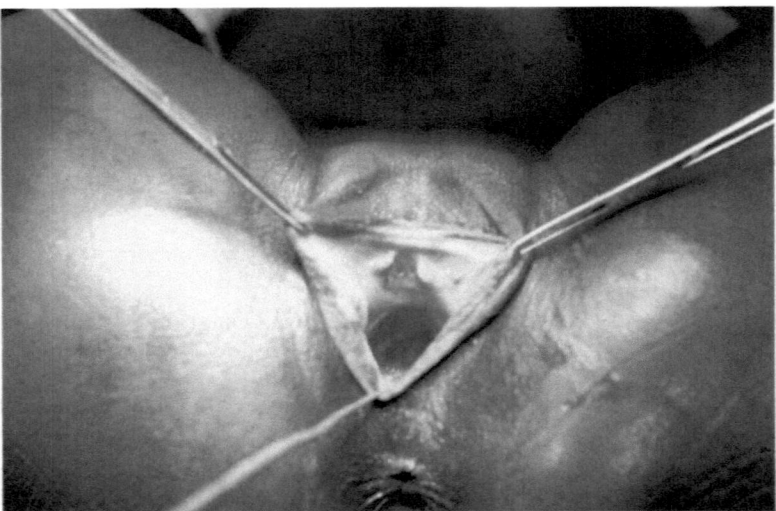

Figure 76 c. The residual fistula after some months of healing—"the urethra has vanished and the examiner looks straight into the bladder"

might contribute significantly to the high incidence of cephalo-pelvic disproportion and other dystocias during labor in primiparae below the age of 15 years. Thompson and Baird (1967) compared childbearing details from Hong Kong, North Borneo, Sarawak and Aberdeen with information from a two-year study in the relatively isolated village of Keneba, Gambia, West Africa, a country without a qualified obstetrician. Socio-economic conditions in these areas differed markedly, with Keneba at the bottom end of the scale, so it was not surprising childbearing in Gambia was both inefficient and dangerous for mother and fetus. Adverse factors included a very early start to child-bearing, poor physique and health of the mother, a wide prevalence of systemic disease especially malaria, and for parts of each year, a relative food scarcity. Little or no qualified medical care was available except in emergency. In all these communities, the mean height of females developing cephalo-pelvic disproportion was lower than the mean height of those who did not, with a critical height—145 cm in Nigeria—below which the risk of major operative delivery for obstruction increased. The use of maternal height as a marker for disproportion was most useful, but of course not absolute. A series in Tanzania showed better living standards affected fetal but not maternal growth, since usually the mother had finished growing by the time she became pregnant.

Yenen (1965) noted most fistula patients originated from a definite area of Turkey near the Black Sea, a region with long-lasting rainy seasons, food deficiencies, and resulting high incidence of contracted pelvis, producing dystocia with increased risk of fistula. Mustafa and Rushwan (1971) reporting 121 fistulae treated in Khartoum, noted that although patients came from all nine Sudanese provinces, 52 came from Daofur province where ante-natal and intra-partum care were inadequate, and women were of short stature with a high incidence of contracted pelvis. Half were under 25 years of age, 70% were primigravid, and the duration of labor had been two to three days. Associated conditions included anemia, malaria, parametritis, bilharzia, vulval and perineal excoriation, calculi and in addition, many had amenorrhea and a recto-vaginal fistula. Harrison (1983), Nigeria stated few Hausa received any formal education, pelvic growth often was incomplete during their first pregnancy and although babies were quite small, disproportion was common. Tahzib (1983), Nigeria, indicated poor childhood nutrition, frequent infections and an early start to child-bearing, often before growth was complete, resulted in nearly 25% of the child-bearing population being stunted, with younger patients tending to have more severe genital tract damage, often associated with recto-vaginal fistula, third degree tear and an increased degree of resulting vaginal fibrosis.

(ii) Fistulae Due to Trauma

In addition to fistulae which occur as a result of spontaneous labor, fistulae also may be produced by direct injury during operative procedures used in endeavors to deliver the child. Destructive operations still are performed in those areas of the world where obstetric fistula is common. Instruments most likely to produce a fistula are the perforator or decapitation hook which may slip and damage the vaginal wall and bladder, or should the cranioclast be applied incorrectly, it can be responsible for extensive bladder and ureteric injury. Kielland or Neville Barnes forceps can be responsible and even the vacuum extractor has been implicated (Akasheh 1966). Especially is delivery hazardous when after prolonged labor, the cervix is not fully dilated, the baby is large and a difficult forceps extraction is employed. Here the cervix might tear to involve large blood vessels and even extend into the bladder.

In 1895, Emmet described in detail the fate of a female delivered by forceps, 12 hours following impaction of the fetal head at the outlet. Three weeks later she became incontinent, and when proper examination could be made after two weeks intensive local treatment, a large fistula was found in which, "all the soft parts had been lost except the fundus of the bladder and a portion of the uterus, while all the urethra, the tissues under the pubes, and for some distance into the bladder above, had sloughed away leaving nothing but the periosteum covering the surface of the bone. The vaginal portion of the recto-vaginal septum had been lost with the cervix uteri, and the whole posterior cul-de-sac. The vaginal canal was only about one and a half inches deep, and continuous with the fistula into the bladder as if the two were one common canal, and through this the inverted bladder, filled with intestines, protruded from the labia". Longaker and Harriman (1927) reported 5% of fistulae seen by them were produced by Kielland forceps, the bladder injury being produced by the anterior blade as traction was applied and the blade rotated over the anterior or bladder area of birth canal. Damage was much less likely if the correct direction of traction was maintained by the operator seated on a low stool. Radman (1961) reporting a 25-year period at his hospital in Los Angeles, detected 23 fistulae of which 15 followed forceps delivery. The operation of symphysiotomy, peculiar to developing countries, also can be a potent cause of vesico-vaginal fistula, and Hartfield (1975) indicated that the fistula probably was due to a clean cut through the tissues, often healing if bladder drainage was instituted. Joyner (1982) reported fistula following symphysiotomy even when standard precautions had been taken, so clearly the procedure was prone to this serious complication.

Cesarian section, whether emergency or elective may damage the bladder or even the ureter. Bladder damage can produce a vesico-cervico-vaginal fistula and this lesion also might follow rupture of the gravid uterus. The emergency nature of a non-elective Cesarian section and the fact that the bladder becomes an abdominal organ during pregnancy, predisposes to bladder injury (Montie 1977). In addition, Cesarian section and operative delivery occurring after unduly prolonged labor does not necessarily prevent fistula development, for often the damage already has been done, or is produced by the surgery when performed by inexperienced surgeons. Bladder adhesion to the lower uterine segment is the rule with repeat Cesarian section and unless the surgeon appreciates this fact, the bladder may be torn when endeavoring to separate bladder and lower uterine segment with a sponge-holder. Sharp dissection which frees the bladder from the lower segment is a safe way to manage the situation, then damage is unlikely. If the bladder is not pushed down sufficiently laterally before entering the lower uterine segment, the ureter may be damaged. The posterior bladder wall can be damaged by suture during closure of the uterine incision after Cesesarian section or the lower segment stump following Cesarian hysterectomy in the management of uterine rupture. Fistula development will be delayed until the damaged bladder wall sloughs. Should the bladder be entered, provided it is closed adequately, and continuous catheter drainage employed for a minimum of 10 days with appropriate antibiotic cover, fistula is unlikely. Spontaneous uterine rupture following obstructed labor may involve a bladder already over-distended with urine and suffering effects of prolonged pressure from the presenting part. Even more likely is bladder damage with rupture of a previous lower segment scar in labor, for the normal connective tissue plane permitting mobility between uterus and bladder is lost, and replaced by adhesions. Rare genital fistulae following Cesarian section are the cutaneous menstrual fistula (Agrawal et al. 1985) and the uretero-uterine fistula (Mahgoub and El Zeniny 1971). Cesarian hysterectomy carries a definite risk of associated bladder damage and fistula formation. Morton (1962) and O'Leary and Steer (1964) reported a large series of patients and found a 2% incidence of bladder damage.

(iii) Social Factors

"The circumstances of child-bearing in Asia and Africa cause obstetric fistula in the same way as they did in Europe and the United States of America over a century ago. It all boils down to gross defects in social, economic and political conditions, and to the inadequacy of health care for most of the population" (Lancet 1981). Predominant factors delaying diagnosis of obstructed labor and allowing its persistence are social, with the root of the problem buried in the traditional custom of early marriage to prevent promiscuity and premarital pregnancy, so females have first babies when pelvic growth still is incomplete. In Northern Nigeria, 65% of patients were primigravid, with nearly half aged 16 years or less. Furthermore parturition is regarded as a normal process not requiring medical attention until complications are at an advanced stage. A most important feature of obstetric fistula is this relationship with a wide range of social, economic and political issues.

Vesico-vaginal fistula ranks still as a major gynecological problem in many developing countries, yet as an indicator of poor obstetric services and low socio-economic status of the community they represent only the tip of an iceberg. It has been well said the incidence of genital fistula in a particular community is an excellent indicator of the quality of the obstetric care available. There is a deep-seated antipathy towards conventional antenatal care and hospital delivery in some countries. Most women of childbearing age are semi-secluded and there are mistaken notions about the pharmacological activity of certain drugs given to women during ante-natal management. In primitive Moslem communities when the family attending the birth realize progress is not normal, the first usual step is to seek aid from a Mallum, an Islamic theologian who practices Koranic medicine. He chalks prayers onto a slate, the writing is washed off into a beaker, and the liquid is drunk as medicine. Kelly (1967) indicated that most women in Nigeria still were delivered at home by native midwives whose qualifications were high parity or age. Frequent vaginal examina-tions were the rule, and with delivery imminent, the patient would be encouraged to push while in the squatting position. After ironing out the perineum which produced enormous vulval edema, fundal pressure was used to assist delivery and pressure would be applied by hands, or by standing or sitting on the patient's abdomen. When all efforts proved ineffective, and the patient was still alive with some money left, then pro-viding relatives and in-laws after consultation agreed it might be worth-while, and it was still daylight, the patient would be transported by bicycle to a main road where an intervillage taxi might be flagged down, or to a church or school where a priest or teacher may have a car to bring the patient to hospital. Findings on admission included enormous vulval edema, gross bladder distension, pyrexia and dehydration. Linke et al. (1971) indicated most births in Rhodesia were attended by an older woman of the family without training in midwifery, and women brought to hospital after prolonged obstructed labor often were critically ill with sepsis, shock, retained necrotic fetal and placental tissue and commonly uterine rupture. Coetzee and Lithgow (1966) reported obstetrical misadventure in South Africa still was the most frequent cause of fistula, confinements usually were conducted by untrained assistants and the unavailability of skilled obstetric care was blamed on inadequate transport and poor communi-cations. The possibility of labor complications causes considerable fear in advance for Hausa women and should a married female become chronically ill she is returned to her parents' home as a charge on her own kin, not in-laws, and ultimately becomes a stranger in her husband's home. Whilst the patient is not blamed for an illness, there is no shame unless it is classed as venereal (Last 1976). In Hausa society a primigravida is confined to her parents' compound and expected to be quiet about her pregnancy and not discuss the forthcoming birth. It is obligatory for a wife to have permission to attend hospital, and should her husband be absent whilst she is in labor, she can not attend until his return. Even when a decision has been made to travel to the hospital, there are great problems for those living in in-accesible villages in remote areas. Especially is this true in the highlands of Ethiopia where a girl in obstructed labor may be carried on a stretcher by relatives or donkey for many miles over a period of days to the nearest road, ultimately to await public transport or attend a local health center. An important root of the problem is the subordinate position of women consequent upon an extreme form of male domination, and clearly the only possible way to improve such attitudes, is by universal education to eradicate mass illiteracy. Northern Nigeria has several primary health centers, maternity centers, dispensaries and a variable level of obstetric care yet fistula is exceedingly common due to the vast distances with poor communications and especially because of mass illiteracy, widespread poverty and harmful tribal customs. Harrison (1980) stated that in 1973, efforts were made to encourage women laboring for more than 24 hours to report to hospital, and hospital deliveries nearly doubled in four years with a striking change in the geographical distribution of vesico-vaginal fistula. Within 50 km of the hospital in Zaria, numbers declined sharply while the proportion of fistulae from other areas increased and by 1977, obstetric fistula virtually had been eradicated from the Zaria area.

A similar pattern has emerged in India. Jaya Rao (1979) said that, "In an unequal world women are the most unequal amongst the unequalled." Poor health and nutrition of Indian women were off-shoots of a deeper and complex malady, namely the inferior status of the female and her expendable nature. Female neglect was evident in all aspects of life, female birth rarely being a cause for celebration. Protein and energy malnutrition were more common amongst females, the literacy rate amongst females was 18% compared to 40% for males and work participation 13% against 52,5%.

(iv) Traditional Genital Tract Injury and Mutilation

A common practice in Nigeria amongst Hausa women is Gishiri cutting made by inserting a large curved knife through the vaginal introitus into the anterior vaginal wall where the cut is made against the pubic bone endangering both bladder and urethra. This cut, utilized in the treatment of a wide variety of gynecological ills and commonly employed during pregnancy and labor, is administered by midwife or witch-doctor. During pregnancy it may be performed prior to labor, at the first sign of uterine contractions or during labor. Gishiri is the Hausa word for salt; but in the context of illness refers to diseases of the vagina and is accepted as an omnibus management for women of child-bearing age irrespective of whether or not they have ever been pregnant. Last (1976) noted that older women had never had Gishiri cutting done to them, yet often insisted younger women endured the treatment when giving birth for the first or second time. Walker (1954) reported a fistula involving the whole urethral length and bladder neck which followed incision of the hymen by a witch-doctor to correct dyspareunia. In the Zaria region of Nigeria, about 10% of fistulae seen at the hospital are due directly to this practice with a further 30% following a combination of the cut with obstructed labor. Patients consider the cut particularly helpful in relieving obstructed labor, treatment of prolapse, and the management of infertility. Patients who have had a fistula repaired successfully following a Gishiri cut have been known to return with a similar fistula after a second cut. Such potentially harmful practices will continue to exist so long as there is inadequate and inaccessible health services. Lister (1975) Zaria, Nigeria commented that the Gishiri cut seemed peculiar to Hausa land and women attending the antenatal clinic and near to term occasionally asked, "if it were not time for the cut to be done?". Many patients were seen exsanguinated with an antepartum hemorrhage from this cause and many cuts were self-inflicted producing excellent "beginner's fistulae". She has described rectal damage, bisection of the uterus and entry into the pouch of Douglas with division of loops of small bowel.

Certain birth canal damage predisposes to prolonged labor and development of fistula, especially female circumcision and inserting caustics into the postpartum vagina. The western world is not well acquainted with the tradition, cultural impact, and complications associated with female circumcision (Cutner 1985). Performed routinely in many parts of the world believing that physical and moral benefits of the procedure include a guarantee of marriage with subsequent economic and social security for a daughter's future, in much of North Africa excluding the Mediterranean littoral, circumcision still is practised widely reaching its zenith in the Sudan, where estimates of incidence range as high as 90%, including such large cities as Khartoum. Although centuries old it differs from other common traditional practices because it has serious physical and psycho-social health implications for both mothers and children. Still it is prevalent, irrespective of improvement in health, education and economic status, and in the past there has been little or limited interest in the subject since it is a sensitive deeply-rooted tradition with which neither governments or other organizations were willing to interfere. Although entangled with beliefs and superstitions of a mystical or religious nature, the varied people who practise circumcision do not conform to a common racial, social or religious background. No continent in the world has been exempt, although in Europe it was confined practically to the Russian Skoptozy, a Christian sect who kept the ritual to ensure perpetual virginity. Reasons put forward for the operation from one community to another have varied widely, but tradition has been the major factor, many societies believing it immoral for a girl not to be circumcised. More than 90% of Moslem females are virginal at marriage and the consequence of not being so are severe in such a society, therefore major forms of circumcision still are performed in Moslem cultures, even though the Koran does not condone the practice (Cutner 1985). Hathout (1963) stated that in some races such as Ethiopians and Hottentots, the operation was performed to excise notable hypertrophy of the labia minora, so furnishing an excuse for the operation on esthetic grounds. There are three methods of circumcision:

1. Pharaonic, so named since it had been seen in some Egyptian mummies leading to the belief it was practised by the Pharaohs (Aziz 1980). However, Rushwan (1982) said there have been doubts raised about the origin of the procedure in ancient Egypt, for the state of preservation of mummies did not allow firm conclusions to be drawn. A lack of well-documented material, has made it impossible to reach a definite conlcusion about the extent or nature of female circumcision in ancient Egypt.

Pharaonic circumcision involves removal of labia minora, most of the labia majora, mons veneris and sometimes the clitoris. Performed usually with a sharp razor, in many instances particularly in rural areas, no anaesthetic is used. The cut edges are stiched together with whatever suture material is available, usually string or hair, and the patient's legs brought together so the wound heals by first intention. The introitus is reduced to the size of a pin-hole, with usually a match stick inserted to allow passage of urine and menses. It is the most widely used method, performed on more than 90% of females. Known also as infibulation, classically the major part of a labium and whole clitoris is removed with the first sweep of the razor, the second excising the corresponding part of the other labium. Infibulation means clamping the two cut skin edges between limbs of a split cane, but modern surgeons use thread and needle aiming to fuse right and left sides, leaving an orifice barely admitting a finger tip. In North and Central Sudan, there has not been an appreciable reduction in this method of circumcision despite a 1946 government enactment making the method illegal, while substituting a lesser procedure known as Sunna. Rather than declining, Nadel (1947) stated that female circumcision was practiced by Arab tribes in the West and South-West of Kordofan (Messirya and Humr) and had spread to their Nuba neighbors (Huddleston 1949) (Fig. 77).

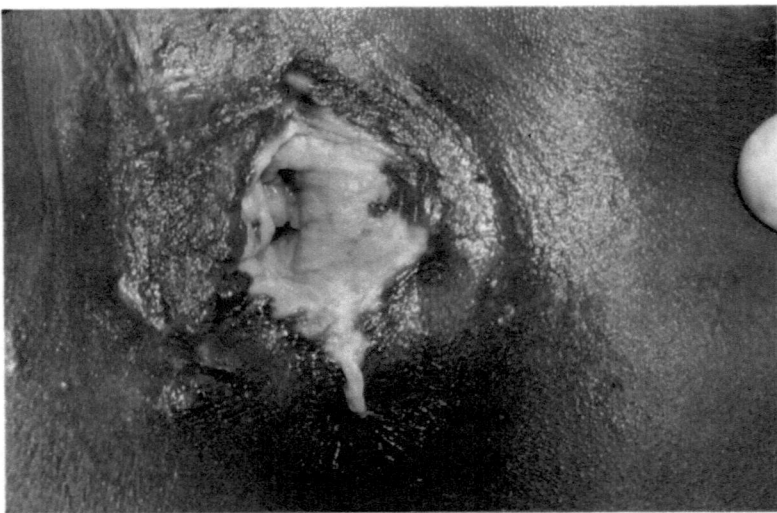

Figure 77. Pharaonic circumcision

2. Sunna. Called the Mohammedan practice since it is thought advised by Islam, only the enlarged clitoris is removed and the stump ligated. It is the type least practiced in the Sudan.

3. Modified Pharaonic is the technique more often used today, and only the clitoris and part of the labia majora is removed. The complications of circumcision are many (Aziz 1980) and include hemorrhage, shock, and retention of urine which is a common problem often requiring de-circumcision and catheterization, and acute infection, the worst of which is tetanus, usually fatal. Injury to neighboring structures especially the urethral meatus together with gross scarring and keloid formation is frequent, also inclusion cysts, vulval abscesses, infertility and the impossibility of adequate gynecological examination are common findings. The legal status or women within Islam dictated by the Koran, indicates clearly the social status of females and furthermore points to the fact, that until the situation changes circumcision will continue. The major source of a Sudanese midwife's income derives from the procedure, and the practice is widespread in East and Central Africa, Sudan, Somalia, Ethiopia, Egypt, Kenya, Chad, West Africa, Nigeria, Togo and Cameroon, also in parts of Asia, Indonesia, Malaysia and amongst the Urabunna Aboriginals of Australia with even occasional cases reported from the United Kingdom, Sweden and Russia.

Circumcision uniformly produces delay in the second stage of labor, managed in hospital by persistent "ironing out" of the perineum by the midwife and eventually after a prolonged period of "head on view" the perineum is incised to allow head delivery. It is usual to make a large midline or mediolateral episiotomy and often an additional incision is necessary anteriorly to permit head delivery. With such traumatized tissues, extension into the anal canal with sphincter disruption may occur readily and accordingly circumcision certainly has a marked influence on recto-vaginal fistula; but probably contributes little to the production of vesico-vaginal fistula.

Inserting vaginal caustics, is a common method of treatment for a variety of gynecological conditions in Western Nigeria, and although the herbal contents may be harmless, the soap base made from palm oil and potash is highly alkaline, causing a severe vaginitis (Lawson 1968). In parts of the Persian Gulf, Arab women are accustomed to pack the vagina with rock salt during the puerperium to shrink it to the nulliparous state, and in some areas, particularly Qatar, the custom has persisted. From the fifth until the twelfth day of the puerperium, balls of rock salt the size of a hen's egg are placed in the vagina by the patient's female relatives (Frith 1960). In Arabia, genital fistulae have followed packing the vagina with salt after labor, and this practice still occurs in some countries around the Arabian Gulf. Salt causes severe chemical vaginitis, and necrosis with sloughing of the vaginal wall after prolonged contact, leading to circumferential contracture of an annular scar causing severe stenosis, dyspareunia, obstruction to the menstrual flow and infertility. Should a patient again become pregnant, the scarring even may be sufficient to cause obstructed labor. Kingston (1957) Qatar, reported a salt-induced recto-vaginal fistula situated about three inches from the anal margin, and mentioned that in cases of complete vaginal atresia due to salt, recto-vaginal fistula can develop above the site of obstruction leading to monthly rectal bleeding. Underhill (1964) Bahrain, mentioned eight genital fistulae in a series with salt-induced vaginal stenosis. Naim and Fahmy (1965) reported six genital tract fistulae complicating salt vaginal atresia, two from Saudi Arabia and four from Kuwait.

(v) The Influence of Bilharzia

Coetzee and Lithgow (1966) discussing a series of 309 fistulae, believed bilharzia never was responsible for failure to close a fistula. A significant proportion of Egyptian fistulae formerly were believed due to bilharzia; but later evidence suggested vesico-vaginal fistula seldom if ever resulted from the disease, although fistula could follow obstructed labor in an infected patient, and for this reason such patients should undergo anti-bilharzia treatment prior to fistula repair, since bladder wall fibrosis un-altered by treatment, could make closure more difficult and healing less certain. Bland (1970) conducted a series of investigations on a group of fistula patients to find that whilst 40 of 60 patients showed evidence of bilharzia infection, only half healed rapidly after surgery, so assumed a probably significant association between bilharzia and failure to heal. It is conceivable s. hematobium could predispose to bladder rupture at the point of fibrosis and thickening, and a case reported in 1949 indicated external trauma could produce intraabdominal rupture of the bladder at such a site. Ova are deposited in enormous numbers in bladder mucosa and submucosa, and not uncommonly also in the muscular and peritoneal layers of the bladder. In chronic cases, sandy patches and granular polypi, together with mucosal ulceration are common, and radiological evidence of bladder wall calcification occurs in 15% of the adult African population, related to the heaviness of egg deposits. Accordingly, fibrous replacement of bladder layers can occur, leading to a small contracted bladder or an atrophic thin-walled dilated bladder, and such an inflammatory response may well impair healing. Repair should be delayed until a proven case of s. hematobium infestation has received full anti-bilharzia treatment. An earlier report by Sandwith (1901) stated that 14% of Egyptian vesico-vaginal fistulae were caused by bilharzia!

(vi) Social Consequences of Genital Fistula

The Hamlins wrote (1974): "To meet only one of these mothers is to be profoundly moved. Mourning the stillbirth of their only baby, incontinent of urine, ashamed of their offensiveness, often spurned by their husbands, homeless, unemployable except in the fields, they endure, they exist, without friends, without hope. No world charities have ever heard of them. They bear their sorrows in silent shame. Their miseries, untreated, are utter, lonely and lifelong."

This disastrous complication of obstructed labor still constitutes a social calamity in most African countries, major problems being the incontinence, childlessness, divorce, and the patient becomes a social outcast with suicide sometimes a terminal event. Attitudes towards them are harsh even though within the family compound the patient is isolated from others, and the initial reaction by husband and family is to offer moral and financial help, nevertheless, ultimately nearly 80% are abandoned. Childless and without hope unless cured, the experience is shattering for these teenaged women

(Murphy 1981). A majority of these young females develop the fistula in their first pregnancy, and most come from poorer subsistence farming backgrounds. These patients are a particularly disadvantaged group since illiteracy in rural areas is widespread. The patient's mother usually remains kind and loving; but other women in the compound resent her presence, smell and incontinence. Islam emphasizes cleanliness especially regarding intercourse, so any affected female is considered unclean and no longer allowed to pray, although in time her condition may come to be regarded as incurable, and resumption of praying permitted. Patients themselves expect to be treated as outcasts, and the shame of the disorder often leads to families denying its existence so the sufferer is not given any chance of treatment. Her only hope of normality is surgical repair, so once aware of this, motivation is strong towards seeking treatment and they overcome incredible obstacles to obtain help.

At the fistula hospital Addis Ababa, Ethiopia, many patients have been on the road for three months or more, travelling quite long distances often accompanied by their father rather than their husband. Within three weeks over 90% of these women are cured; but quite obviously the real need for such patients is prevention and the major factors of improved transport including in the future air ambulance evacuation, better health care and a change in attitude toward women will take time, money and universal education. Unfortunately Walker (1954) found no evidence to suggest frequency of fistula had diminished by improving social and medical conditions and Murphy and Baba (1981) stated that in the previous ten years problems of rural health care delivery in the third world had received more attention than before; but to be effective, knowledge of particular problems at the local level, and an account of the life experiences of people seeking help were paramount. They found provision of health care services in villages of northern Nigeria were negligible, local people regarding the hospital only as a place to die, so traditional health medicine was more accessible and its practitioners more familiar to the people. It was rare to meet a literate fistula patient, since lack of education in itself deterred people from attending hospital, particularly when they are made to feel stupid and when hospital staff were from an alien culture with differing traditions, customs and language. Observations made on village visits confirmed general comments about rural health care in the majority of third world countries being a picture of deprivation. There was a lack of health services, those that existed were under-manned and ill-equipped and basic amenities such as electricity and public transport were rare. Of particular concern was lack of encouragement for girls to attend school and an absence of adult literacy classes, since a mother's lack of education was a most important socio-economic factor affecting perinatal mortality. They believed health education programs relating to obstetric and child-care practices could be directed usefully towards older women, since it was clear these senior women were decision makers in matters relating to every day life in the family compound.

In a study of traditional birth attendants and their potential to be improved by training programs, Maglacas and Simons (1986) indicated the difficulties encountered in various countries, and emphasized that success with such programs could be achieved only after a thorough understanding and appreciation of local customs, superstitions, beliefs, folklore and ritual relating to child-birth combined with adequate literacy instruction to ensure the information was being understood.

Pathology of Obstetric Fistula

Obstetric fistula occurs as a result of pressure necrosis produced by long and difficult labor, or by attempts, either abdominal or vaginal to effect delivery in the course of this labor. Less commonly, fistula may follow operative delivery during normal pregnancy or normal labor.

(i) Pressure Necrosis

Fistula site is determined by the level at which the presenting part impacts, and this may be the pelvic brim, pelvic cavity or outlet. The genital tract, urinary tract, anal canal and rectum all may be involved. Typically the vagina has a dusky discolored appearance following delivery, and by the second day, the epithelium is purplish or black with a clearly delineated area of necrosis. Between the third and fifth day, the anterior vaginal wall and bladder floor begin to slough, and the patient becomes incontinent of urine (Longo 1964). Genital tract damage may involve uterus, cervix or vagina and rectum, and in worst cases, all may be affected with the uterus ruptured, and cervix and vaginal wall eventually sloughing. When brim impaction occurs before full dilatation, necrosis of cervix, bladder and ureter is likely, and later in the pathological process, large amounts of grossly infected and necrotic tissue—a mixture of cervix, vagina, bladder and rectum—may be discharged through the introitus (Fig. 76 B). Parke Gray (1970) noted obstetric fistula resulted from obstructed labor, yet in the circumstances in which it occurred, study of obstructing mechanisms was precluded, although it seemed unlikely the bony pelvis was the sole responsible factor in all, since after successful fistula repair, many females in their next pregnancy, were delivered vaginally. Hamlin and Nicholson delivered half their cured patients by Cesarian Section and half vaginally, indicating the pelvis was adequate for vaginal delivery in many who previously had developed a fistula when labor had been prolonged. It is important to emphasize that such patients must be supervised closely in a well-equipped labor ward with facilities available for Cesarian section should it prove necessary. Many obstructed labors seen in Addis Ababa were delivered vaginally after catheterization, even though some progressed to fistula formation. Linke et al. (1971) reported most Rhodesian births were managed by older women without midwifery training and after admission to hospital the history and findings were quite typical. A still-birth had occurred at home after one or two days of labor, the bladder was grossly distended and there was marked labial edema with a large perineal tear. Some of the worst injuries occurred with babies weighing less than six pounds. The bladder wall is subjected to two opposing forces—mechanical pressure from the impacted presenting part on one side, and hydrostatic pressure from unrelieved retention of urine on the other, emphasizing that factors which produce vesico-vaginal fistula need not be recurring.

Urinary damage may involve ureters, bladder or urethra, the size of the defect depending upon the level of obstruction and its duration. Former opinion believed the ureter was protected in protracted labor because of its upward displacement above the pelvic brim; but Mahfouz (1938) disproved this theory with postmortem studies in ten women who had died undelivered with a ruptured uterus. In most, the trigone and distal ureter had been subjected to direct compression against the pubic symphysis, showing that when the cervix was not entirely effaced and retracted, the distal ureter was liable to damage.

The most usual urinary fistula involves bladder and bladder neck in the midvaginal area and in many, part of the urethra also is involved. This should be hardly surprising since in obstructed labor, when the bladder rises above the pelvic brim the urethra follows, and with brim obstruction, bladder neck and part of the upper third of the urethra usually are at risk. When the presenting part impacts in the pelvic cavity or outlet, the entire urethra is threatened, and may slough completely. In certain patients, annular sloughing of the bladder neck may occur blocking the internal urethral orifice, with the urethral stump separated from the bladder by a plug of dense scar. In worst examples of distal obstruction, the vagina may slough completely healing to a narrow gap surrounded by scar, criss-crossed by fistula tracts. Similarly, the anal canal or rectum can be involved, and rectal injuries may follow pressure necrosis of the posterior vaginal wall and neighboring rectum during obstructed labor, the fetal head compressing these structures against the sacral promontory. A high recto-vaginal fistula due to compression opens into the posterior fornix; but a similar defect may be produced by an extensive third degree tear involving the whole posterior wall, up to the cervix. The more usual recto-vaginal fistula follows neglected third degree tear or a tear recognized and sutured, but healed inadequately. Third degree sphincter involvement with great tissue deficit also may be due to sloughing following obstructed labor.

Fistulae can be mobile or fixed, and sited centrally or laterally; but some lie concealed within scar tissue and may escape detection. On occasion, multiple fistulae occur, e.g. a uretero-vaginal fistula in the vault and a urethro-vesico-vaginal fistula on the anterior vaginal wall. Fistula edges may be thick, or thin and sharp, and size may vary from a tiny hole hardly admitting a fine probe to a large gap caused by total destruction of bladder base and urethra. As mentioned already, in many patients, cervix and vaginal vault slough leaving a mass of dense scar tissue surrounding a large bladder defect, and in such cases, the ureteric orifices usually are to be found at the fistula edge or even displaced outside it, in scar tissue.

(ii) Healing Phase

For many weeks after bladder or rectal damage, edges of the communicating passage are grossly infected, and necrotic debris continues to be discharged. Healing is by secondary intention, the persisting inflammation encouraging growth of granulation tissue infiltrated by many cells, predominantly fibroblasts. These connective tissue cells contract, gradually reducing the size of the defect and epithelium regenerates from vagina and bladder or vagina and rectum. Eventually, necrotic material at the surface—the eschar—is discharged, and cross-union of the two epithelia follows. Bladder epithelium regenerates very rapidly, experimental evidence showing just how quickly and completely this can occur. Following total cystectomy in dogs, Bohne and Hettle (1955) placed an acrylic mould into the resulting extraperitoneal space, and within five weeks a thick-walled inflammatory pouch lined by granulation was in place, by six to ten weeks the pouch was lined by transitional epithelium, and at fourteen to sixteen weeks, the pouch wall contained fibrous tissue, giant cells and smooth muscle bundles.

Fistula may be defined as an abnormal connection between two epithelial surfaces, and with continued scar contraction, the defect if small, may even close spontaneously; but in all patients the defect will diminish

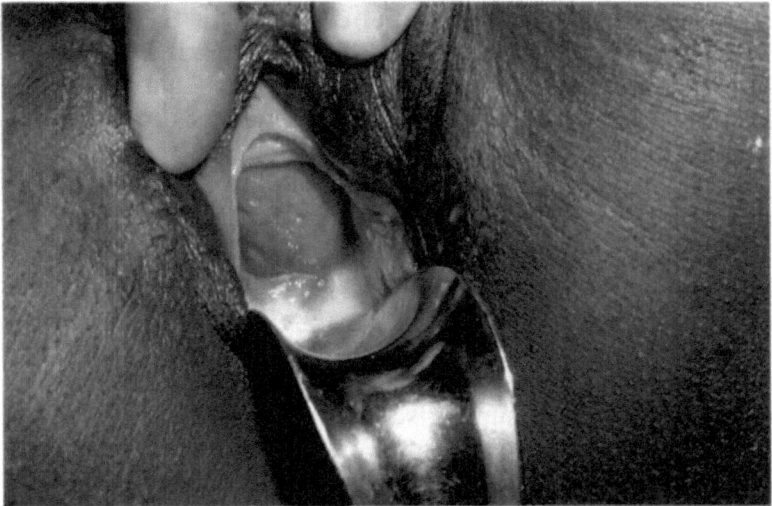

Figure 78. Bladder prolapsing through a large fistula

gradually, epithelial cross-union and the size of the tissue deficit being major reasons for persistence. Associated with scar contraction is scar adhesion to underlying tissues producing gross vaginal distortion with thick fibrous bands in various situations, and commonly a large annular constriction in midvagina. To be complete, the healing phase occupies a period of ten to twelve weeks. Whilst scar tissue is maximal at and about the fistula tract, nevertheless there is not a sudden cut-off point between normal and scarred bladder wall, the fibrous tissue replacement extending for an appreciable distance into tissues well away from the fistula, the extent depending upon the degree of bladder wall injury which occurred when the fistula was produced. This important fact must be borne in mind when argument arises about scar excision during fistula repair, for obviously if all scar tissue were removed, a much larger defect would result. Scarring and contraction occurring with a large vesico-vaginal fistula, often are associated with a tendency for the anterior bladder wall to prolapse through the defect and appear in the vagina as a reddened mass of tissue (Fig. 78). A further and most important effect of scar contraction is involvement of the uretero-vesical junction in a significant number of patients. Lagundoye et al. (1976) reviewed intravenous pyelograms performed routinely on 216 patients with vesico-vaginal fistula following obstructed labor. Half the patients showed normal pyelograms; but marked changes in others included varying degrees of calyceal abnormality, ten patients with nonfunctioning kidneys, hydro-ureter present in 34%, medial deviation of the terminal ureter in 10% and four had developed bladder calculi. There is a high risk of renal morbidity in patients with obstetric vesico-vaginal fistula due most probably to scar contraction which results in a rigid ureteric orifice, stenosis of the lower ureter, or medial deviation of the terminal ureter. With grosser degrees of tissue deficit and scar replacement, adhesion to the bony pelvis is the rule, particularly to periosteum on the inferior margin of the ischio-pubic ramus on either side, and the back of the bodies of the pubic bones. In addition, with large fistulae and the passage of time, phosphatic con-cretions about the vulval area and within the bladder as calculi, are com-mon. Failure to achieve surgical repair means the whole healing process must begin again, each intervention leaving a greater residue of scar tissue with further diminution in blood supply, so prospects for success recede further with each failure. The duration and completeness of the healing phase are vital pieces of information when deciding to intervene and attempt closure. Three months is the commonly accepted time interval for all in-flammatory changes and scar contraction to have subsided; but while the healing phase is continuing, in general, surgery is regarded as unwise with an increased risk of failure. Nevertheless many pressures face the surgeon, and temptation to intervene before the healing phase is complete may be great, yet it must be remembered always, that the first attempt at closure offers the greatest chance of success, so careful timing is essential to gain maximum advantage. Despite an increased risk of failure with earlier in-tervention, nonetheless attempts have been made to speed up the healing phase using cortisone as an anti-inflammatory agent. Collins et al. (1952, 1957, 1971) reported 38 vesico-vaginal fistulae including some due to ob-stetric injury and most were operated on within 30 days of diagnosis—one third within 14 days—after 10 days oral therapy with cortisone. The ra-tionale for such therapy was the marked clinical improvement gained in patients with chronic pelvic inflammatory disease ("ligneous pelvic cellu-litis"), when treated with oral cortisone which "experimental evidence showed to inhibit fibroplasia, to increase growth of tissue macrophages in tissue culture and prevent or reduce tissue reaction to chemical irritants". Surgery performed after cortisone therapy showed "a marked reduction in vascularity, the acute exudate was more plastic, the tissue planes were easily dissected and the sutures held". They reported a primary success rate of 72.4% and of eight failures, five were cured at a second operation and three at the third. Experienced fistula surgeons would expect a primary closure rate between 90 and 100% preferring to delay intervention until local tissue reactions have ceased. Failure to close a fistula is a great emotional let-down for the patient, so all effort must be directed at gaining a very high primary closure rate, and the most certain way to achieve this is by thorough observance of surgical principles laid down so long ago by James Marion Sims. In spite of this widely held conservative point of view, some surgeons (Fearl and Keizur 1969) have advocated more selective intervention determined by the cause of the fistula, believing tissue reaction after surgically produced fistulae to be much less than that following obstetric trauma and so, in theory recovery should be more rapid. Again, in 1979, Persky et al. advocated intervention with surgically produced fistulae once the diagnosis was confirmed. They used a transvesical approach and following closure, reinforced the repair with peritoneum or omentum. A longer waiting period was necessary only when managing obstetric fistula, for this was produced by pressure necrosis and sufficient time must elapse to allow delineation of viable tissues, discharge of slough and completion of scar contraction. They were successful with six of seven cases. Taylor et al. (1980) used Phenylbutazone and antibiotics to reduce associated inflammation and avoid several months delay.

(iii) Associated Diseases and Conditions

Malnutrition, intercurrent infection and anemia commonly are associated in patients with genital fistula. The anemia may follow malaria, intestinal parasites, schistosomiasis or various hemoglobinopathies such as sickle-cells anemia. Whilst varying degrees of protein malnutrition are common in much of Africa, at the fistula hospital in Addis Ababa, the general condition of patients is good, for the local diet of tef and wat is rich in protein and iron, when adequate food supplies are available. Important associated conditions include foot-drop from obstructed labor, amenorrhea, other menstrual abnormalities, and mental depression with an occasional history of attempted suicide. Sinclair (1952) reported 20 cases of maternal obstetric palsy and indicated foot-drop was due to injury of peripheral nerves in the lower extremeties during labor, and in most reported cases usually prolonged labor in a primigravida had been terminated by difficult forceps delivery. It was a matter of some interest that while foot-drop was presumed due to nerve compression during difficult or obstructed labor, there were no records of the lesion being associated with vaginal fistulae, where certainly there had been prolonged pressure by the presenting part in the lower pelvis. Likewise it had not occurred with breech presentation. Naidu (1962) in a series of 208 fistulae reported six in whom "foot-drop palsy" was associated, due he believed to the ravages of obstructed labor. Hamlin and Nicholson (1986) indicated foot-drop was a relatively common occurrence in association with fistula and in none of their patients, had forceps delivery been employed.

There are definite changes to pubic bones and symphyseal cartilage in patients with obstetric vesico-vaginal fistula, produced by vascular obstruction and thrombosis because of obstructed labor. Cockshott (1973) reviewed pelvic radiographs of 312 patient with obstetrically produced vesico-vaginal fistula and in general, the patients had small pelves; but additionally, 32% showed pelvic abnormalities including bone resorption, pubic separation greater than one cm. and marginal fractures with bony spurs due possibly to muscular avulsion. In patients with chronic fistulae, especially those resistant to surgical correction, common findings were gross bladder neck scarring and urethral destruction with pubic periosteum forming the fistula boundary, and in this group, there was bony obliteration of the symphysis, consequent upon interruption to the blood supply of the symphseal cartilage by the previous obstructed labor. Naidu (1962) stated that "amenorrhea was the rule in most cases of fistulae" and when the opportunity presented, the smooth, pearly, polycystic ovaries present in many patients were subjected to wedge resection with resumption of menstruation. In some, menses resumed following correction alone. Hudson (1970) indicated that traumatic amenorrhea followed sloughing of the entire endometrium, and hematometra might occur should some endometrium remain in the upper uterus; but sometimes amenorrhea was secondary to the poor general condition of the patient, corrected when her health improved. Hamlin and Nicholson (1986) stated that amenorrhea was not commonly associated with fistula in Ethiopia.

Bieler and Schnabel (1976) studied 11 patients with menstrual disorders dating from obstructed and prolonged labor and their results indicated that menstrual disturbance after such a labor was associated with an upset of different hypophyseotrophic areas of the hypothalamus.

Associated recto-vaginal fistula, secondary hemorrhage, loss of anal sphincter tone, foot-drop and necrosis of symphyseal cartilage also were reported by Linke et al. (1971).

7

Management of Urinary Fistulae

Clinical Features

(i) Classification

Marion Sims (1852) classified urinary fistulae by their relative position dividing them into:

1. Urethro-vaginal where the defect was confined to the urethra.

2. Fistulae situated "at the bladder neck or root of the urethra, destroying the trigone."

3. Fistulae involving the body and floor of the bladder.

4. Utero-vesical where the opening communicated with the uterine body or cervix—although he confessed he had never seen such a fistula.

Mahfouz (1930) reported 300 fistulae dividing them into seven anatomical groups: vesico-vaginal, vesico-cervico-vaginal, urethro-vaginal, vesico-cervical, vesico-uretero-vaginal, urethro-cervical, uretero-vaginal. This classification although acurate anatomically, was too complex to be accepted widely, and in 1945 Benion Thomas suggested only three groups—juxta-cervical, midvaginal and juxta-urethral—as being far more practical. Krishnan (1949) added a fourth group termed "the combined fistula". McConnachie (1958) offered a classification based on an experience with 300 fistulae and used the following terms: "grade of fistula" which depended whether normal healthy tissues and sphincters were present, together with ease of access, and "type of fistula" dependant upon size. He distinguished 15 different varieties of fistula, far too involved for general acceptance. Chassar Moir (1961) commented that an injury so variable in form and degree as vesico-vaginal fistula, led enthusiasts to evolve complex classifications in attempts to cover each anatomical possibility; but his view was that such comprehensive systems had no great practical merit, so put forward three simple anatomical subdivisions.

1. High fistulae which involved the trigone well above the urethro-vesical junction.

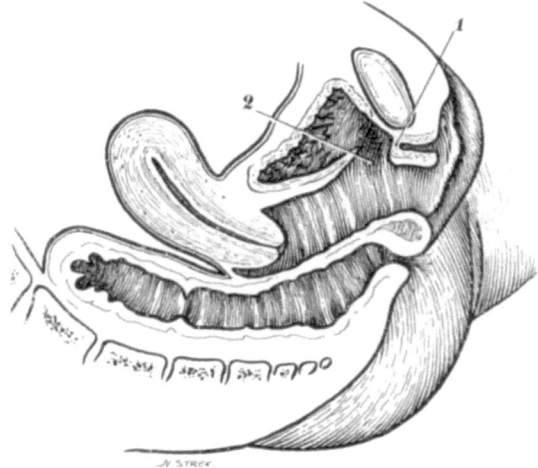

Figure 79. The circumferential fistula of Chassar Moir with bladder and urethral discontinuity (*1*) urethral block, (*2*) fistula. (From Mahfouz)

2. Mid-level fistula involving the urethro-vesical junction.

3. The urethro-vaginal fistula.

This classification was entirely practical, and in 1965 he added "the circumferential fistula", which resulted from extensive sloughing of the bladder neck on both pubic and vaginal sides so a circumferential sloughing with subsequent discontinuity of urethra and bladder occurred, the intervening tissue being only epithelium which had grown over and become adherent to periosteum on the back of the pubis. He preferred to distinguish this fistula since it presented a particular challenge to the surgeon, because of extreme difficulty with exposure and technical problems with closure (Fig. 79). Bird (1967) divided fistulae into anatomical types similar to that of Benion Thomas, and of 69 vesico-vaginal fistulae, 14 were circumferential. Lawson (1968) offered a practical classification covering more variations than the scheme of Chassar Moir.

1. Juxta-urethral which involved bladder neck and upper urethra together with damage to the sphincteric mechanism, and fixity to bone. This defect could be confined to the urethra with total urethral loss.

2. Mid-vaginal without involvement of either sphincter or trigone, and it was unusual for this fistula to be tethered to bone.

3. High fistula or juxta-cervical, opening into the anterior fornix or cervical canal with the possibility of distal ureteric involvement.

4. Massive fistula, a combination of all three with extensive tissue loss. The ureteric orifices commonly would be involved at the fistula margin, and bladder may prolapse throught the defect.

Hamlin and Nicholson (1969) simplified the classification still further, relating anatomical varieties to difficulties of operative correction, and recognized six main varieties:

1. Simple vesico-vaginal fistula.
2. Simple recto-vaginal fistula.
3. Simple urethro-vaginal fistula.
4. Difficult high recto-vaginal fistula.
5. Vesico-uterine fistula.
6. "Difficult urinary fistula", a complex of several grave injuries which occurred together and included:

(a) total urethral destruction and its replacement by scar and epithelium, densely adherent to the retro-pubic periosteum,

(b) extensive sloughing of bladder neck and trigone with one or both ureteric orifices opening directly into the vagina,

(c) extensive scarring which distorted and narrowed the vagina, and bound the bladder remnant high up to the ischio-pubic rami and pubic bones.

This difficult fistula involved every part of the lower urinary tract and daunted the heart of most observers who saw it for the first time.

A brief review of these classifications shows clearly that too detailed a subdivision is unhelpful in the clinical setting for usually there is overlap of one fistula type with another, and often as in the massive or difficult fistula, all the divisional features are represented. The important features of each fistula are:

(i)   the anatomical site of the damage,
(ii) the size of the defect,
(iii) scarring.

Accordingly a further simplification into small, medium and large fistulae, based on the realities of surgical correction is proposed. Typically the small fistula lies in the anterior vaginal wall, does not involve bladder sphincter or urethra, is not tethered to bone, and surgical correction is relatively easy (Fig. 80).

The middle-sized fistula involves a large area of the anterior vaginal wall, the urethro-vesical junction is lost together with part of the proximal urethra, and adhesion to bone is usual. One or both ureteric orifices will be near the fistula edge, and even may be displaced outside it (Fig. 81).

The large fistula affects a significant proportion of bladder floor, vesico-urethral junction and commonly the entire urethra. The anterior vaginal wall is replaced by massive scar tissue, so upon examination of the patient, one looks straight into the bladder. Ureteric orifices are always near the

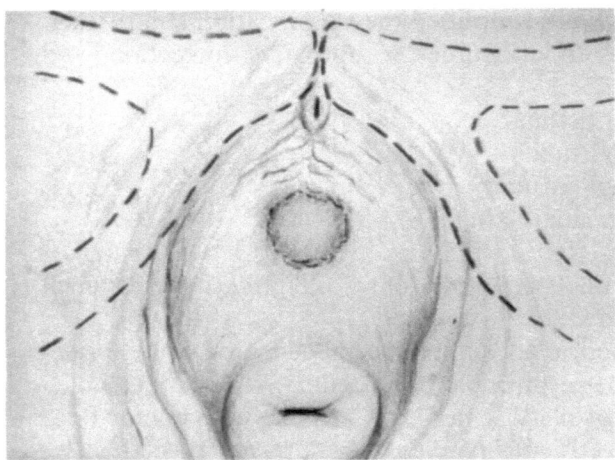

Figure 80. Line drawing depicting the small fistula—central situation, minimal tissue deficit, and scarring without bony adhesion

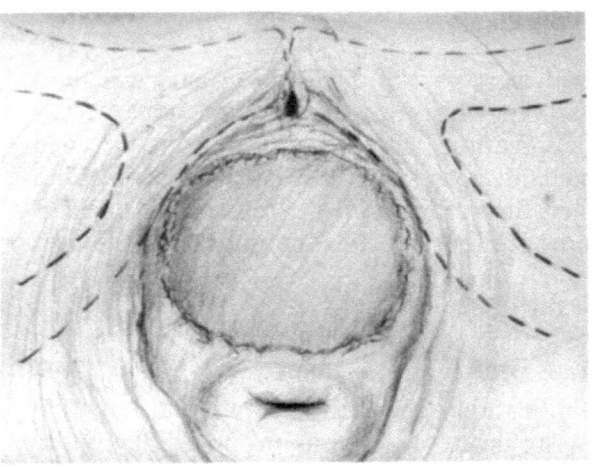

Figure 81. Line drawing showing the middle size fistula—increased tissue deficit with scarring and the likelihood of ureteric involvement together with moderate bony adhesion

fistula margin or displaced externally, inevitably there is extensive adhesion of the bladder remnant to the inferior margins of the ischio-pubic rami, and the site of the former urethra is replaced by scar tissue (Fig. 82).

(ii) Symptoms

Primary symptoms of bladder damage present during the puerperium as dysuria and painful micturition. Blood and mucus soon appear in the urine associated with a raised temperature and signs of general and local sepsis.

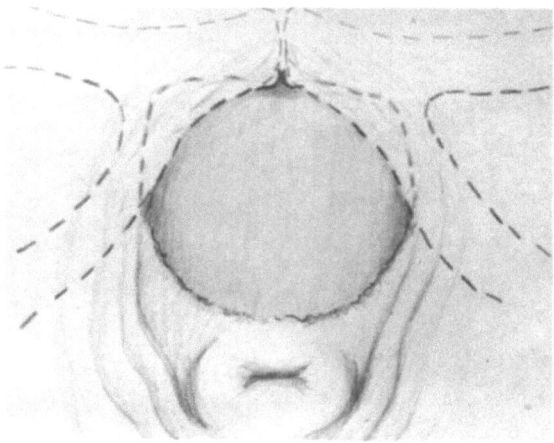

Figure 82. Line drawing of the large fistula with massive tissue loss, scarring, bony adhesion, and the ureteric orifices may lie near to the fistula edge or even outside it

Incontinence occurs when the slough begins to separate, and usually this takes about a week. Should the fistula be due to trauma, then incontinence appears immediately. It must be made quite clear that incontinence of urine following labor is not necessarily due to fistula, and this must be clarified during investigation. Constant dribbling of urine associated with poor hygiene soon produces vulval dermatitis, vulval hair becomes covered with incrustations, and quickly the effects of a urinary fistula on the patient's morale become marked for the offensive nature of the problem compels her to lead a solitary life.

(iii) Diagnosis and Investigation

It is wise always to assume there is something unusual about each patient with a fistula, and to make a thoughtful and thorough examination (Scott Russell 1966). Accuracy is essential; but usually the diagnosis can be made comparatively easily. An obvious loss of urine through the defect may be witnessed, and the fistula itself palpated, enabling site, size and degree of scarring to be assessed. Confirmation is made by passage of a sound through the urethra, to be seen or palpated in the vagina (Fig. 83 a, b). Small granulated regions should be considered as possible fistulous openings, and watched carefully for urinary leakage, then the area must be examined meticulously using a fine vaginal probe after inserting a sound into the bladder. Felix Platter (1597) first mentioned visual diagnosis of a bladder tear and its confirmation by passing a probe. Pinaeus (1650) used a silver probe passed through the urethra to the bladder, where it was detected by the index finger, or another probe inserted into the vagina. Roonhuyse

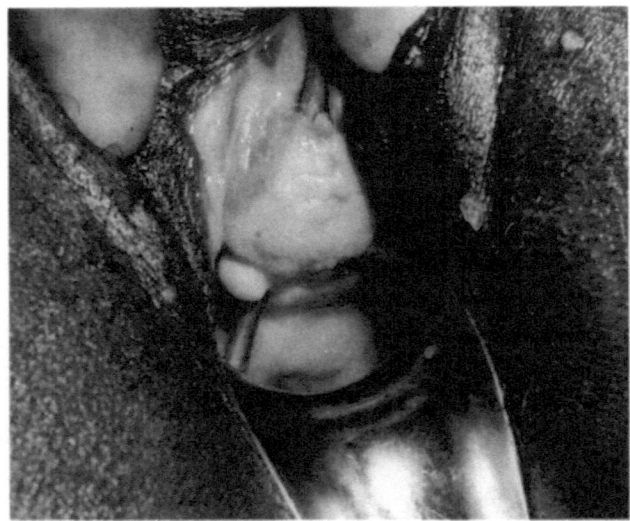

Figure 83 a. Metal sound passed through the urethra into the midvagina. Cervix can be seen in the upper vagina

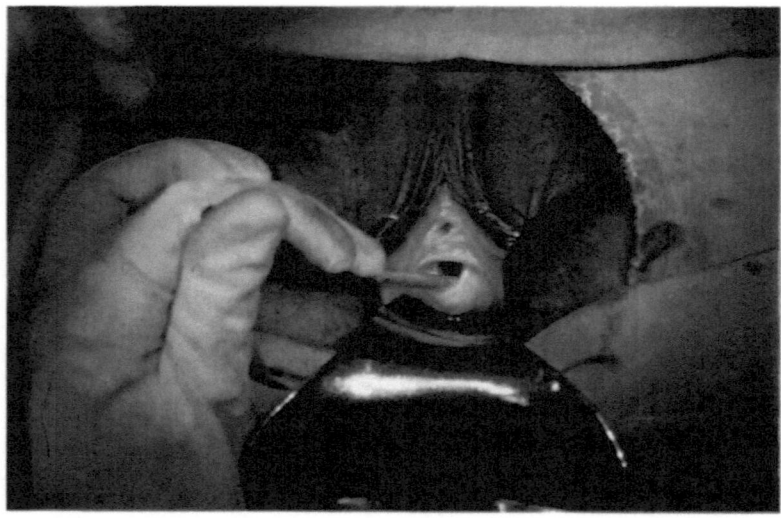

Figure 83 b. Sound in mid-vaginal small fistula

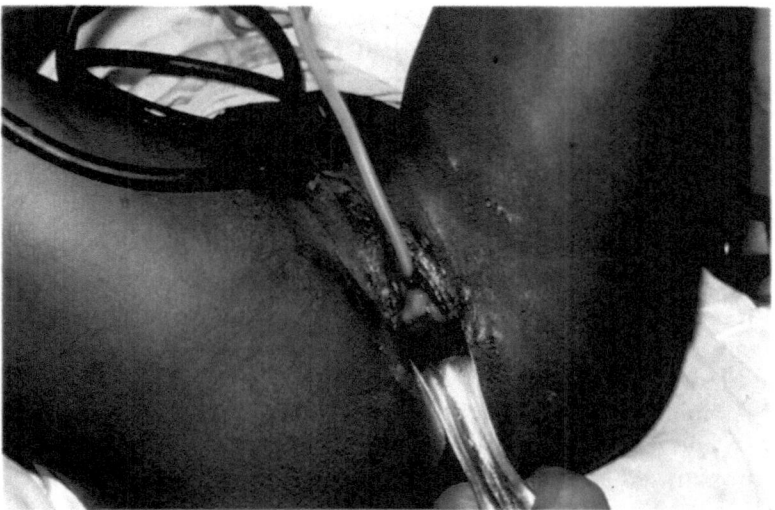

Figure 84. Dye entering the vagina through a fistula

(1663) confirmed the presence of a fistula by railroading two catheters, one through the bladder and the other through the vagina and also described visual diagnosis using a speculum. Present day diagnosis of fistula site using intra-vesical dye began with Voelter (1679) who injected barley water along the urethra and observed whether or not it appeared in the vagina (Fig. 84). When a fistula is suspected: but not obvious at routine clinical examination, the bladder can be filled with dye and three white swabs placed one below the other in the vagina. This test will help distinguish ureteric, vesical and urethral fistulae. The patient walks about and after a period of time, the swabs are examined. If the vault swab is soaked with clear urine, a uretero-vaginal fistula probably is present, whereas a colored wet vault swab means a vesico-vaginal fistula. A colored wet swab at the introitus suggests either a urethro-vaginal fistula or urethral incontinence. Even if dye leaks into the vagina, it does not exclude absolutely the presence of a uretero-vaginal fistula or stress incontinence. With some vesico-uterine fistulae it is necessary to apply traction to the cervix to see whether or not dye leaks from the cervix (Ward 1985). Massee et al. (1964) used air instilled into the bladder to aid diagnosis of the small fistula. After filling the vagina with warm water, air bubbles may be observed—the "flat tyre" technique. Should a uretero-vaginal fistula be suspected, further special investigations are necessary for confirmation. Cystoscopy, intravenous pyelogram and perhaps a retrograde pyelogram are required to elucidate special facts about each fistula, necessary before thoughts of surgical correction are entertained. Cystoscopy may be done without anesthesia; but for a detailed bladder examination particularly with the possibility of multiple fistulae or of a small fistula hidden in an area of scar tissue, general anesthesia and exaggerated lithotomy position are necessary. The possibility of a double fistula uretero-vaginal and vesico-vaginal, or vesico-vaginal and urethro-vaginal—must always be considered. If the fistula is large and it is difficult to maintain bladder distension, a vaginal swab supplemented by a gloved vaginal finger may enable cystoscopic examination to be completed. To facilitate localization of a small fistula at operation, Massee et al. (1964) suggested, "that a silk thread could be passed through the fistula from the bladder during cystoscopy and then knotted loosely over the perineum." As mentioned previously, Lagundoye et al. (1976) carried out intravenous pyelography on a large group of women with obstetric fistulae and demonstrated urinary tract abnormality was present in approximately 50%, so this investigation, when possible, should be performed before surgery is contemplated.

Important details in diagnosis are:

1. Anatomical Facts

1. Site and size of the fistula into the vagina, its relation to the cervix, bladder, urethro-vesical junction and urethra, and should cervix be involved, then the external os should be identified.

2. The number of fistulae.

3. Patency of the urethra.

4. Relationship of ureteric orifices to the fistula, and their proximity to the fistula edge is an essential piece of information. In larger fistulae, one or both ureteric orifices can lie outside the fistula edge, and this possibility must be clarified with certainty, early on during reparative surgery.

2. Pathological features

All these features are emphasized following previous attempts at surgical correction, and the more attempts made, the more apparent are these changes.

1. The amount of tissue deficit.

2. The extent of scarring at the fistula edge, and degree of associated vaginal fixity and stenosis.

3. Adhesion of the fistula to bone—the ischio-pubic rami and the pubic bones.

4. Bladder inversion through the defect.

5. The presence of bladder calculi.

6. Progress of epithelial healing in the bladder and vagina is gauged by the return of normal epithelial appearances; but after frequent attempts at surgical repair, return to normal is much delayed. The assessment of normality is made by periodic vaginal inspections and cystoscopic examination of the bladder. The major indices of normality are:

(a) loss of tissue edema, with return of normal epithelial color,

(b) softening and return of tissue mobility,

(c) a decrease in inflammatory reaction shown by diminution in the blanching test—compression of the vaginal epithelium with the tip of a uterine sound produces marked blanching in inflamed tissues, diminishing as healing progresses.

7. The assessment of renal function.

8. Vulval and vaginal cleanliness must be restored prior to any surgery.

9. General examination should exclude common associated problems of malaria, anemia, bilharzia and various parasites.

Consideration of all these factors enables forward planning to commence, both in terms of general and local preparation, and the decision about an appropriate time for surgical intervention. General diseases, especially bilharzia and malaria, must be treated, and local vaginal cleanliness achieved by simple hygiene, especially mechanical scrubbing and washing, and intra-vaginal douches. With long-standing fistulae, calculi must be sought and removed. Urinary tract infection is not a problem before surgery because of free urinary drainage but requires appropriate prophylaxis after fistula closure.

Fistulae Involving the Urinary System — Clinical Groups

(a) Vesico-vaginal fistula without urethral involvement.

(b) Vesico-vaginal fistula with partial or complete urethral destruction.

(c) Vesico-cervico-vaginal fistula.

Surgical Correction

(i) Prophylaxis

Reginald Hamlin put the matter succinctly, when he described the causes of obstetric fistula as obstructed labor and obstructed transport, and accordingly prophylaxis should be directed to these two major problems. Lister (1986) posed the question: "What can be done to decrease the incidence of this very distressing condition and cut the enormous fetal and maternal wastage?—more hospitals, health centers, proper communications, roads and adequate transport and sufficient doctors gradually are coming, being the obvious solutions, but these factors are not the immediate answer to the problem. The real answer comes within the wide term of education of the patient, husband, relatives and influential people at the village level. Most fistulae occur as a result of unrelieved obstructed labor and the Nigerian primigravida's labor should not last longer than 24 hours and the multigravida half that time. Relatives should be made to realize these facts and bring all women to hospital who are undelivered after 24 hours. The family should be educated to appreciate that certain women are high risks patients—short young girls, elderly primigravidae, grand multiparity, patients with previous still-births and those who have had operative deliveries or a repaired vesico-vaginal fistula in the past. If all these women would come to hospital early in labor or even attend an antenatal clincic, then fistulae in many countries would become things of the past."

St. George (1969) West Indies, indicated that deep transverse arrest of the fetal head was more common in a primigravida with an android pelvis and primiparae were permitted to labor for much longer by their family, because of their youth, and accordingly any resulting fistula was extensive. After prolonged obstructed labor and following delivery of the child, treatment with antibiotics, continuous bladder drainage, vaginal douches and sofra-tulle packing minimized local sepsis and assisted devitalized tissues to recover with a minimum of fibrosis and fixity, so with later attempts at cure, the layers could be dealt with much more readily.

Bladder injury during Cesarian section demands prompt recognition and careful management. The realization that bladder integrity has been breached is most important, and proper investigation must ensure the site and dimensions of the defect. Sterile milk or dilute methylene blue may aid identification and once limits of the defect are known, a water-tight double-layer closure together with adequate bladder drainage and antibiotics are necessary for 10–12 days. Hutch et al. (1970) advocated purse-string closure of such defects, but the general view believes double-layer Lembert-style closure excluding bladder mucosa is more appropriate and Benson et al. (1955) made the point that bladder mobilization usually is required to allow double-layer closure without tension. In addition to bladder drainage, suprapubic drainage of the cave of Retzius is necessary.

(ii) Difficulties Associated with Urinary Fistulae

Sir Reginald Watson-Jones (1946), emphasizing the great importance of controlled treatment of fractures, remarked, "Bones are filled not with red marrow; but with black ingratitude" and the essential sense of this aphorism can be applied with an equal impact to underline the meticulous care necessary for successful fistula management.

The nature of the injury which caused the fistula, the type of fistula and its location, are the main factors determining the results of attempted repair (Carter et al. 1952). Chassar Moir (1955) and Foda (1959) stated that fistula size was no indication of difficulty of closure and indeed some of the largest were surprisingly easy, even the association of a large fistula with prolapse of the bladder through the fistula, posed few technical problems. Whilst many supposed the bladder would be incapable of regaining its normal function after incontinence present for years, Moir indicated this was not true, and duration of the fistula had little relevance to its curability, with bladder capacity often returning to normal quickly after closure. Two most important factors which could militate against successful outcome were the amount of tissue deficit, and the presence of dense fibrosis with bony adhesion to the rami and body of the pubic bones. Either complication if extreme could make functional cure almost impossible, although substantial improvement often might be obtained with residual "stress incontinence" less distressing than the previous constant wetness. Ability to mobilize grossly scarred tissues adequately without destroying blood supply, and then to be able to close them carefully in layers without tension, were vital prerequisites for successful repair.

Associated vaginal stenosis usually can be overcome by adequate incisions. Urinary infection is not a problem with large fistulae due to free urinary drainage and infection becomes a problem only following successful closure of the fistula with the need for prolonged catheter drainage. Infection may be a problem with multiple small fistulae and inadequate bladder drainage, particularly if phosphatic concretions are deposited, resulting in bladder calculi. Concurrent rectal lesions complicate the problem of bladder fistula, and in general the rectal defect should not be attempted until the bladder has been closed. It may be unwise to attempt correction of the two fistulae simultaneously, since the necessary tissue borrowing may lead to breakdown of the bladder repair (Lawson 1977). On the other hand, Hamlin and Nicholson (1986) stated that it was their usual practise in Addis Ababa to close vesico-vaginal and recto-vaginal fistulae at the one operation.

Scarring produced by repeated operations particularly near the bladder neck may result in a rigid, patulous internal urinary meatus densely adherent to bone, resulting in severe incontinence even should successful closure be achieved.

(iii) Methods Available for Surgical Correction

1. Cauterization.
2. Vaginal surgery.
3. Abdominal surgery—transvesical extraperitoneal,
                         —transvesical intraperitoneal.
4. Combined vaginal and abdominal surgery.
5. Colpocleisis.
6. Ureteric transplantation.
7. Unorthodox procedures.

Cauterization

Sims (1852) said: "Cauterization has but little to boast of in the way of success. Very small fistulous openings occasionally have been cured by application of the nitrate of silver, a catheter being retained in the bladder; but, in fistulas of any size, it has proved entirely abortive." Cauterization destroyed epithelial fusion between bladder and vagina allowing normal healing to occur, but unless the fistula was pin-hole in size, the method was unsatisfactory and tended to make the problem worse. When cautery failed, the outcome was greater tissue deficit with even more scarring.

Vaginal Surgery

This was the initial and sole surgical route employed in surgical attempts to correct bladder fistula until 1890 when Trendelenburg published attempts to repair vesico-vaginal fistula using a suprapubic approach. In all large series of obstetric fistulae from many countries, the vaginal approach has been the method of choice and for a variety of reasons. Undoubtedly this approach was safer for the patient and for future bladder function, and suturing through the vagina was more adequate since dissection could be wider, and firm union achieved with more perfect hemostasis. Using the proper technique and avoiding tearing bladder edges, postoperative bleeding with clot formation was virtually negligible (Foda 1959).

However it must be emphasized that a versatile approach to the surgery of fistula is vital, ultimate decisions depending upon fistula accessibility. Whenever a fistula can be reached through the vagina, this should be the preferred route; but some prefer an abdominal approach when the fistula is tethered high and there is difficulty making it accessible by pulling down the cervix or vaginal vault. Clearly the level of expertise of the vaginal surgeon plays a major role in choosing the approach. The vaginal route allows choice of lithotomy, left lateral and reverse Trendelenburg positions with various points in favor of each, and the vaginal approach particularly suits massive fistula with bladder prolapse since the prolapse is corrected in the knee-chest or reverse Trendelenburg positions and in lithotomy it can be reduced using a small bladder pack. Counsellor and Haigler (1956) gave many reasons favoring a vaginal approach; but particularly since most obstetric fistulae were vesico-vaginal and after mobilization the surgeon worked with the injured tissues in plain view. Also, convalescence following vaginal surgery was much shorter and less disabling. Ward (1986) with an experience of nearly 2,000 genito-urinary fistulae expressed the view that repair by a vaginal approach still was the most applicable technique and used by her in more than 1,300 patients.

If a vaginal approach is selected, two techniques are available to deal with the fistula. Saucerization, the method popularized and publicized by Sims, nevertheless had its beginnings in 1663 when the technique was described by van Roonhuyse. Later workers—Fatio (1675), Schreger (1817), Mettauer (1840), Hayward (1839) and Wützer (1852) used and embellished the technique which entailed excision of the scarred fistula margin; but involving only vaginal wall. The excision extended through the vaginal wall in a sloping fashion down to but excluding bladder mucosa, then the defect was closed with full-thickness sutures—differing slightly with each surgeon—which passed through the vaginal wall excluding bladder mucosa. The alternative method of layered repair although attributed to Mackenrodt (1894), had commenced at a much earlier date and extended by succeeding surgeons—Dupuytren (1829), Lamballe (1834), Hayward (1839) and Maisoneuve (1848). In this technique, bladder and vagina were separated, allowing sufficient mobility for the bladder defect to be closed without tension. Presently, the majority of vesico-vaginal fistulae are closed employing the method of layered repair—known also as flap-splitting or dedoublement.

Abdominal Surgery—the Transvesical Extraperioneal Approach

Miller (1935) stated that although interest in the suprapubic approach developed slowly, progress had been steady, and presently it ranked second in popularity. A gradual favoring of the approach was attributed to the fact that most fistulae occurring in the western world, followed surgical trauma particularly total hysterectomy, and frequently were much less accessible than those resulting from parturition. Another obvious reason for increased interest in the suprapubic route was the involvement of urologists more commonly than formerly. Kirwin and Lowsley (1935) reporting an unusual fistula complicated by bladder eversion and managed by a transvesical extraperitoneal approach, declared "vesico-vaginal fistula to be a urologic lesion" offering a challenge which the urologist had been slow to take up. In general, when the uterus still was present, the transvesical extraperitoneal route was preferred which allowed ureteric catheters to be passed under vision. If the uterus had been removed, the alternative approach was transvesical intraperitoneal, splitting the bladder in the midline down the level of the fistula.

Earlier doyens of fistula surgery such as Moir would have nothing to do with the transvesical approach, and indeed there has been prolonged argument—much of it unpleasant—about relative merits of gynecologists and urologists and their approach to the problem of vesico-vaginal fistula. Moir (1966) had nothing to say in favor of the transvesical approach. If the fistula could be closed transvesically, he was sure it could be repaired more easily and more certainly through the vagina. However he agreed the extraperitoneal route had a role on rare occasions (less than 5% of his cases) although technical difficulties would be encountered from scar tissue which fixed the fistula to the back of the pubic bone and rami; but generally this could be overcome by sharp dissection. Counsellor and Haigler (1956) agreed the abdominal approach probably was best when the fistula was very high with difficulty in exposure, and particularly should it be complicated by the presence of a recto-vaginal fistula. Nevertheless it was hard to rationalize going through the top of an organ to repair a hole in the bottom of it, and they made the point that the female bladder irritated by a suprapubic tube for any length of time, never was completely comfortable in the future. Stephen (1978) reported 78 difficult vesico-vaginal fistulae treated in Nepal and believed Chassar Moir's gloomy opinion about the transvesical approach probably was not wholly warranted; but judging by his many failures it seems his vaginal technique was not comparable to that of Chassar Moir. Really it is a truism to suggest the urologist being accustomed to opening the bladder prefers to attack a fistula from this angle, and Sargent (1955) suggested the woman with a vesico-vaginal fistula was lucky to be repaired at the hands of a urologist, since he didn't cause the fistula and therefore was not under any distracting embarrassment, also he was completely at home inside the bladder being familiar with both the anatomy and surgical principles involved. He advocated the extraperi-

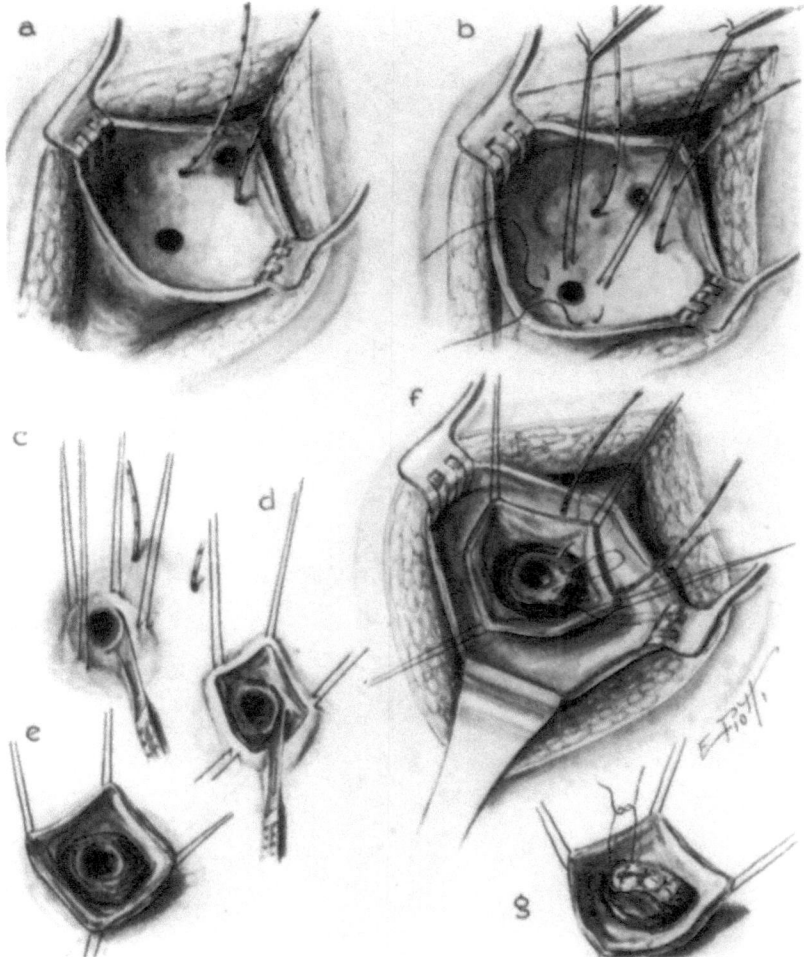

Figure 85. Cystotomy followed by elevation of the fistula with traction sutures, then free separation of bladder from vagina, and the vaginal defect closed. Note ureteric catheters. (From Phaneuf and Graves)

toneal procedure after packing the vagina with gauze and inserting retrograde catheters, then the bladder was opened, the tract excised completely and the healthy bladder mobilized widely. After wide excision of devitalized scar, and bladder closure, a peritoneal flap was interposed between bladder and vagina. Phaneuf and Graves (1949) advocated intravesical closure for the high fistula difficult of access by the vaginal route. they emphasized wide   mobilization   of   the   bladder   particularly   laterally

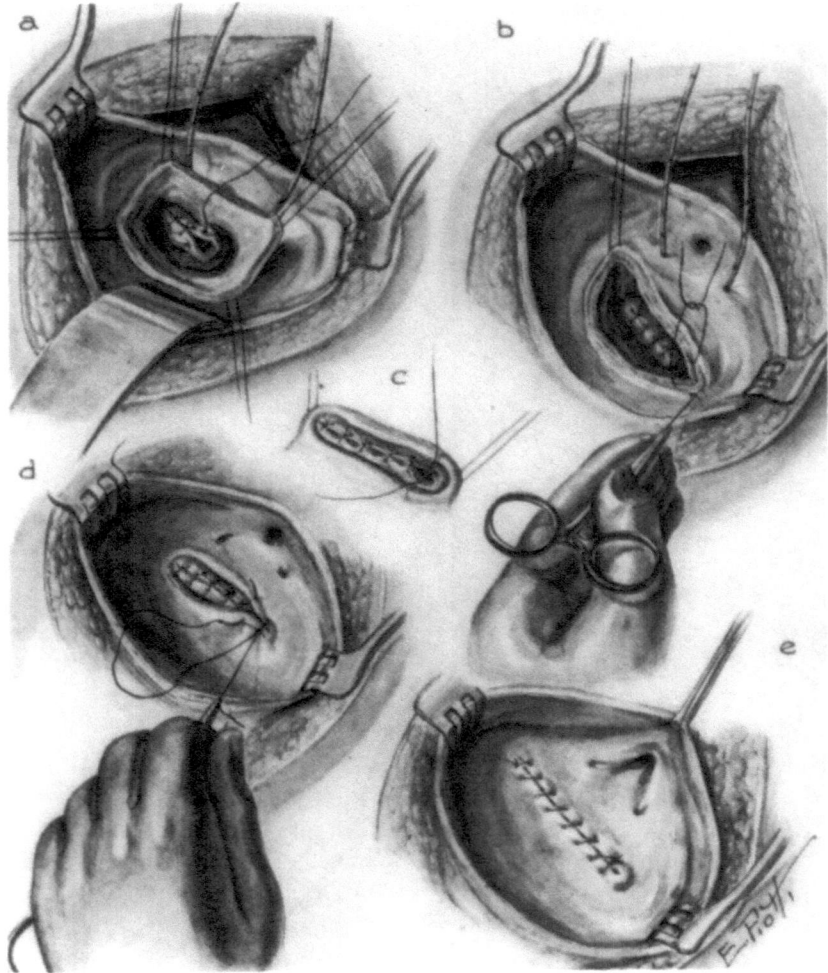

Figure 86. The vaginal defect closed by a second layer of sutures, and then bladder wall also closed in two layers. (From Phaneuf and Graves)

prior to opening, then ureteric catheters were passed and careful note made of the position of the internal urethral meatus. Placing traction sutures about the fistula, the fistula margin was incised around the circumference, and bladder and vagina separated widely. Following vaginal and then bladder closure, a suprapubic mushroom catheter was employed for bladder drainage (Figs. 85, 86).

Transvesical Intraperitoneal Approach

This route, suggested originally by von Dittel (1893) allowed wide separation of bladder from vagina at the site of the fistula, enabling each defect to be closed separately. In 1914 the route was revived by Legueu who reported success in 1929 with 24 patients. With the patient in extreme Trendelenburg position, an incision in the median line extended through the posterior wall of bladder and vaginal vault, exposing both fistulous openings. In a majority of patients since the fistula was midline, the openings were exposed by this incision. The bladder and vagina were separated by sharp dissection until both openings were isolated completely, the bladder mobilized on all sides at a distance from the fistula, then both bladder and vaginal openings were closed with interrupted catgut sutures, keeping the suture lines of each as far apart as possible and the peritoneal edges were approximated with fine catgut. The importance of postoperative bladder drainage was emphasized. This technique combined the procedures of Trendelenburg and von Dittel. Dorsey (1960) reported 17 cases cured by this one operation and believed it was applicable to the high fistula which lay in a narrow, fixed vaginal vault, since attempts to mobilize the bladder from the vagina without entering the peritoneal cavity were extremely difficult. The advantage of a bladder incision right down to the fistula meant an excellent and continuing view of ureters, fistula, trigone and bladder neck was obtained (Figs. 87 a–d). Mack (1966) emphasized the relative ease of a transvesical approach compared to difficulties of access encountered with the transabdominal approach. Bladder separation could begin well out in healthy tissues, then carried towards the fistula once a clear line of demarcation between vagina and bladder had been demonstrated. Usually it was possible to raise an ample healthy bladder flap with a good bood supply even if a vaginal flap was more difficult to obtain. Transvesical surgery minimized ureteric damage as the orifices were visible throughout, nevertheless it was most important to be certain the orifices were not near the fistula edge, since they could be at risk when raising flaps or at fistula closure, and required preliminary reimplantation to a higher level.

Linke et al. (1971) Rhodesia reporting on large obstetric fistula advocated this approach. Ureteric catheters were inserted and a full-thickness flap of posterior bladder wall above the fistula area was fashioned to rotate into the trigonal defect and after extensive mobilization of the anterior vaginal wall to separate bladder and vagina, transverse closure of the anterior vaginal wall was effected without tension. It was then possible to

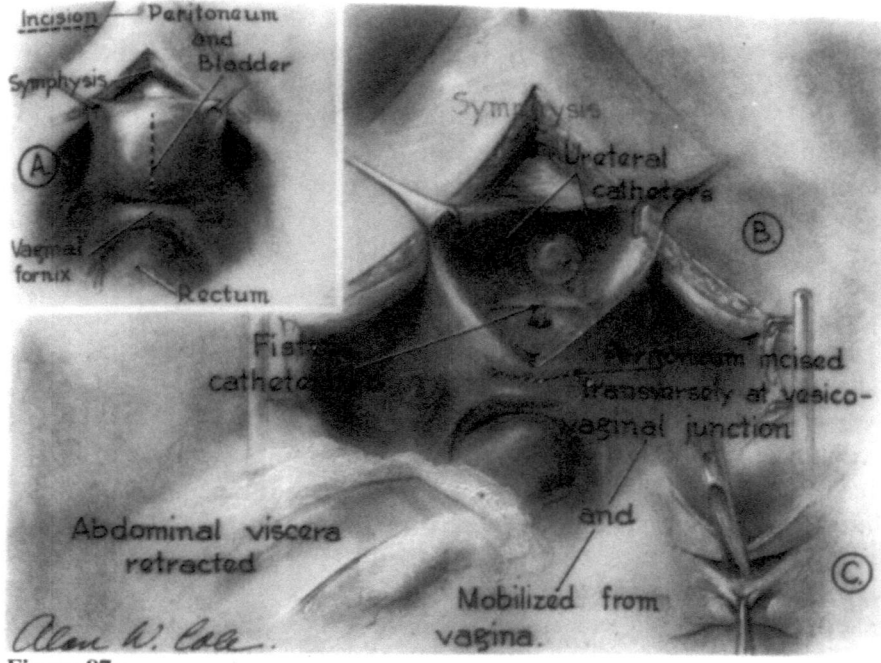

Figure 87 a

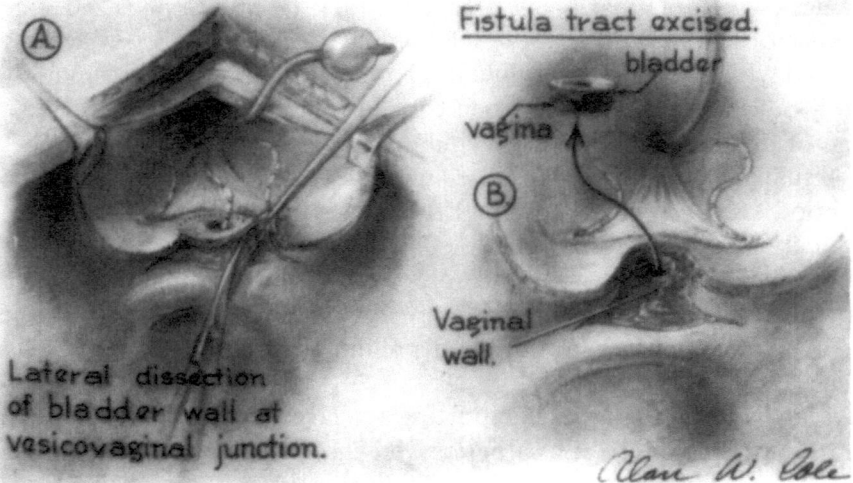

Figure 87 b

Figures 87 a, b. Elevated bladder incised in the midline exposing the fistula, then catheter placed. Mobilization of bladder from vagina with excision of fistula track

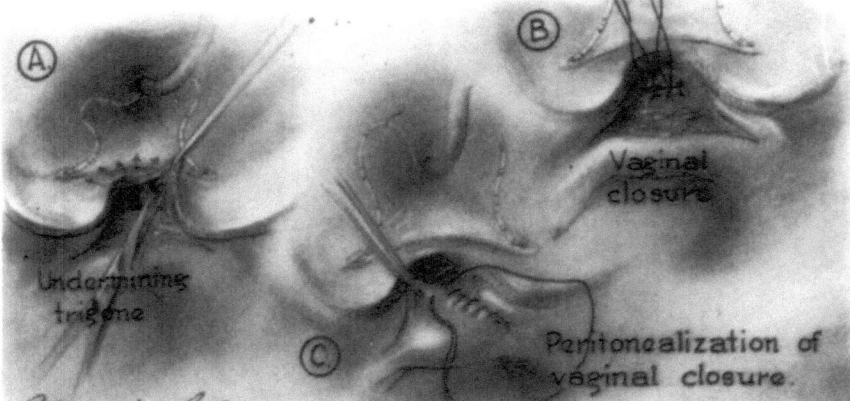

Figure 87 c

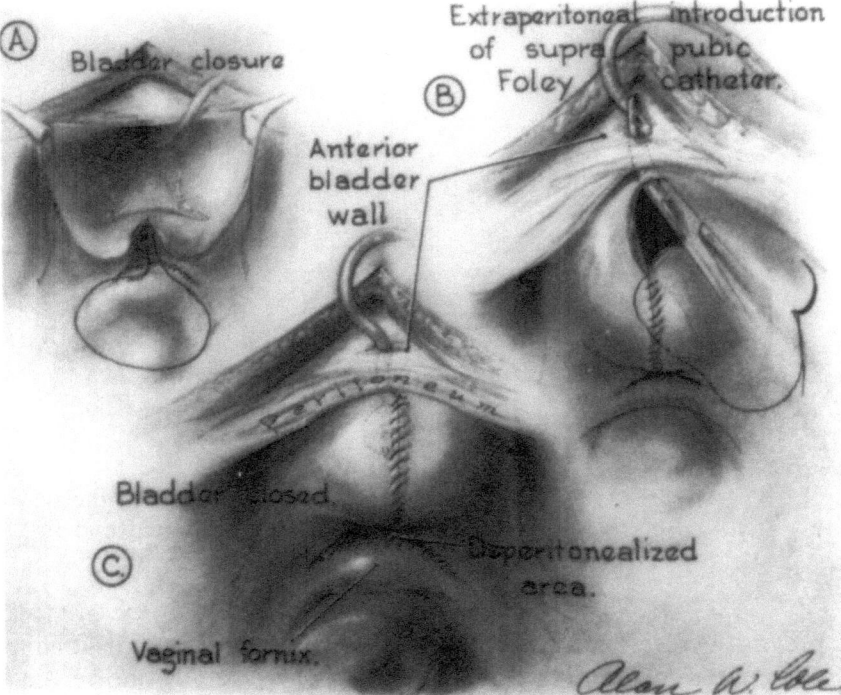

Figure 87 d

Figures 87 c, d. Vaginal defect closed and covered with peritoneum followed by closure of the bladder defect. (From Dorsey)

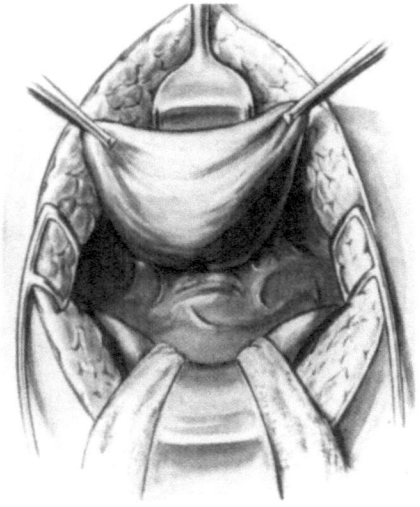

Figure 88 a. Extraperitoneal wide bladder mobilization

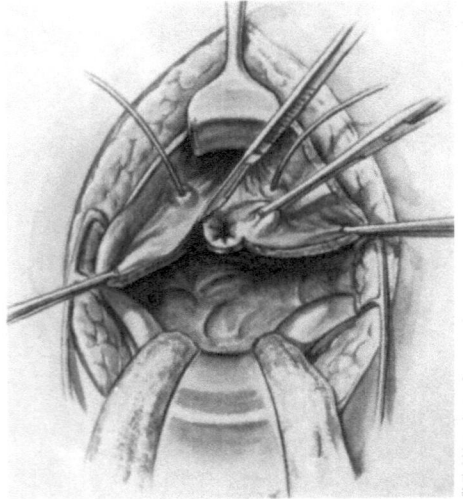

Figure 88 b. Bladder bisected to the fistula, ureteric catheters inserted and fistula track excised. (From O'Conor)

rotate the previously fashioned posterior bladder wall flap into the trigonal defect. A suprapubic tube remained in situ for two weeks. O'Conor et al. (1973) advocated suprapubic closure of vesico-vaginal fistula as the ideal technique, whether performed extraperitoneally or transperitoneally. The key step bisected the bladder to the fistula, then wide bladder and vaginal mobilization permitted tension-free closure. Stay sutures placed every few centimeters on either side of the incision allowed bladder wall elevation, improving exposure considerably. The fistula track was excised completely and the bladder mobilized widely from the vagina, then after vaginal closure, the suture line was reinforced by a fat or peritoneal graft. Bladder closure began at the apex of the incision, using a continuous suture including all muscle layers. Usually splinting ureteric catheters were inserted to minimize risk of injury or damage, and bladder drainage was effected by suprapubic catheter with occasionally a urethral Foley catheter (Figs. 88 a, b). The urethral catheter was removed on the fourth or fifth day, and the suprapubic on the 14th; but should suprapubic drainage persist for more than 24 hours, the urethral catheter was reinserted. Ward (1980) performed transvesical closure on 251 occasions in a series of 1789 fistulae, selecting this approach for the inaccessible vesico-vaginal fistula or the vesico-uterine fistula. More recently (1985) at University Hospital, Khartoum, transvesical intraperitoneal closure was witnessed, the technical problems encountered were many and included difficulty of access with a very low fistula, scarring from previous Cesarian sections, and most importantly a flimsy posterior bladder wall, inevitable with a very large fistula. As a preliminary, the Foley catheter and two ureteric catheters were passed into the bladder, then at laparotomy following division of the vesico-uterine peritoneum, bladder and genital tract were separated to the fistula. The bladder was opened in the midline, the ureteric orifices identified and catheterized, using indigo carmine for any identification problems. The bladder defect was closed knowing the ureters were safe, then the vagina, and an omental graft was fashioned and placed across the front of the uterus and sutured to the site of bladder wall closure. The procedure was eminently suited to high vault fistulae difficult to reach from the vagina in females in whom the uterus was present and needed to be retained; but with lower fistulae near the bladder neck, access was difficult and uncertain.

Combined Abdomino-Vaginal Approach

Roen (1960) stated many standard techniques of fistula repair failed, leading to greater difficulties at subsequent procedures; but a combined abdominal and vaginal approach virtually assured fistula closure at the first attempt. Beginning with a vaginal approach, the patient was positioned in extreme lithotomy and guy sutures inserted for traction on the fistula, then the bladder and vagina were mobilized adequately. A layer of tissue under the vaginal wall was approximated with "00" C.C.G. similar to the method of closure employed with the saucerization technique, then the vaginal epithelium was closed. Placed in the supine position, the bladder was distended

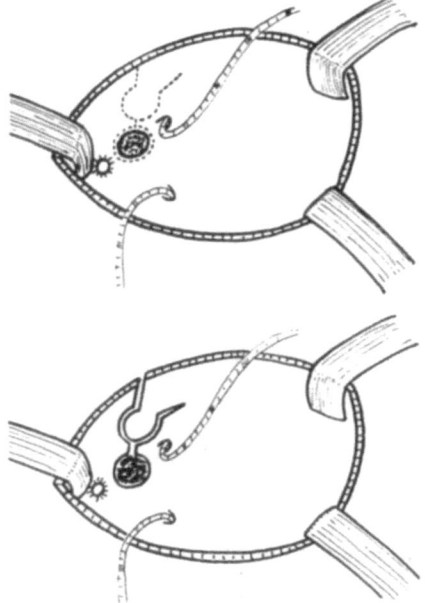

Figure 89 a. Flap raised from the lateral bladder wall to fit the trigonal defect after fistula excision

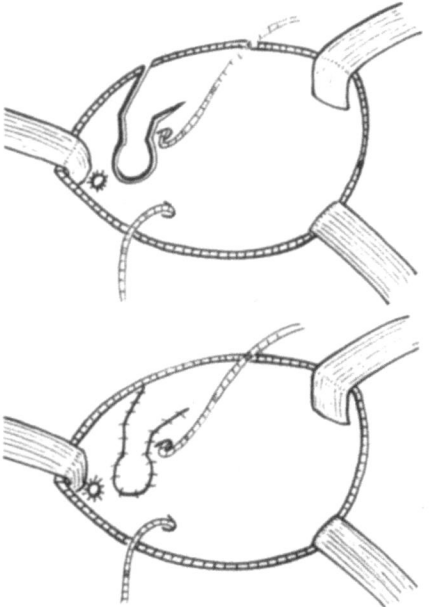

Figure 89 b. Bladder flap advanced to fill the defect

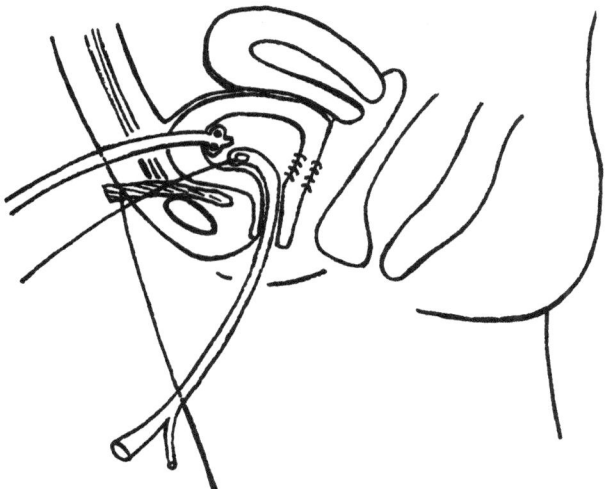

Figure 89c. Bladder drainage by suprapubic and urethral catheters with the tip of the urethral catheter suspended to avoid pressure on the repair. (From Su)

with a self-retaining ballon catheter to aid ready identification, then the bladder was opened. The fistula edges were excised, the bladder wall undermined for a short distance, and the bladder wall defect closed in two layers—muscular and mucosal. A suprapubic cystostomy tube drained the bladder, and the patient was nursed face downward for dependant bladder drainage on a split mattress for 10 days. Weyrauch and Rous (1966) used the combined technique in difficult instances when unsuccessful attempts had left a mass of chronically infected scar tissue surrounding a persistent fistula. After mobilizing the bladder apparently adequately at the vaginal approach, later during the transvesical stage of the procedure, the limited separation between bladder and vagina could be appreciated. A Foley bag of appropriate size was passed through the fistula and inflated, enabling the fistulous area to be drawn down to the surgeon. The fistulous tract was excised, and a wide area of adjacent vaginal wall mobilized from the bladder. Extraperitoneal entry into the bladder was effected, the Foley catheter was changed around enabling the bladder to be elevated and the bladder side of the fistulous tract divided at right angles to the vaginal incision, to avoid overlapping the future suture lines and both defects were closed. They advised removal of vaginal sutures at about ten days so the epithelium had no opportunity of growing along the suture lines and perhaps producing persisting pin-point fistulae. Su (1969) in addition to the combined approach, advocated raising a flap with a rounded tip from the lateral bladder wall which was advanced towards the trigone, the tip fitting the defect (Figs. 89 a–c). Clark and Holland (1975) suggested proper indications for the combined approach were very large fistulae unsuitable for vaginal closure, failed repair in patients with massive scar tissue around the fistula, fistula close to or involving a ureter, difficult vaginal access and if other urological or abdominal surgery was required. Taylor et al. (1980) reported nine large vault fistulae healed successfully by synchronous combined transvaginal-transvesical repair and regarded it as the technique of choice for large postoperative fistulae because of the advantages it conferred. Tissue positioning for accurate closure was enhanced and omental or muscle grafting and ureteric reimplantation away from the fistula edge could be added to the procedure.

Colpocleisis

Sims (1852) referred in contemptuous terms to the operation of Vidal for an "obturation of the vulva" whereby bladder and vagina became a giant compound receptacle for urine and menstrual secretion. He said it was an idle waste of time to dwell longer on means so perfectly ineffectual, not to say mischievious. Simon (1856) used high transverse obliteration of the vagina, and although opposition to colpocleisis was voiced during the later years of the 19th century, its elimination did not occur until Coffey made his great contribution to ureteric transplantation. Simon practised circular denudation of the vagina "at a place situated next to the defect" then sutured the wound surfaces by means of sagittally applied stitches—a transverse closure. The inevitable diverticulum formed was small and the lower vagina remained functional. The method was simple yet effective since the suture line was free of tension. Simon performed the operation 12 times with 12 cures. Whilst we may look with intolerance upon the operation today, it should be remembered that once this operation gave great benefit to women with an incurable fistula. Using this procedure, Blaikley (1965) safely closed some very difficult fistulae with minimal discomfort for the patient. He described one 3 cm defect with hard scar tissue about it, and continuous with a large defect in the posterior wall of the urethra. Two flaps of vaginal skin hinged at the lateral margin of the fistula were rotated through 180° facing the bladder and sutured in the midline filling the large opening. All remaining vaginal skin was removed as a sleeve and the vagina obliterated completely beneath this repair. The patient was continent at night; but occasionally damp during the day. In a further case, Blaikley used the posterior vaginal wall to close the bladder defect making a transverse incision across the posterior wall opposite the lower margin of the fistula, then removed all the vaginal skin below it is a sleeve. Suturing the lower end of the remaining skin to the lower margin of the fistula, the bladder neck and upper urethra were reconstructed over an indwelling catheter, and the lower vagina obliterated by bringing the levator ani muscles together. He reported seven patients in whom colpocleisis had been used for a double fistula, the upper vagina remaining as a passage between bladder and rectum, a point of great importance being that the lower limit of the rectal fistula should be below that of the bladder and if necessary, the rectal fistula was enlarged downward as a preliminary step. Postoperatively, urine was voided by the urethra and anus; but normally feces was not passed by the urethra. All the skin from the remaining vagina was removed as a sleeve, but two small flaps back and front were preserved, turned upwards and sutured together to bridge the floor of the channel connecting bladder and rectum.

Transplantation of Ureters

Lawson (1978) stated diversion of the urinary stream seldom was necessary and should be regarded as a confession of defeat, to be undertaken only when the most experienced operator available could not achieve continence with a reconstructive procedure. The most important indication was total destruction of urethra and bladder neck, with no viable tissue available for reconstruction. In such cases the bladder opened directly into the vagina, the back of the symphysis was bare, covered only by a thin bloodless sheet of scar tissue from which reconstruction of a urethral tube controlled by an effective sphincter was impracticable. The level of continence attainable after successful fistula closure using a gracilis muscle graft was difficult to assess. Foda (1959) performed ureteric transplantation in 16 of 220 patients with urinary fistulae and in ten it was the only possible treatment whilst in others, one or two trials of vaginal surgery had convinced him of the probable ineffectiveness of further attempts. Humphries (1961) noted an extraordinary improvement in the physical and mental state of African patients following ureteric transplantation, transforming them from outcasts to becoming socially acceptable. Major contraindication to the procedure were an irreparable recto-vaginal fistula and loss of tone or incontinence of the anal sphincter. In the series reported by Foda, three associated recto-vaginal fistulae were corrected satisfactorily two months following transplantation. In the series of 1,789 cases treated by Ward (1980) 26 ureteric transplantations were performed although in a majority, fistula closure had been successful but did not achieve urinary control. Lawson (1977) reported 30 diversions in 377 patients, but commented that increasing experience made the need for diversion less frequent.

Unorthodox Approaches

Freund (1895) succeeded in closing two large vesico-vaginal fistulae utilizing the body of the inverted uterus delivered through the posterior fornix into the vagina, and then stitched to the anterior vaginal wall. Dudley, Chicago (1886) closed a large intractable fistula making a semi-circular denudation on the inner surface of the bladder extending from one fistula margin around to the other, then attached the denuded surface to the anterior part of the fistula, and Kelly (1896) closed a very large fistula in the following fashion: A crescentic incision was made around the posterior two thirds of the fistula facilitating wide bladder separation from the vagina and then by blunt dissection, the bladder was detached from the cervix up to the peritoneum and widely on both sides. The ureters were catheterized. A strip was removed around the remaining one third of the fistula on the vaginal surface down to the mucosa of the bladder and urethra, then that part of the bladder freed from its attachments behind was drawn forwards, and applied accurately to the immovable anterior one third. Each suture caught the under surface of the muscular coat of the bladder, turning the cut edge up towards the newly formed bladder, and in the same fashion the urethral orifices fixed at this edge were turned into the bladder. Macalpine (1940) described an ingenious method utilizing the upper vagina to form a bladder extension and so close the fistula. The procedure divided

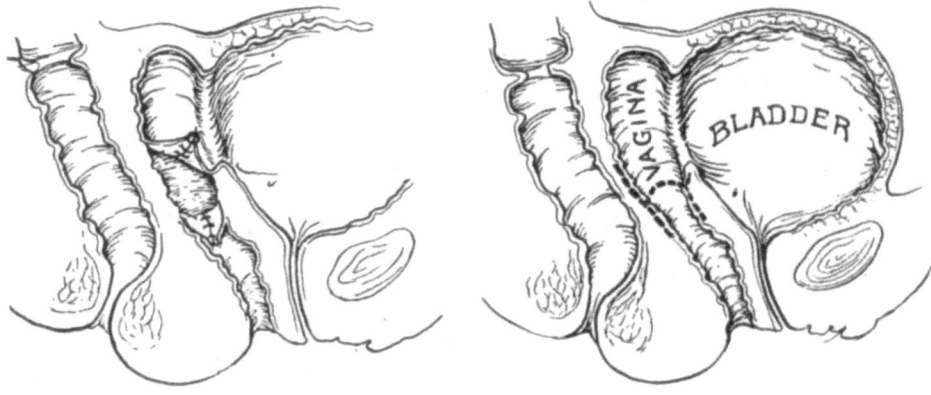

Figure 90 a   **Figure 90 b**

Figure 90

a Large vesico-vaginal fistula with the line of the flap indicated

b Flaps lifted and sutured. (From Macalpine)

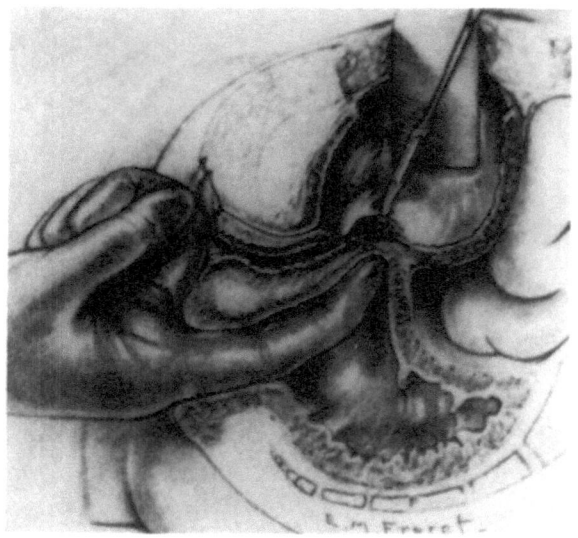

Figure 91. The posterior vaginal wall pushed against the fistula to outline the disc. (From Marshall)

the vagina across, the line of section lying about 2 mm below the lower fistula lip and it began on the posterior wall which was steadied and elevated by transfixion sutures (Fig. 90 a). When the anterior wall was reached, the fistula margin was drawn forward directing the incision behind and below the edge of the opening. All vaginal coats were divided, the edges above and below the incision were undermined and elevated for a third of an inch, and both vaginal sections were sutured to close off the fistula above, and create a new vaginal vault below (Fig. 90 b). Macalpine believed vaginal mucosa stayed healthy even when continuously sodden with urine. Twombly and Marshall (1946) devised a technique for difficult vesico-vaginal fistula in which a button of posterior vaginal wall epithelium was cut to fit the defect in the anterior vaginal wall. Opening the bladder and exposing the fistula, the bladder and anterior vaginal wall were mobilized then the assistant, with a finger in the rectum, pushed the posterior vaginal wall into the defect allowing a pattern of the defect to be cut through the bladder (Fig. 91). The posterior vaginal wall disc was sutured to bladder mucosa and the surrounding vaginal wall to the mobilized anterior vaginal wall, resulting in partial colpocleisis. Marshall (1979) reported success with 24 of 27 patients.

Greenslade (1969) successfully closed a low vesico-vaginal fistula after three failures of orthodox methods. Essentially he employed an orthodox bladder wall closure in layers; but supported by a wide pad of posterior

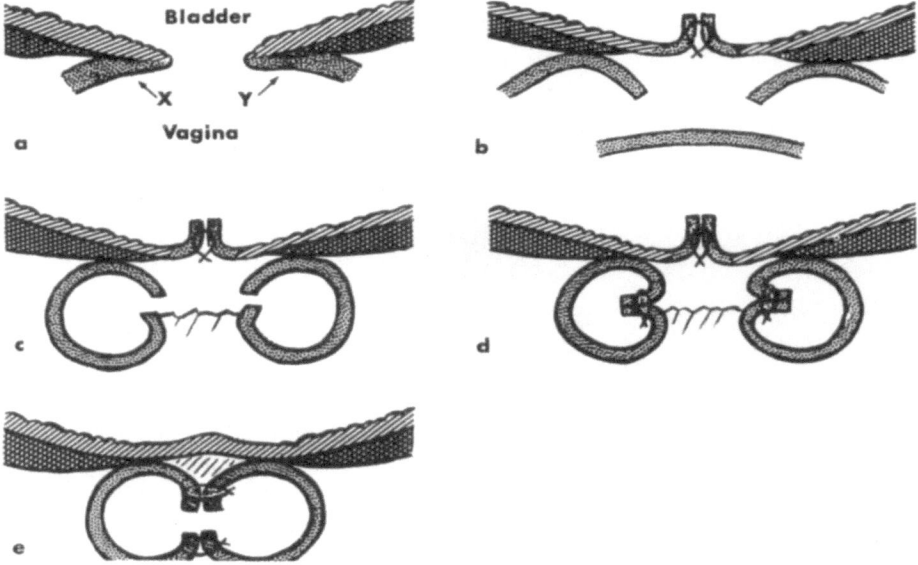

Figures 92

a, b The anterior vaginal wall around the fistula incised at (X) and (Y) then inverted to close the bladder defect

c, d Midline incision in the posterior vaginal wall, then anterior and posterior walls united to produce a median septum

e Vaginal septum divided. (From Greensade

vaginal wall brought up to the anterior wall as a median septum similar to the Le Fort colpocleisis. The mucosa of the anterior vaginal wall surrounding the fistula was incised and inverted closing the defect, then the posterior vaginal wall incised in the midline and the edges of the anterior and posterior vaginal walls united on either side to from a median septum. Three months later, the vaginal septum was divided well posteriorly, to leave a firm tissue pad supporting the fistula repair and reconstitute the vaginal canal (Fig. 92 a–e). This simple two stage repair brought a fresh pad of non-tense tissue with a new blood supply from the posterior vaginal wall and avoided superimposed suture lines.

(iv) Choice of Surgical Approach

A majority or either simple of difficult urinary fistulae can be managed using a transvaginal approach. Selecting the abdominal approach for such fistulae reflects the skill, experience and preference of the surgeon, and those with wide experience with the surgery of obstetric fistulae usually select a vaginal approach. Chassar Moir (1966) valued this route so highly "that I no longer regard any vesico-vaginal fistula as incurable. We need neither colpocleisis as a makeshift treatment nor laparotomy as a means to cure the fistula—a means that serves that serves its purpose well but does endanger the patient's life. The vaginal method as described by me is the natural way of operating on vesico-vaginal fistulas, combining a successful outcome with a riskless performance."

Principles of Vaginal Closure

Fistula surgery is difficult and demanding and success will be gained only by meticulous attention to detail, for the tissues are scarred with a poor blood supply leading to slow healing in addition to tissue loss of greater or less degree. For these reasons, the best chance of surgical success is at the first attempt, so everything related to the surgery must be right or made as right as conditions permit. Nothing must be withheld at this first attempt and every principle of diagnosis, preoperative, intra-operative and post-operative care must be observed—these principles laid down so long ago by many surgeons of world renown have survived the great test of time, so meddling with them or attempting to circumvent them usually brings its own penalty. Slavish devotion to detail is not required; but an intelligent appreciation of the many important details, most certainly is. One could draw an analogy between difficulties of fistula surgery and winning the America's Cup by the 12-meter yacht, Australia II captained by John Bertrand. That goal was achieved by the captain, crew and ancilliary team giving "their best shot" in each race, and that same attitude is what makes for success in fistula surgery so nothing that will help favor success, can or should be omitted. Despite the best care failures will occur still, for the nature of the tissues precludes 100% success; but the greater the attention to detail, the more likely the success, and those great characteristics displayed by James Marion Sims—persistence, tenacity and humility—still are a necessary part of the make-up of the fistula surgeon today.

1. Immediate Preoperative Requirements

The time chosen for intervention should be well away from the menstrual period—a point made first by Atlee (1860)—for the tissues become unduly vascular and engorged near this time, making dissection more difficult. Should the patient be menstruating when admitted to hospital, then surgery

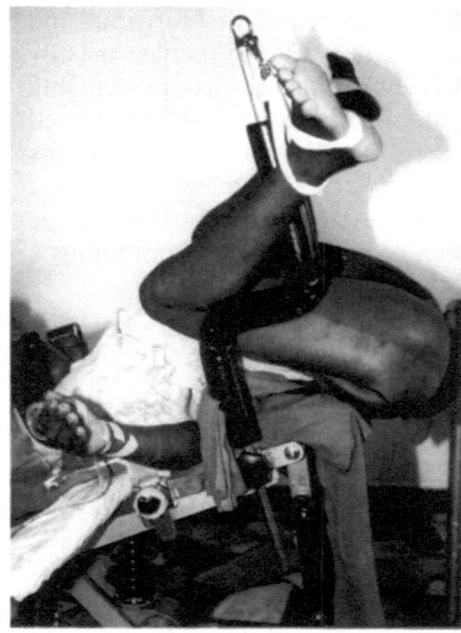

Figure 93 a. Exaggerated lithotomy position and Trendelenburg tilt with the buttocks protruding. (Courtesy Fistula Hospital, Addis Ababa)

should be deferred. For similar reasons, the oral contraceptive pill should cease several weeks before surgery. Blood group and hemoglobin should be known and blood must be available for replacement in patients requiring extensive surgery with grafting.

2. Adequate Exposure

(a) Anesthesia. Depending on availability, either low spinal or general anesthesia is suitable.

(b) Position on the operating table. A majority of surgeons favor an exaggerated lithotomy position for all bladder fistula surgery; but some prefer the reverse Trendelenburg (prone or knee-elbow or knee-chest) position (Figs. 93 a, b). Barnes and Martin (1949) used the prone position for all patients, preferring the fistula on the floor of the operating field rather than the roof. Others (Lawson 1978, Ward 1985) use the position with all bladder neck fistulae, and with all high and relatively inaccessible fistulae. Kelly (1986) in a series of 406 fistulae, employed the postition on 15 occasions only. The exaggerated lithotomy position implies that the patient's buttocks protrude over the end of the operating table, with enough Trendelenburg tilt employed to make the anterior vaginal wall perpendic-

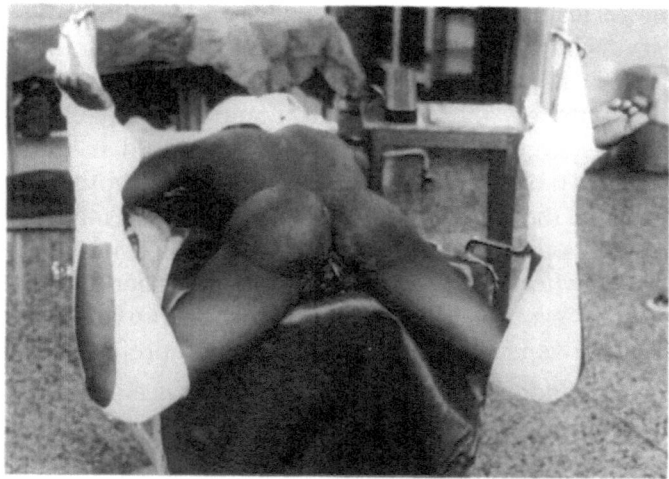

Figure 93 b. Reverse Trendelenburg position

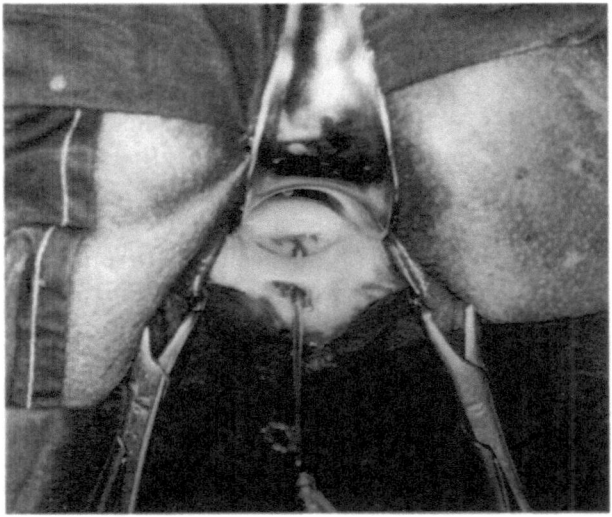

Figure 93 c. The fistula on the floor of the operating field using the prone position. Sound is seen in the urethra passing through the fistula. (Courtesy Ann Ward, St. Luke's Hospital, Nigeria)

ular to the surgeon's line of vision. Gynecologists are used to lithotomy position for vaginal surgery which is a distinct advantage, rather than the unfamiliarity of the knee-elbow position where the anatomy is "upside down" (Fig. 93 c); but undoubtedly the adjustment would come quickly with experience. Bladder inversion with a large fistula is reduced in the knee-elbow position; but it may be reduced by a small pack in lithotomy position, until mobilization of the bladder has been completed. Finally, bleeding during surgery runs away from the site of dissection with the patient in lithotomy position, whereas it accumulates in the bladder in the knee-elbow position. In either case, suction will keep the operative field clear, so the choice of position depends really upon individual preference.

(c) A properly focused and adequately bright theatre light is essential, many surgeons employing both a head lamp and magnifying operating glasses for enhanced clarity of the limited operative field.

(d) Vaginal access—a variety of speculums are necessary depending upon the degree of stenosis and include the Auvard self-retaining speculum, small and large Sims speculum and a range of Deaver speculums. Vaginal access may be improved by episiotomy; but with gross degrees of scarring, the Schuchardt incision or modification may be necessary.

(e) The labia are stitched back with "00" silk, and when feasible the fistula should be drawn towards the vaginal introitus, using four guy sutures of "00" chromic catgut inserted about the periphery of the fistula (Fig. 94); but in so many large obstetric fistulae, scarring and adhesion inhibit vaginal mobility in varying degrees. Judd (1920) used a small curved hemostat passed through the urethra and into the vagina through the fistula to depress it and aid exposure of the fistula for commencement of dissection. Taylor et al. (1967) passed a Foley catheter from the vagina into the bladder through the fistula and when inflated it provided an excellent instrument for traction and exposure. The idea originated with Falk and Kurman (1963).

(f) Proper instruments. Essentials include a range of sharp pointed scissors and fine-toothed dissecting forceps of adequate lenght so the surgeon's hand does not obscure the surgical field, a long-handled Bard Parker scalpel with no. 11 blades, fine Allis forceps and skin hooks, a small neurosurgical sucker, and a range of fine needle-holders together with "00" chromic catgut and "00" nylon sutures on small curved strong needles. An ideal suture of "00" CCG with an especially strong curved needle is made by Ethicon, Scotland (serial number W 565) and is recommended.

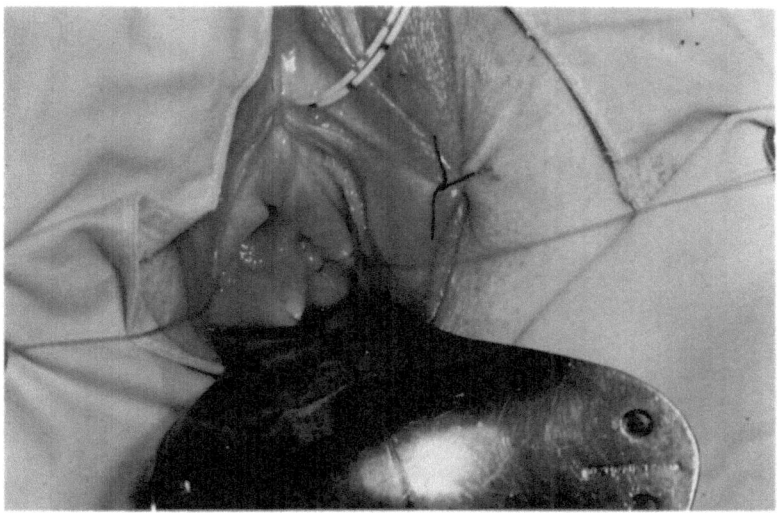

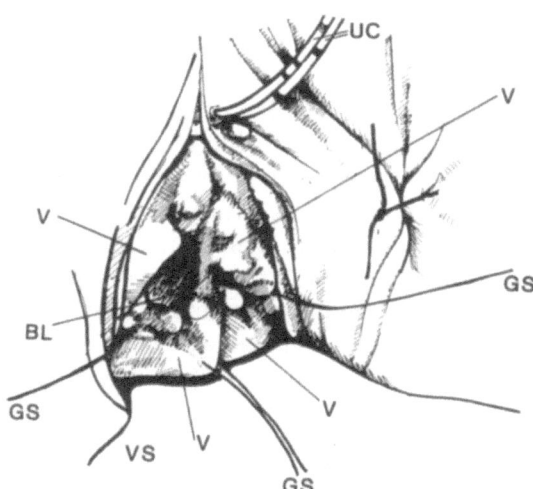

Figure 94. Labia stitched back and guy sutures exerting traction

3. Assessment Under Anesthesia.

All preoperative impressions should be confirmed and if necessary ureteric catheters passed.

4. Mobilization

The primary object of mobilization is to free bladder from the vaginal wall, and flap-splitting is the standard procedure. Steadying the fistula with either

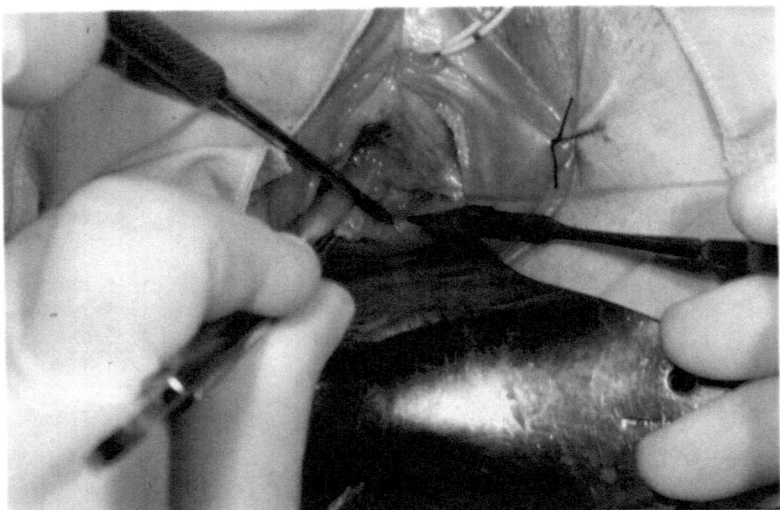

Figure 95 a. Mobilization using dissectors, no. 11 blade and sucker

guy sutures, Allis forceps or transfixion with the point of no. 11 scalpel blade, the junctional zone between bladder and vagina is incised, beginning where access is easiest. The freed vaginal skin edge is held by Allis or long-toothed forceps and incision of the junctional zone continued. Once the circular incision is complete, extensions of 1–2 cm are made anteriorly and posteriorly at 6 o'clock and 12 o'clock through the full thickness of vaginal wall. The judicious use of suction enhances speed and accuracy, and progressive undercutting to free bladder from vagina is achieved using the 11 blade and sharp scissors. The blade steadies the tissue whilst long-toothed forceps pick it up, then the knife divides it. Ultimately mobilization must be sufficient to allow bladder closure without tension, for tension means failure so larger defects require most extensive mobilization (Figs. 95 a, b). Chassar Moir (1961) and Lawson (1967) warned against excessive dissection because of possible interference with blood supply in the vaginal flaps, so flap-splitting should be adequate rather than excessive. Special attention must be directed to lateral extensions of the fistula, particularly bony adhesion at the ischio-pubic rami. All such attachments must be freed, using sharp scissors aided by palpation and finger pressure between bladder and vagina. The finger detects ridges of scar tissue and areas of adhesion which need division, so the next scissor cut can be directed with accuracy. Clegg (1979) Rhodesia, favored finger palpation to identify fibrous strands

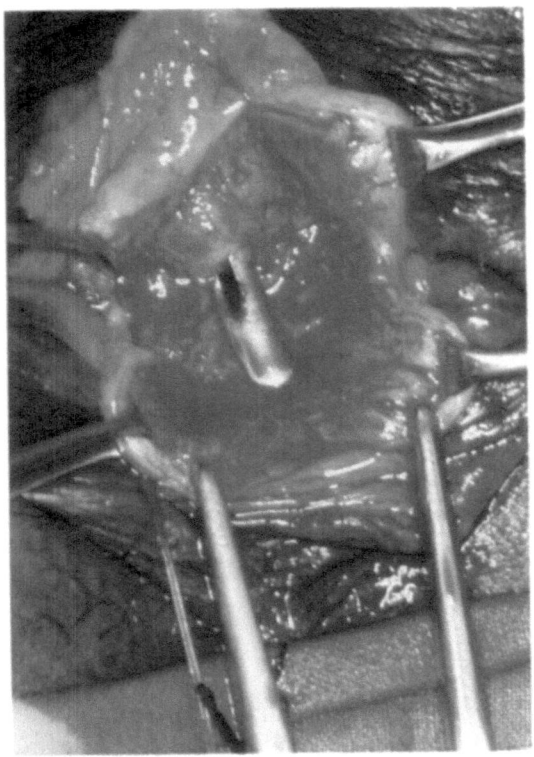

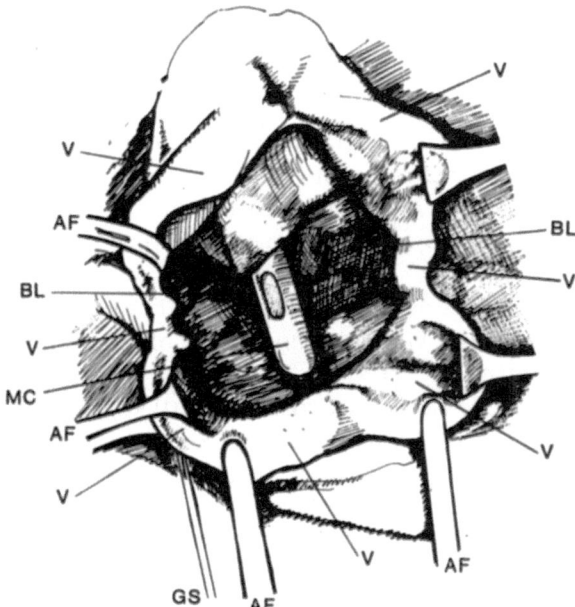

Figure 95 b. Mobilization completed with a small fistula

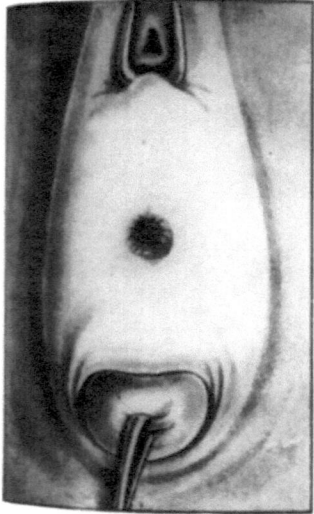 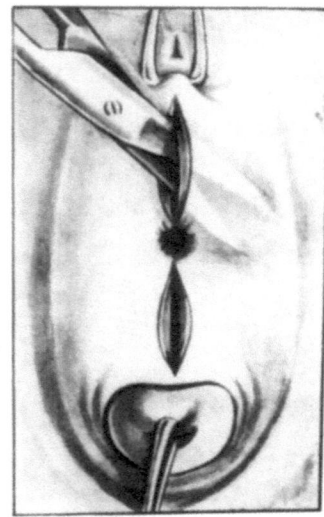

Figure 96. The incisions made, the scissors separate bladder from vagina. (From Benion Thomas)

requiring division, and digital dissection to extend further the exposed cleavage plane. Great care is necessary when the fistula involves partial urethral loss, since the tissues are more flimsy, and dissecting vaginal wall from underlying urethra must proceed with caution, aided by a catheter in the urethra. Bladder eversion can be restrained by the assistant or use of small bladder pack until mobilization is complete. Once cicatricial scar has been freed and adequate mobilization effected, the bladder defect contracts becoming smaller than it appeared previously. Even with proper mobilization, single layer closure usually is all that can be expected with large fistulae; but double layer over-lapping closure is the ideal to be attained with smaller defects.

The more usual method of flap-splitting commences at the fistula edge by separating the junction of bladder and vagina, then freeing bladder and vagina in all directions away from the fistula.

Benion Thomas (1945) quoting Crossen and Crossen (1930) suggested alternative methods of flap splitting, one which proceeded from the margin of the fistula towards healthy tissue and the other from healthy tissue toward the fistula, and although not much mention was made of the latter method and it was used infrequently, it seemed the more sound technique. It can be difficult to find a plane of cleavage between vaginal wall and bladder and searching for it through scar tissue at the fistula margin can be a problem, and it is easier to find it at a place remote from the fistula. An incision was made from below upward to the fistula, through vaginal skin and then from the fistula toward the cervix. The depth of incision was the same as for colporrhaphy and the points of Mayo scissors curved on the flat thrust into the fascial space between the bladder and vagina, easily separated the two by opening and closing the scissor blades (Fig. 96). Finally, bladder and vagina were held only by the adherent fistula margins, and the next step cut through the fistula margin cleanly with a sharp knife and released the bladder. The method left a clean-cut orifice in the bladder, much more fit for suturing than the usual lacerated edge.

5. Excision of Scar Tissue

This separate heading is included to emphasize the point, that scar excision is never—repeat never—necessary. This step, emphasized in many gyne-cological textbooks, has been copied it seems from one publication to another; but never from the pen of an experienced fistula surgeon. Admittedly, there is some controversy on the point; but the Hamlins dealing with over 10,000 genital fistulae, teach that excision of bladder scar tissue only makes the present tissue deficit even greater, leading to a more difficult and hazardous closure, and in addition creats unnecessary bleeding which hinders closure and allows the bladder to fill with blood. One need only review the pathological process involved in the appearance and subsequent course of a fistula, to appreciate that the bladder wall for some distance around a fistula is infiltrated heavily with scar tissues with an associated decreased blood supply, so clearly, further excision at the fistula edge can remove only a small area of affected bladder wall. Such remarks carry added weight when dealing with a radio-necrotic fistula. McCall and Bolten (1957) stated categorically that, "at no time must tissue be removed and every fistula operation must be planned to use all available tissue. Surgery should not add to the deficiency, and indeed some fistulae became incurable because too much tissue was removed at preceding operations". Hadley et al. (1984) said success with closure was possible without excising a fis-tulous tract and in addition to this being unncessary, excision caused ex-cessive bleeding, damage to either or both ureters and made a small fistula large with increased difficulty of closure. Foda (1959) in a large series of fistula repairs commented that, "during a vaginal approach I found paring of the fistula edges to be harmful, since it results in a wider opening should the first attempt fail, thus reducing the chances of final cure. The unpared edges do not in the least interfere with proper healing, and on the contrary, bleeding from the edges may be a menace during and after the operation. The unpared edge provides a point d'appui for adequate suturing."

6. Care of the Ureters

Ojo (1967) stated a common reason for damage to ureters in Nigeria was ligation during vesico-vaginal fistula closure. Although a majority of fistulae were midvaginal or juxtaurethral, well clear of the bladder trigone and repair carried little or no chance of ureteric injury, nevertheless many fistulae were high juxta-cervical or vesico-cervical involving bladder trigone, therefore the ureters were exposed to risk. With excessive scarring and poor access, localizing the ureteric orifices was difficult, and he concluded catheterization was imperative in such patients. One must go further and declare that whenever there is any likelihood of ureteric involvement, either during bladder mobilization or bladder closure, the ureters must be catheterized.

With small fistulae, when preoperative investigations have demonstrated the ureteric orifices well clear of the defect, catheterization is unnecessary; but with a small surgically-produced vault fistula, even though a retro-trigonal position of the fistula tract is usual, with any encroachment onto the ureteric orifice area, preoperative catheterization is essential. Most obstetric fistulae are large or very large and the likelihood of ureteric

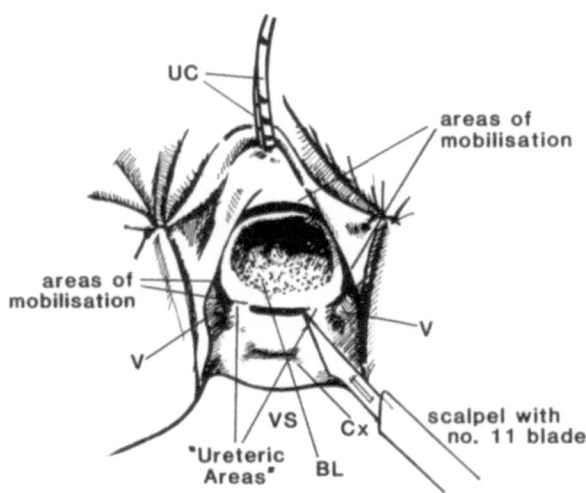

Figure 97. Diagramatic representation of areas to be mobilized and "ureteric areas" to be avoided until the ureters have been indentified and catheterized

involvement at or near the fistula edge or outside it, *must be presumed in each case until disproven.* Early on in dissection, the orifices must be identified and catheterized. Accordingly, with a middle-sized fistula, mobilization proceeds superiorly, laterally and centrally, carefully avoiding the lateral angles of the defect near the cervix (Fig. 97). It is most important the bladder should be mobilized centrally from the cervix. Pockets of freedom produced by this preliminary mobilization, aid eventual ureteric orifice identification, by freeing the bladder; but with large fistulae, identification often can be made before any attempt at mobilization begins.

Methods of Ureteric Orifice Identification

1. After preliminary mobilization has been completed, the terminal ureter and orifice may be palpable. Eversion of the lateral angle of the fistula might enable the orifice to be seen with the possibility of passing a fine probe gently through the orifice, particularly if the probe lies flat on the bladder mucosa and is passed with great care in the anticipated line of the distal ureter, in several areas (Figs. 98 a–c).

2. With a very large fistula, or when probing is unrewarded, 5 c.c. 0.5% indigo carmine injected intravenously will produce the tell-tale blue dye within five minutes and identify both orifices.

3. If the dye investigation should fail, a second indigo carmine injection or even a double dose together with 10 mg of intravenous Lasix usually will finalize identification.

When both ureters have been catheterized, bladder mobilization can proceed and be completed with safety. The catheters are drawn through the urethra by artery forceps to remove them from the operative field.

7. Bladder Wall Closure

Although there are no fixed rules to be followed, usually the bladder is closed with interrupted sutures of "00" chromic catgut, ("00" extrachromic W565 Ethicon with a very strong needle is recommended), whilst observing the following principles:

1. A Foley 12 self-retaining catheter is inserted and the balloon filled. Formerly, vaginal cystotomy above the site of fistula closure was advocated frequently as a method of bladder drainage. Falk and Tancer (1957) discussing urethral reconstruction, repair of vesico-vaginal fistula involving the bladder neck, and excision of a broad-based urethral diverticulum, concluded in these specific indications where continuous bladder drainage was necessary and use of a catheter inadvisable, vaginal cystotomy was

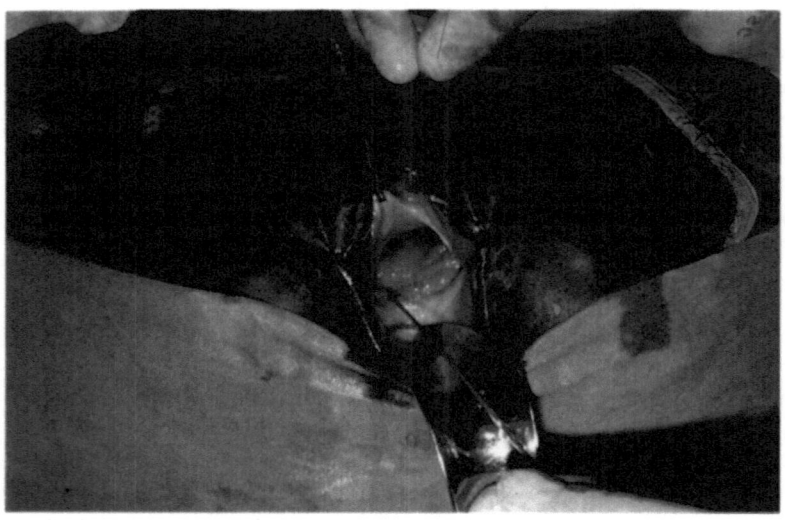

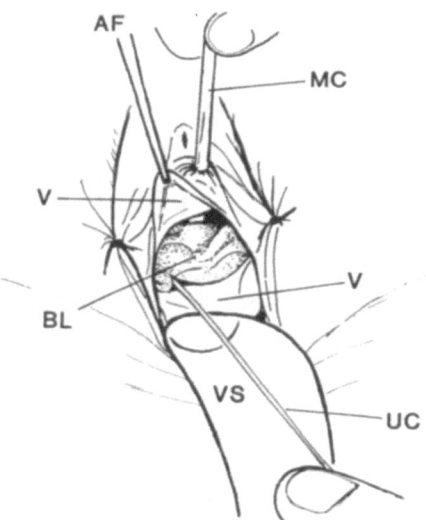

Figure 98 a. Preliminary ureteric orifice identification and passage of a ureteric catheter

complicated much less than suprapubic cystotomy. Introducing a Kelly clamp throught the fistula to that portion of the bladder nearest the cervix, the blades were opened and a vertical incision made into the bladder. The scalpel blade was grasped by the clamp and the clamp advanced through the cystotomy opening to take the catheter and pull it into the bladder. The time for catheter removal was never later than the 14th day, to avoid epithelialization of the cystotomy opening. Chassar Moir (1966) wrote of

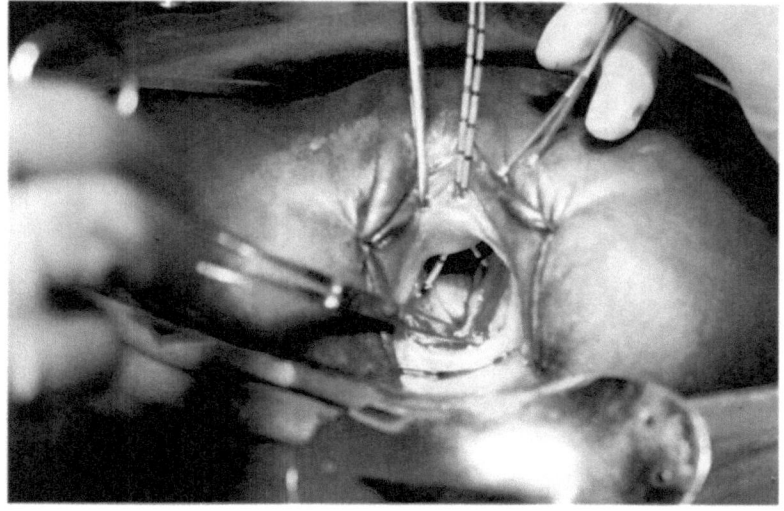

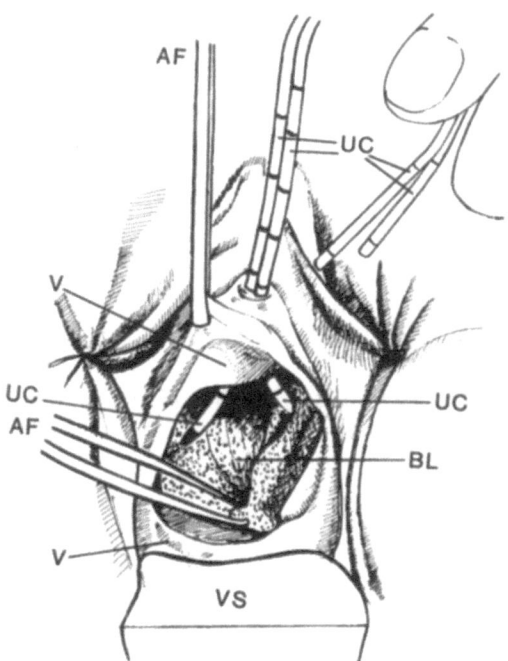

Figure 98 b. With both ureteric catheters in place, bladder mobilization proceeds

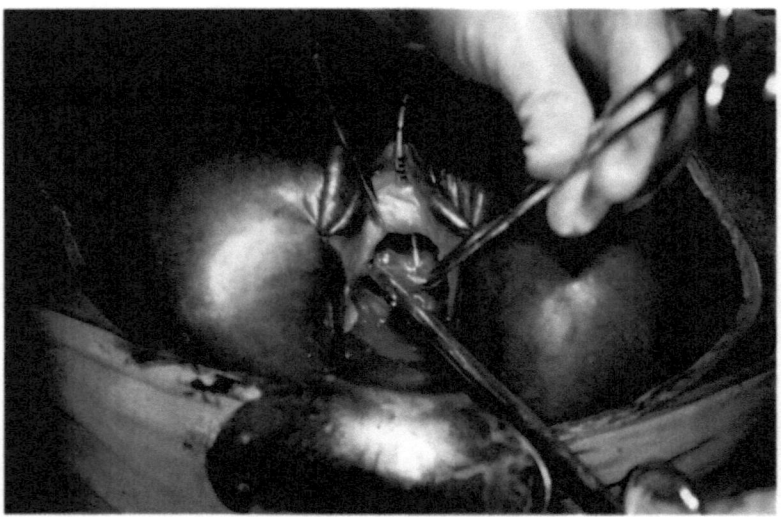

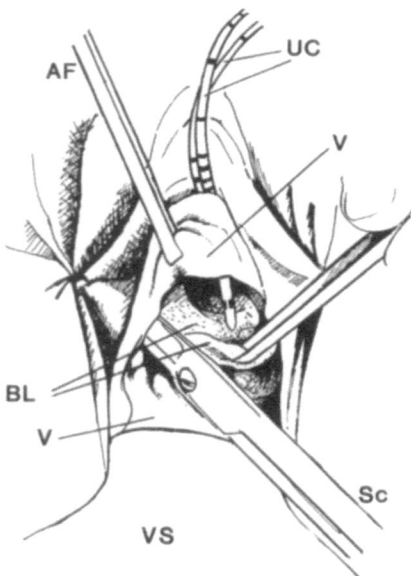

Figure 98 c. Scissors free bladder adhesions to the pubic ramus

the advantages of vaginal cystotomy and regarded it as a neglected method, but emphasized that after the removal of the catheter, some days of urethral drainage would be required to allow spontaneous closure. Falk and Tancer (1969) again suggested vaginal cystotomy to drain the bladder after correction of a urethral fistula, to avoid an indwelling catheter. The popularity

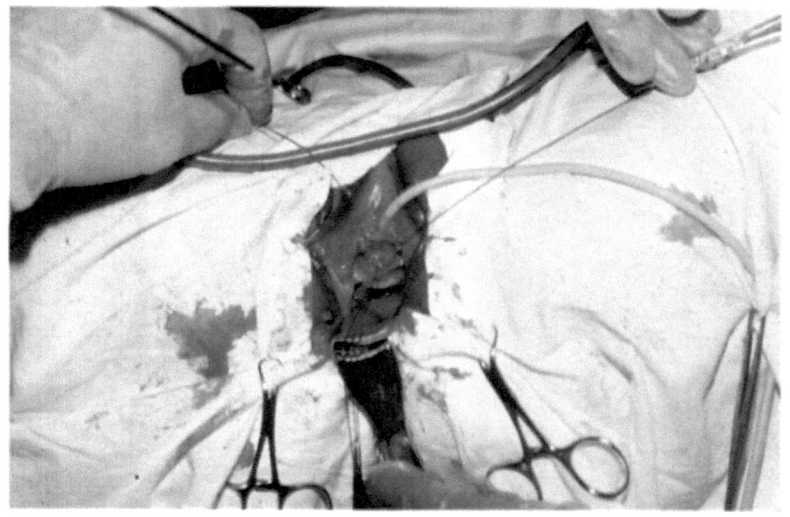

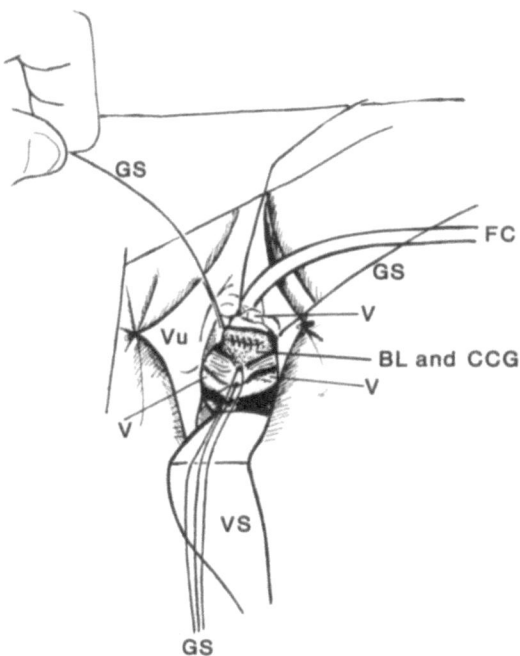

Figure 99. Completed closure of a small bladder defect

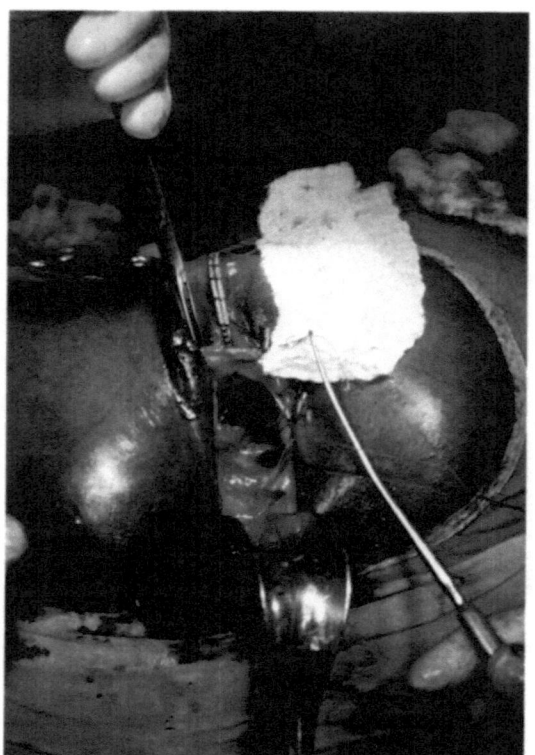

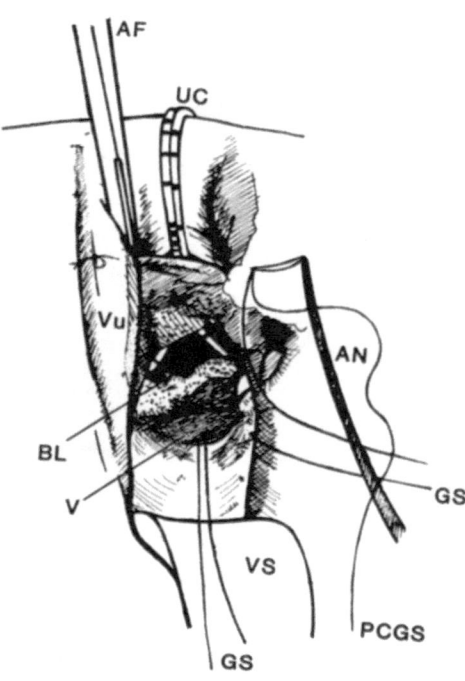

Figure 100 a. Aneurysm needle loaded with "0" plain catgut ready to insert the stabilizing suture, attaching bladder wall to the periosteum of the pubic ramus

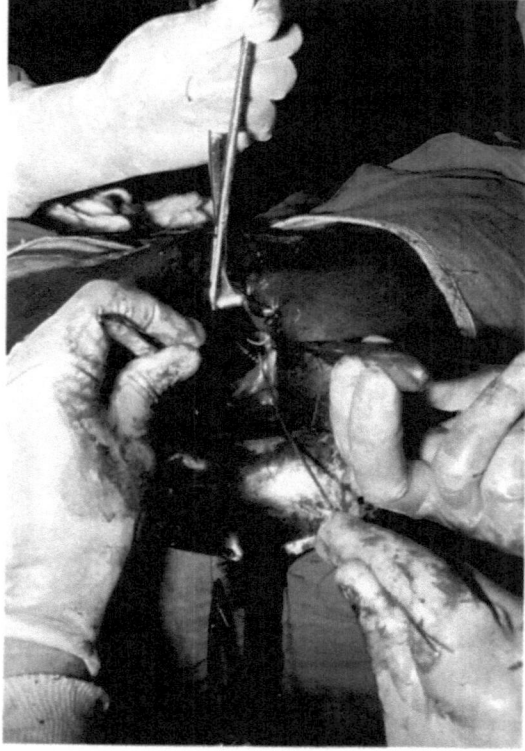

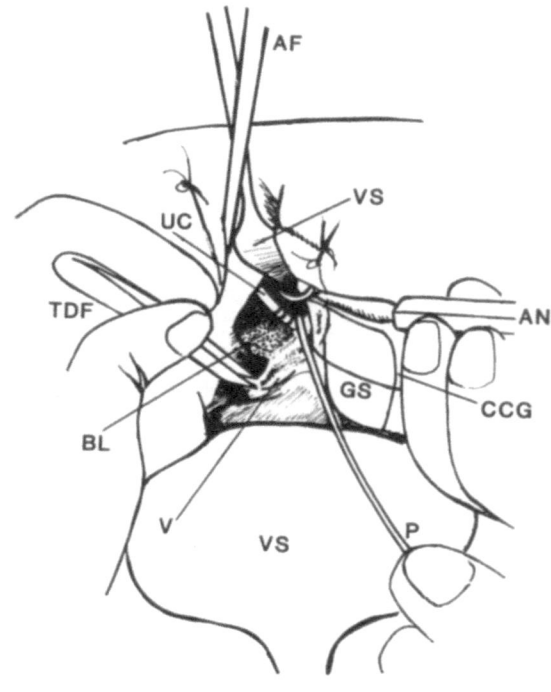

Figure 100 b. Inserting the stabilizing suture

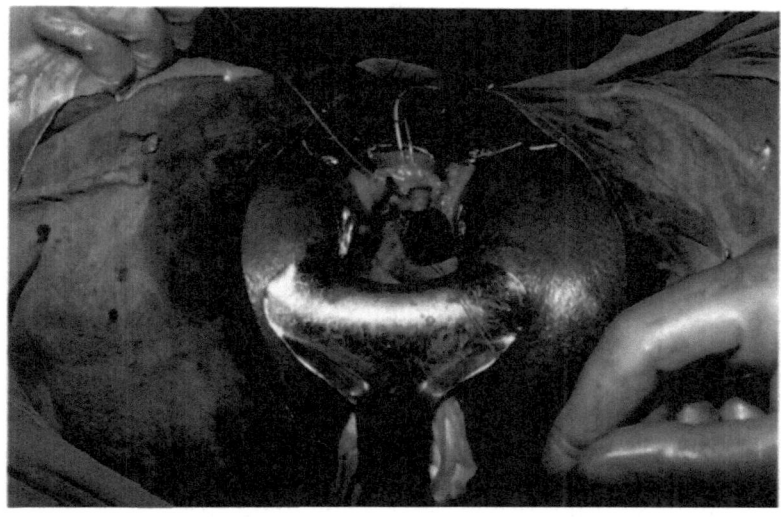

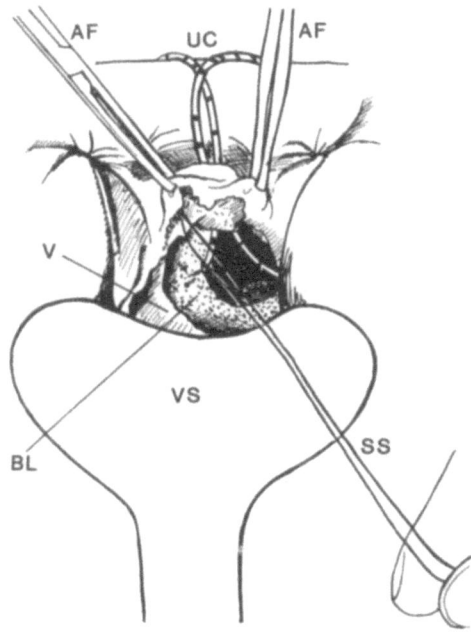

Figure 100 c. The suture tied, anchoring bladder to the pubic ramus

of vaginal cystotomy has waned with the efflux of time, and virtually no fistula surgeons now employ this method of drainage since objections to a small indwelling urethral catheter seem largely theoretical.

Some believe suprapubic drainage essential when bladder neck and urethra have been repaired, and others like Waghmarae and Handscomb (1968), Kenya obtained improved results in the management of obstetric vesico-vaginal fistula by combining suprapubic and urethral drainage through a single catheter.

2. With a Foley 12 catheter in place, the fistula limits are defined and the bladder mucosa inverted by interrupted sutures passing through muscle and submucosal layers only, avoiding the bladder lumen. Wide bites are necessary to avoid tearing out, and sutures should ensure apposition without strangulation. Never should the surgeon forget these tissues have been subjected to excessive trauma, and even through they appear nearly normal, always they are far from it—healing will be slow with blood supply much less than usual, so tight suturing is unnecessary and dangerous (Fig. 99).

3. Prior to beginning closure of larger fistulae, the lateral edges of the bladder defect are identified on either side, and the bladder wall immediately lateral to this fixed to the periosteum of the ischiopubic ramus of that side. A small aneurysm needle picks up periosteum with "0" plain catgut and then bladder wall immediately lateral to the fistula. This important and key step in large vesico-vaginal fistula closure, stabilizes the bladder against the rami, minimizing postoperative movement of the recent bladder suture line (Figs. 100 a–c).

4. Bladder wall closure commences laterally and moves centrally, either in the natural transverse direction or in the antero-posterior direction should this seem more appropriate. Lawson (1978) stated that bladder defects should be repaired transversely since vertical repair might distort the underlying trigone, and crowd the ureteric orifices together in the midline. Whilst this certainly may be true, in such instances one may not have the choice of transverse closure if a watertight junction is to be achieved and of course with any risk to underlying ureters, clearly catheters must be inserted preoperatively. Lawson also mentioned avoiding deep stitches lateral to the fistula in case one may include the intramural ureter, and again, in case of a doubt such as this, the procedure should not commence without catheterization of the ureters. Occasionally a combination of transversely placed sutures laterally, with centrally sited antero-posterior sutures, will be the best method of dealing with a large defect. The important principle to be remembered and re-emphasized is that there must never be any tension on the suture line (Fig. 101).

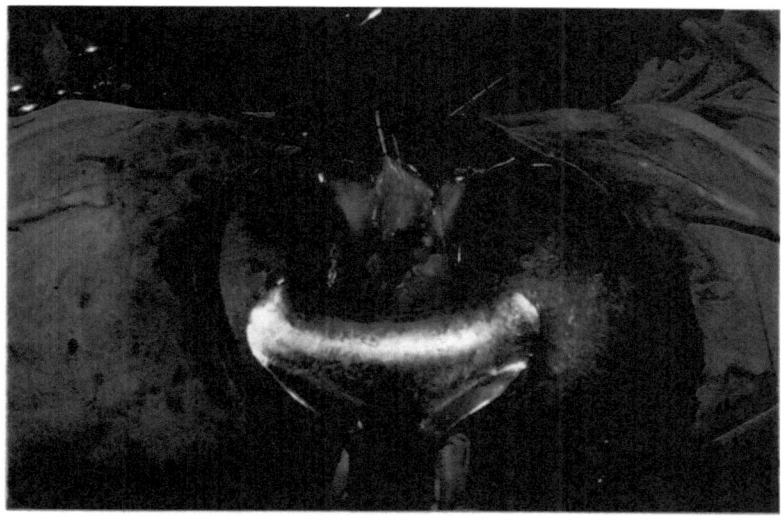

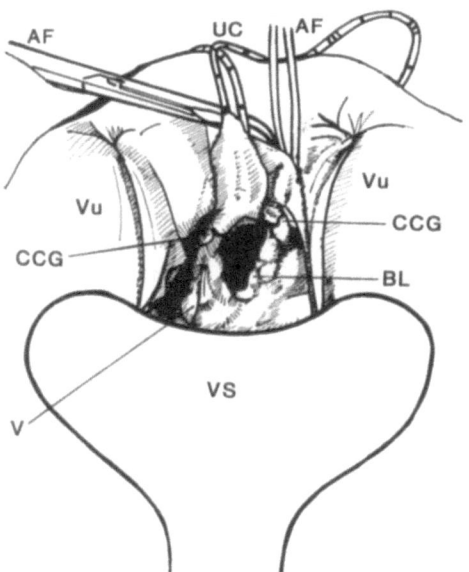

Figure 101. Large fistula partly closed horizontally at the lateral extremities—the central defect to be closed vertically

5. Usually it is not possible to insert a double layer of sutures, the outer overlapping the inner; but at several points along the suture line this may be achieved. Apajalahti (1931) reported results of treament in 200 urinary fistulae and claimed a key point in the surgical technique was the quadruple layer closure used since 1915. The layers were bladder wall, two

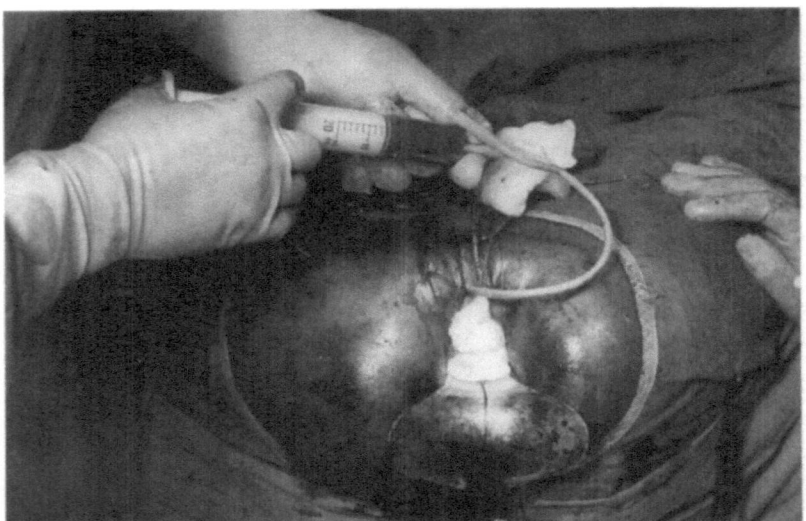

Figure 102. Injecting methylene blue into the bladder to confirm water-tight closure

connective tissue layers and then vagina. Similarly, Barnes and Martin (1949) advocated wide mobilization so five or six layers of sutures could be used to build a thick mass of tissue between bladder and the vaginal wall and whilst the principle is admirable, in practice, with large obstetric fistulae such an ideal usually is quite impossible. It would be applicable only to a very small fistula and then unnecessary. Similarly, the technique of Mayo (1916) wherein circular dissection around the fistula elevated the vaginal mucosa for about $^1/_4$ inch and formed a cup or funnel-shaped opening projecting into the vagina. Ingeniously, with a ligature carrier, the suture was passed via urethra and bladder then into the vagina through the fistula so the long suture could then pull the cup into the bladder allowing closure of the defect from the vagina. This inkwell procedure of Charles Mayo clearly is applicable to only very tiny fistulae.

6. Following fistula closure, the patency or otherwise of the suture line always must be tested by injecting methylene blue solution into the bladder through the catheter. Moderate pressure on the bladder can be applied, and any leaks detected require extra sutures (Fig. 102).

8. Grafting

Historically, placing a graft between bladder and vagina is a relatively recent innovation, yet it ranks equally in importance with other principles of fistula closure. Some form of grafting should be employed during the closure of every fistula, for there is no point in saving the technique for future surgical attempts, and there can be no doubt the graft enhances the quality of fistula closure and makes successful outcome more likely. There are several theoretical reasons why grafting is so valuable:

1. It helps plug minor defects in the suture line.
2. It beings a fresh blood supply into an area of poor quality tissues.
3. Most imporantly it keeps the healing bladder and vaginal wall apart, limiting greatly any opportunity for cross-union during the healing phase.

The two grafting techniques employed are:

a) Martius graft.
b) Gracilis muscle graft.

The Martius graft.

The Martius fat graft should be employed with all fistulae excluding the very small, and the very large with urethral loss when of course it would be inadequate. It may be taken from the greater labium of either side, or in some instances from both sides. A vertical incision on the external surface of the labium is followed by careful separation of the underlying fat from the skin to develop a discrete, elongated centrally situated fat graft, without buttonholing the introital skin. The upper extremity of the graft is freed from the overlying undivided labial skin—length according to need—then folded back and freed from deeper attachments. Free bleeding from the donor site following elevation of the graft is controlled by artery forceps and ligation, then hemostasis is achieved by pushing a gauze swab firmly beneath the upper skin hood. The pedicle is elevated to the posterior end of the vulval incision where the inferior hemorrhoidal vessels enter, then with curved artery forceps, a tunnel is developed from the donor site to the site of fistula closure (Figs. 103 a, b). Some pressure is required, but the technique is facilitated and virtually bloodless providing the forceps follow closely against the inferior surface of the bony ramus. Once the initial passage has been forced, opening and closing the forceps makes the track adequate to allow passage of the graft. The tunnel must not exert undue pressure on the graft for fear of interference with blood supply. Several anchor sutures of "00" chromic catgut are inserted into the vaginal submucosa ready to receive and fix the graft, then the tip of the graft is grasped by slender curved forceps, introduced from the bladder side. Assisted by pressure from the donor side with a finger, fine-toothed forceps or curved artery forceps, the graft is drawn through the tunnel to the closed bladder defect (Fig. 103 c). Occasionally traction on the fundus of the graft

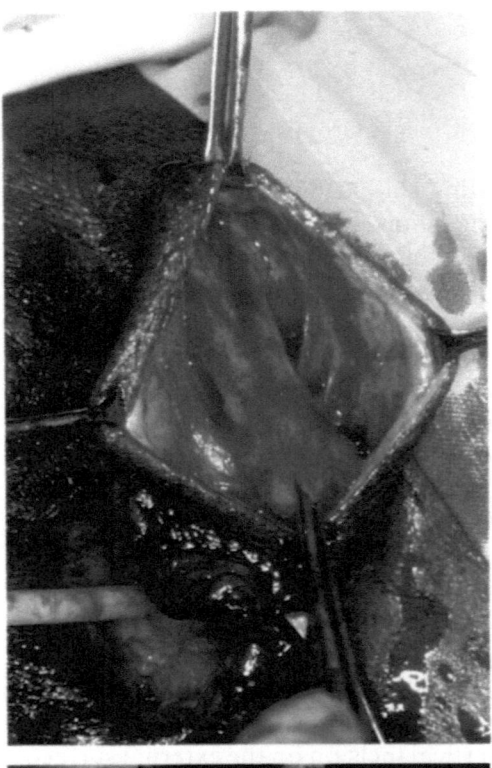

Figure 103 a (i)

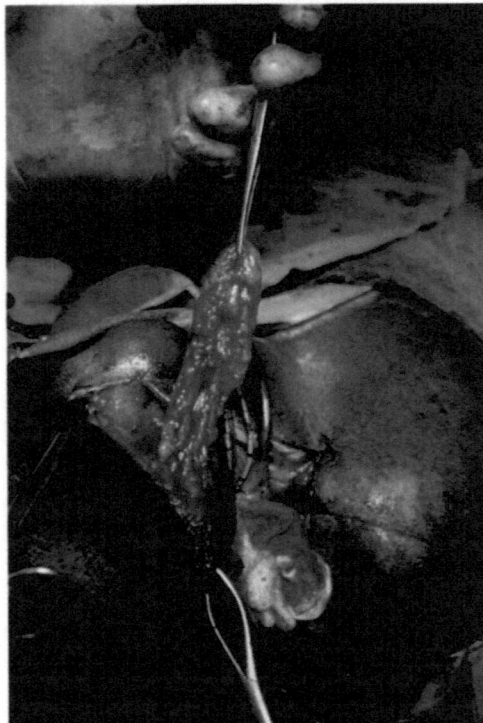

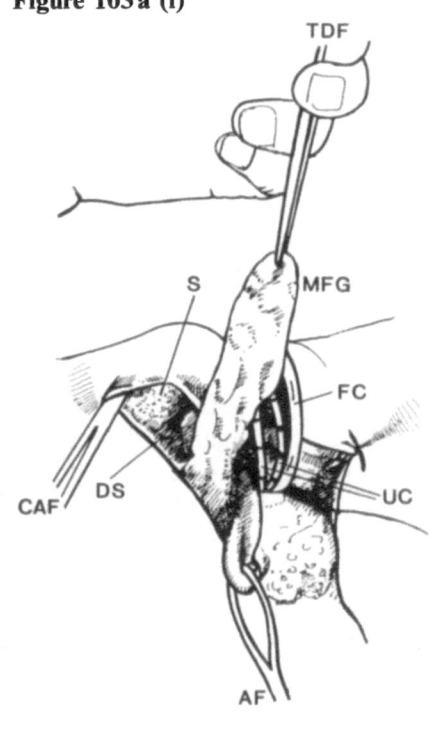

Figure 103 a (ii)

Figures 103 a, b. After the development of the pedicle fat graft (i) and (ii), curved artery forceps fashion a tunnel from the site of fistula closure to the donor site

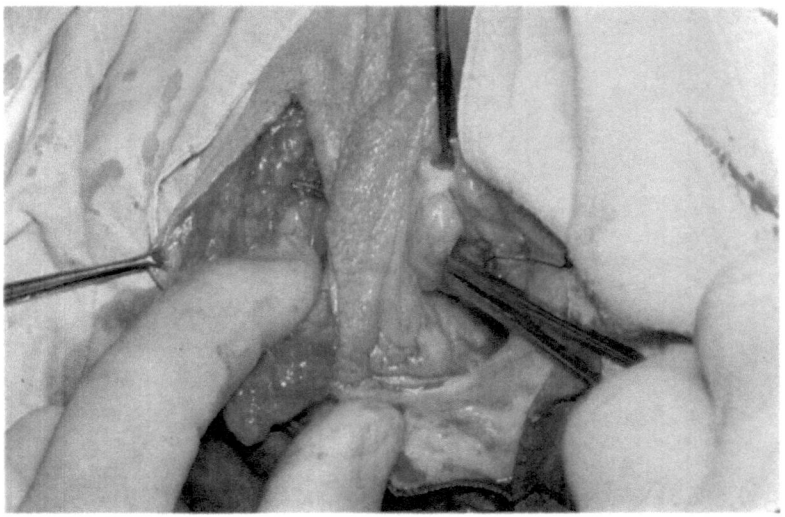

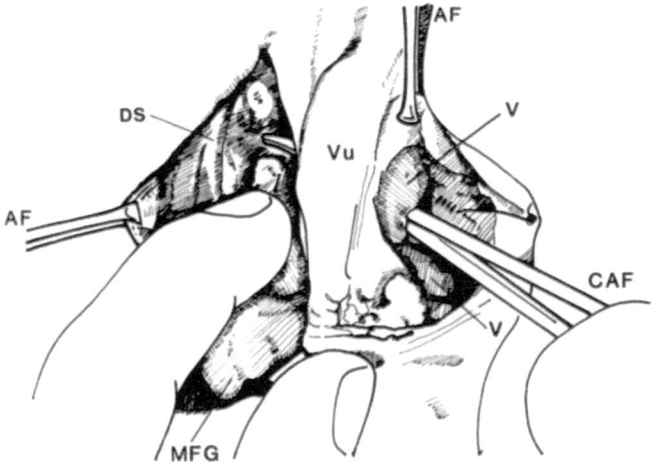

Figure 103 b

by suture may be more appropriate and often necessary in a small female with a narrow pelvis and limited access. At this stage, the track may require some enlargement to ensure that the graft lies easily within it without constriction, then the graft is anchored by the waiting sutures (Fig. 103 d). The gauze swab can be removed from the donor site and by this time, usually bleeding has ceased; but any remaining must be controlled since hemostasis is essential. Dead space at the graft site is eliminated in the following manner:

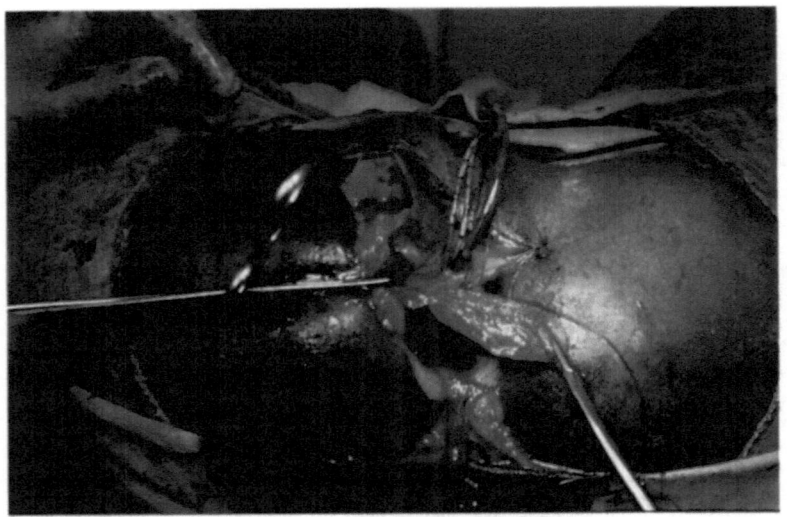

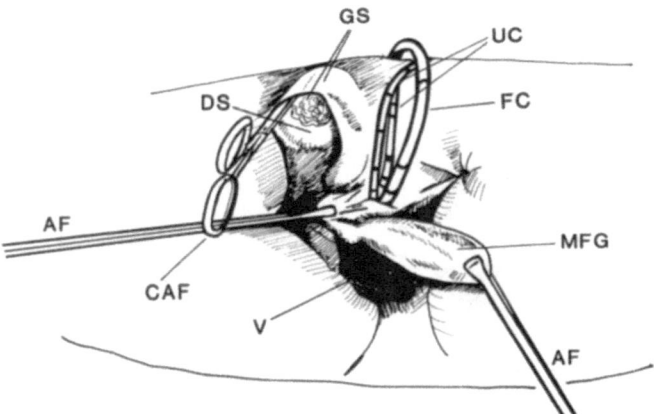

Figure 103 c. The Martius fat graft drawn through the tunnel

1. The subepithelial and deeper tissues are drawn together without penetrating the overlying skin, using a series of interrupted "0" plain catgut sutures.

2. Large skin needles carrying no. 1 nylon are passed deeply from side to side beneath the graft site. Usually three or four are required.

3. The vulval incision is closed using horizontal mattress sutures of "00" silk, or "00" Vicryl, which incorporate deeper layers.

4. A roll of gauze the length of the wound, 1–2 cm in diameter, is laid

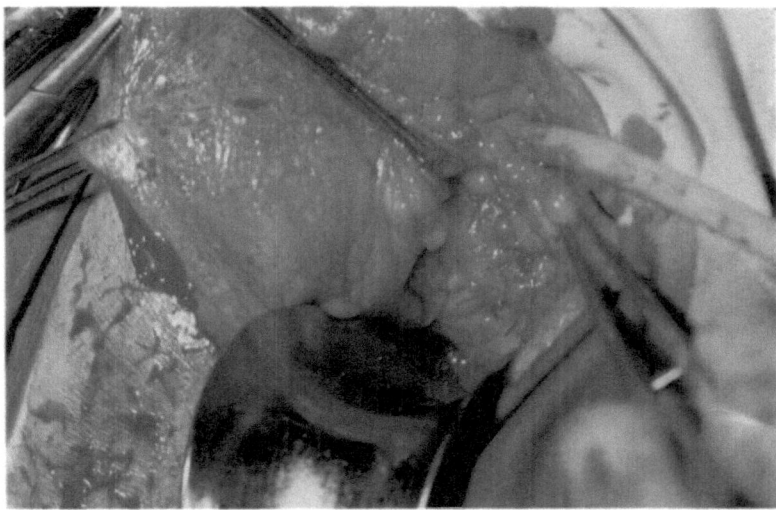

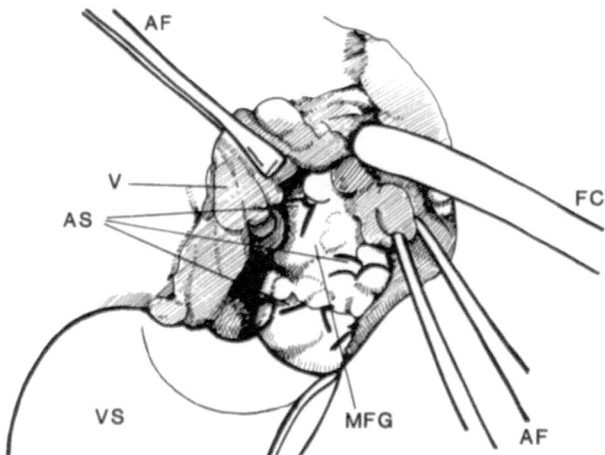

Figure 103 d. Graft fixed over closed bladder defect with anchor sutures

upon the suture line and fixed firmly against the wound by the deep nylon sutures. Experience has demonstrated this haemostatic technique to be superior to suction drainage, promoting rapid healing with an excellent cosmetic result (Fig. 135 a, b).

The Gracilis Graft

This technique described originally by Garlock (1928) and further embellished by Ingelman-Sundberg (1950, 1954), was simplified by Hamlin and

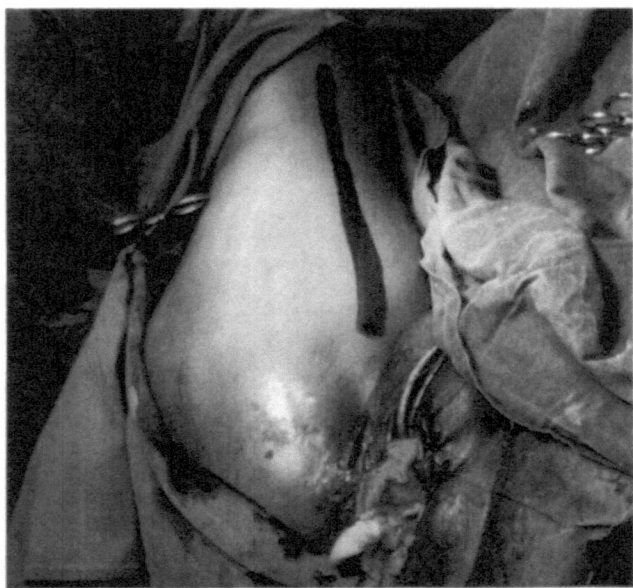

Figure 104 a. Surface anatomy of the gracilis muscle marked with dye

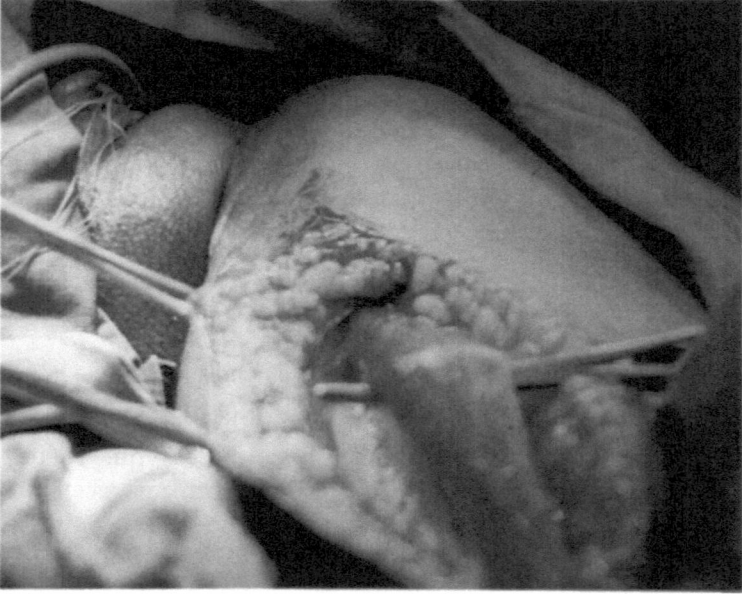

Figure 104 b. Gracilis muscle elevated. Foley catheter and anchor sutures seen near the vulva

Nicholson (1969). Garlock commented that although principles of fistula surgery were well-established, even when the principles were followed, not uncommonly a case would not respond to treatment, and recurrences developed necessitating repeated surgery, yet still the fistula might recur. He cited one report where 18 operations failed to effect a cure. Barring the presence of constitutional disease, the cause for recurrence seemed to be local. Each operative attempt caused more tissue slough and so a vicious circle was established.

The Hamlin-Nicholson gracilis muscle graft is required in the correction of many large fistulae, especially those involving urethral reconstruction. A bilateral Martius graft could be used; but the gracilis is essential in very large fistulae with gross fibrosis and great tissue loss. The surface anatomy of the muscle is a line between the pubic tubercle and the medial edge of the patella, and a long incision in the lower two thirds of the thigh reveals the flat muscle enclosed by deep fascia (Figs. 104 a, b). Easily mobilized from its deep fine attachments, the tendon is freed, isolated then divided as near the tibial condyle as possible. The technique is comparatively bloodless. Both blood and nerve supply enter the upper one third of the muscle, so care is required during mobilization to ensure these connections remain intact. The subcutaneous tunnel beneath the labium must be large to allow free passage of the muscle, the muscle tendon is attached to the cervix and anchor sutures fix the belly of the muscle over the site of fistula closure (Figs. 105 a–d). The long wound is closed following hemostasis using a fat suture of 1 plain catgut which incorporates deeper tissues, then the skin is sutured with horizontal mattress sutures of "00" silk. After wound closure a firm dressing with a crepe bandage covers the whole length of the wound, and suction drainage is unnecessary.

9. Closing the Vaginal Skin

Where vaginal skin flaps are adequate after proper mobilization, the skin wound can be closed with "00" monofilament nylon inserted as vertical mattress sutures incorporating the underlying grafts and helping to eliminate dead space. Just enough tension is required to bring skin edges into apposition without strangulation, and the number of sutures is recorded as a check against their future removal (Fig. 106). Skin deficit often can be a problem especially with fistulae large enough to require a gracilis muscle graft, and a labial skin flap can be raised from the lesser labium of one or other side and laid over the muscle or fat graft, as a full thickness skin graft (Figs. 107 a, b). The resulting vulval defect can be closed independently or by incorporating it with the episiotomy closure.

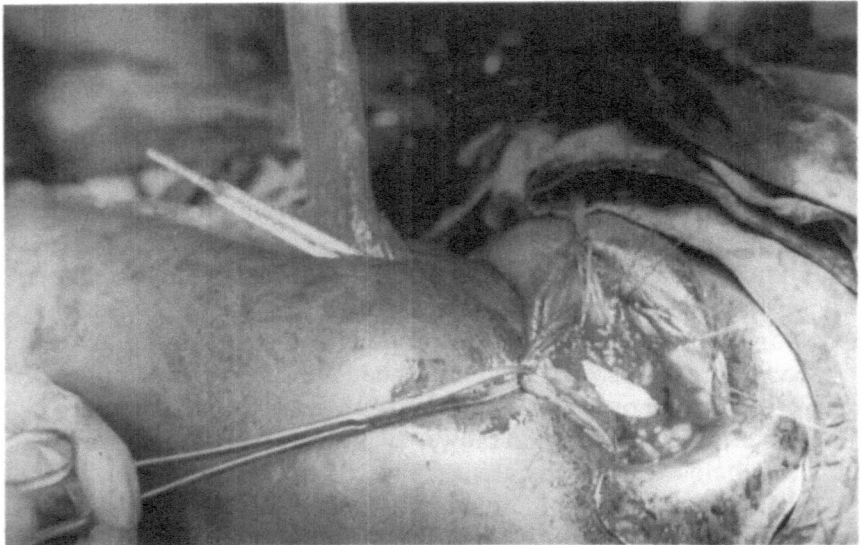

Figure 105 a. Muscle elevated and subcutaneous tunnel created

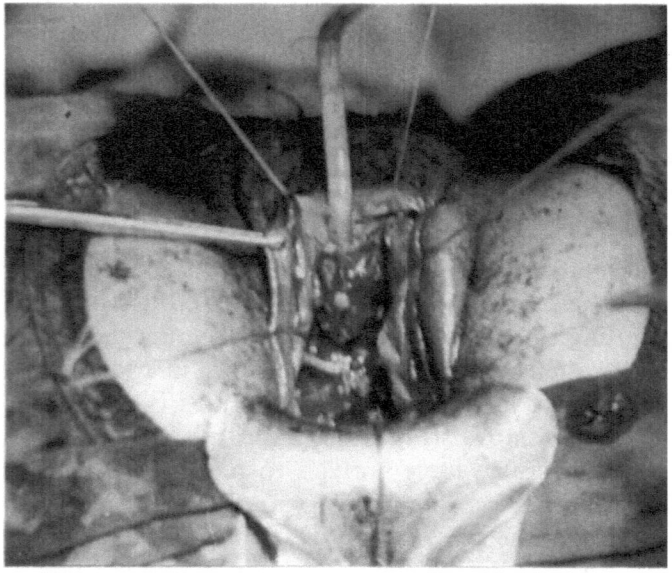

Figure 105 b. Fistula closed and anchor sutures in readiness

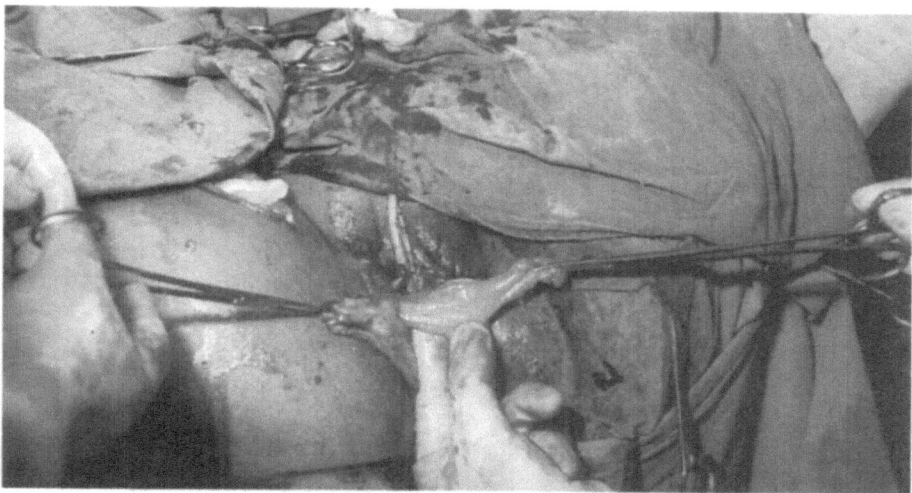

Figure 105 c. The muscle graft passed through the sublabial tunnel into the vagina

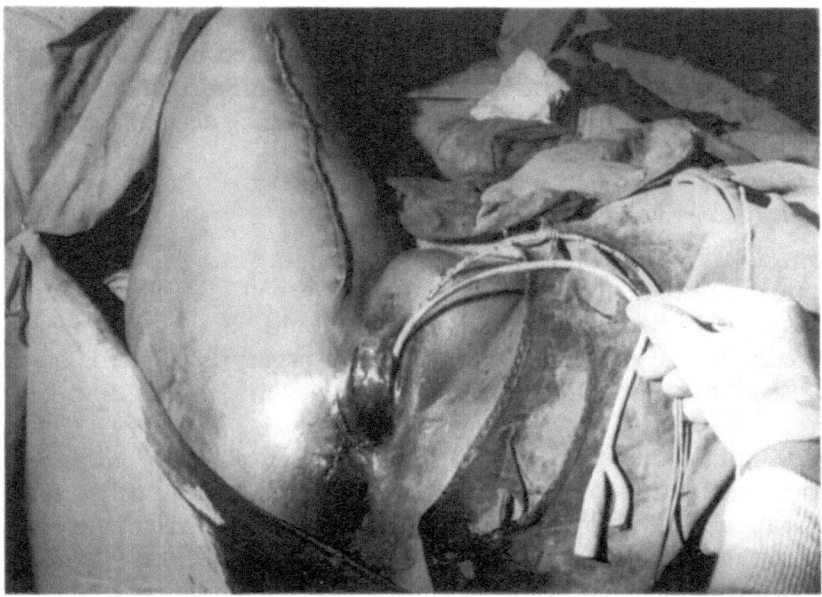

Figure 105 d. Operation concluded—thigh wound closed, labial skin flap covers the muscle graft, and episiotomy of access closed. Note Foley catheter and two ureteric catheters

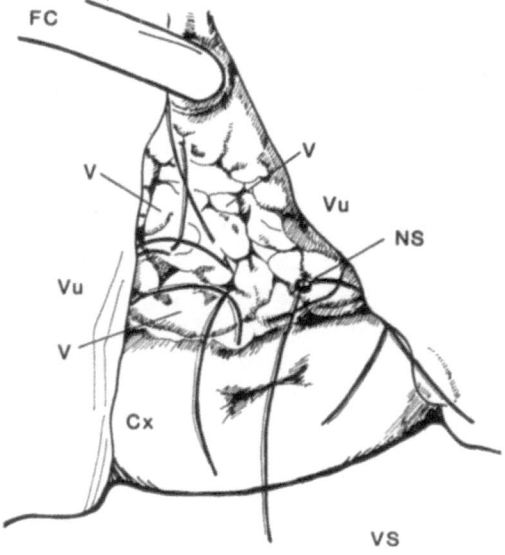

FC

V

V

Vu

NS

Vu

V

Cx

VS

Figure 106. Vaginal skin closed over the Martius graft using "00" monofilament nylon sutures

10. Vaginal Pack

The vagina is packed gently but firmly with gauze soaked in paraffin oil or vaseline, and the pack remains for 48 hours. This important step encourages various layers of the repair to adhere, minimizing dead space and hematoma formation.

11. Postoperative Management

Immediately following surgery, urine should be draining from all catheters employed, and if not, 10 mg Lasix given intravenously will start the flushing action through the catheters. Bladder washout should be avoided unless absolutely necessary—usually blood loss during surgery is minimal obviating the risk of clot in the bladder. The two important principles to be observed are:

1. The bladder must be kept empty during the healing phase.

2. Antibiotics are required to prevent urinary tract infection, but *only* after closure of the fistula and so long as the catheter is required. The catheters are strapped to the patient's leg with waterproof adhesive tape and allowed to drain freely into bedside bottles—one for each catheter employed. Some surgeons prefer to suture the catheter to the inferior border of the pubic symphysis even when inflation of the catheter bulb is not hazardous to the line of repair (Ward 1985). A nurse cares for the patient continuously until

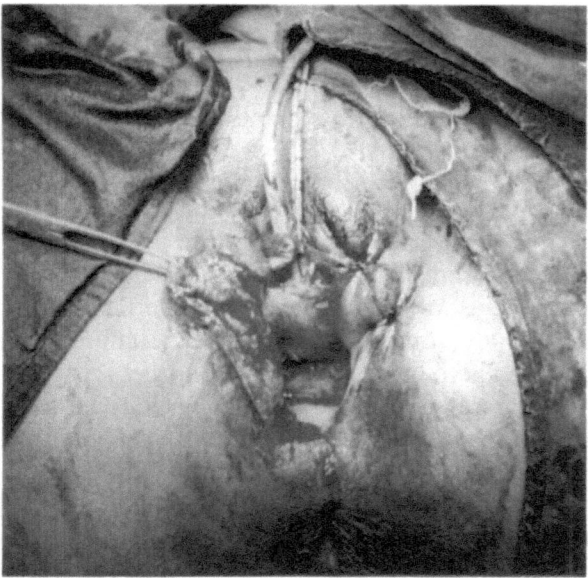

Figure 107 a. Labial graft prepared to cover gracilis graft

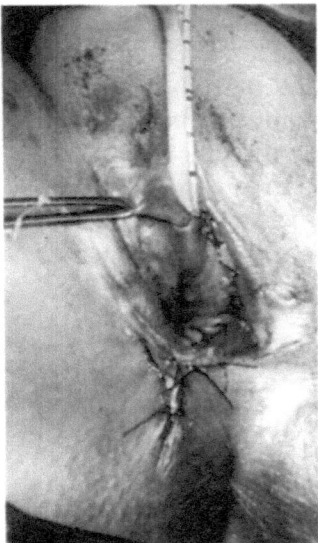

Figure 107 b. Flap fixed over the graft

she has recovered fully from the anesthetic and is able to understand what is happening. This precaution minimizes any risk of the patient interfering with catheter drainage. Suction is not employed for it has inherent problems. The nurse in charge of the patient on hearing the suction machine which seems to be working adequately, may presume all is well without checking drainage and an obstruction in the early healing phase means certain failure. Under no condition must the free flow of urine be hindered by any obstruction whatever to the catheter. Once the patient is wide awake, she watches the Foley catheter, having been instructed in this role prior to surgery. Should the patient have any doubt whatsoever about efficacy of drainage, the moment she reports any concern, the catheter is changed, immediately and without question. There is no need for the surgeon to be notified. A high fluid intake is necessary, and the vaginal pack together with the vulval pressure pad dressing are removed at 48 hours. The length of urinary drainage depends on the size of the fistula, the quality of the tissues and problems that were encountered with closure. These tissues heal slowly, so rarely should the period of drainage be less than 10 days. Large fistulae need a minimum of 14 days. If ureteric catheters have been employed, they should remain in situ for 8–10 days to allow meatal edema to subside, and the Foley stays in for a total of 14 days. During the entire period of catheter drainage, an appropriate urinary antibiotic is necessary. When the catheter is removed, usually there is no difficulty with voiding; but the patient is observed carefully and would be catheterized at 4–6 hours, depending on fluid intake should she not be able to void. In practice, voiding usually occurs easily, and providing volumes of 100–200 c.c. are voided, no further checks are necessary. The patient remains under supervision for a further 24 hours, a specimen of urine is taken for bacteriological examination and the antibiotic ceases. Upon discharge from hospital, the patient is advised to use Acijel vaginal jelly ($^1/_2$% lactic acid) and avoid intercourse until the postoperative visit in one month, when the nylon sutures are removed.

Vesico-vaginal Fistula Associated with Partial or Complete Urethral Destruction

The addition of partial or complete urethral destruction to a vesico-vaginal fistula has been regarded always as a serious complicating factor difficult to correct. Emmet (1895) described a new method for treating an "Incurable Vesico-vaginal fistula" and described the findings in his patient: "All the soft parts had been lost except the fundus of the bladder while all the urethra, the tissues under the pubes and for some distance into the bladder has sloughed away, leaving nothing but periosteum covering the surface of the bone. The vaginal canal was about one and a half inches deep and was continuous with the fistula into the bladder as if the two were one common canal." This is an excellent description of the "difficult fistula" of the Hamlins, a type still seen commonly in Ethiopia. Emmet, although previously successful with urethral reconstruction in 1862, realized the technical difficulties of obtaining enough tissue with which to make a new urethra, and the functional problem of continence control since there "was little or no muscular structure, there can be no relative power beyond the mechanical effect gained by extending the new urethra to the clitoris".His solution was to cease any urethral reconstruction but simply bridge over the fistula and insert suprapubic drainage through an epithelialized cystotomy.

Noble (1901) cited Emmet's six or seven successes and his intention not to attempt the procedure again, the two cases of Olshausen, and three reported by Baker-Brown. Olshausen had two successes and Baker-Brown (1863) presented a mixed bag of urethral damage and achieved continence in all three, two by direct repair and one in which he fashiond a new urethra using a trocar. The patient described by Noble had suffered 11 previous attempts at closure and examination showed "the entire anterior wall of the urethra was gone and a fistula existed involving the neck of the bladder".Mobilizing flaps of tissue on either side of the midline, these were united over a catheter, at the same time closing the bladder fistula. An effort was made to reconstruct the urethro-vesical sphincter during closure. The failure which followed, he deemed due to tension on the suture line. At the 14th operation, he mobilized urethral flaps more widely, closed them over the catheter as before and applied a flap fashioned from the left labium minus over the raw surface and well back into the vagina. This time the closure succeeded; but a vaginal tampon was necessary to achieve reasonable continence. Gray Ward (1923) stated that when the complication of urethral destruction was added to the difficulties of extensive vesico-vaginal fistula, a problem resulted to try skill and ingenuity to the utmost. No two cases were exactly alike and improvisations in technique were necessary to meet differing conditions. Ward's patient with a large fistula and absent urethra was dealt with by a two-stage procedure. The fistula was reduced in size leaving a defect corresponding to the urethro-vesical junction, and at the second procedure a tunnel was made deep to the scarred urethral remnant and a flap, cut from the anterior vaginal wall with its end attached to the vesical opening was drawn through the tunnel to form a new urethra (Figs. 108 a, b). The procedure concluded using a

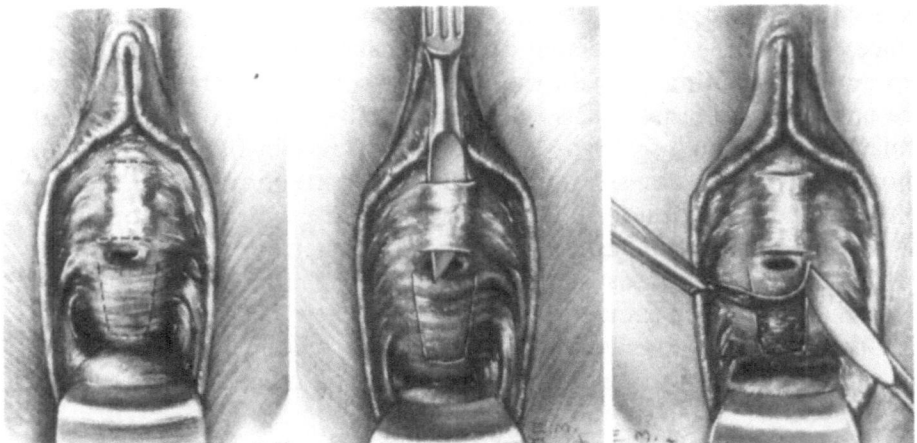

Figure 108 a. Urethral reconstruction outlining a vaginal wall flap above the bladder fistula, then drawing it through a tunnel deep to the former urethra

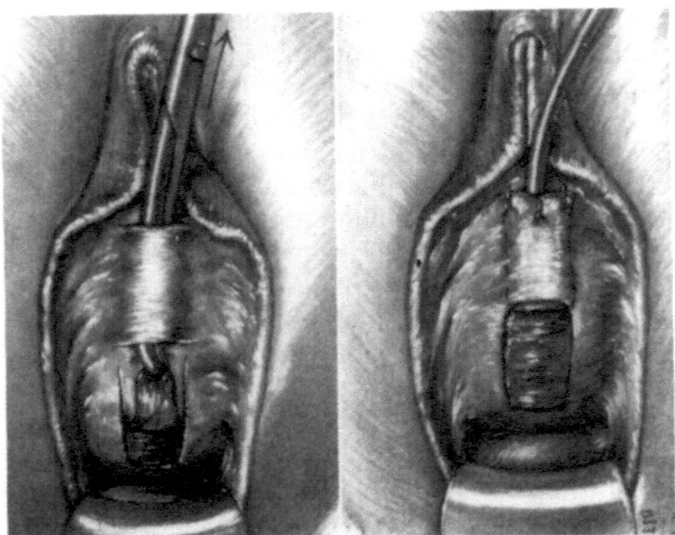

Figure 108 b. The flap forms the new urethra, and the catheter maintains patency

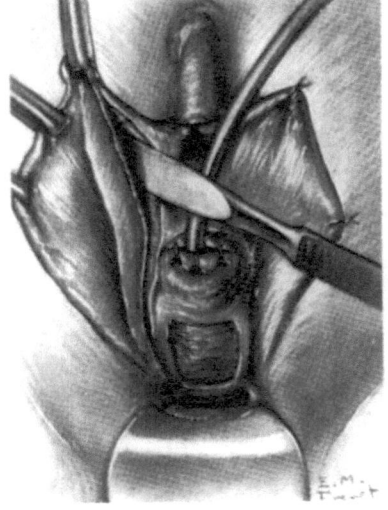

Figure 108 c

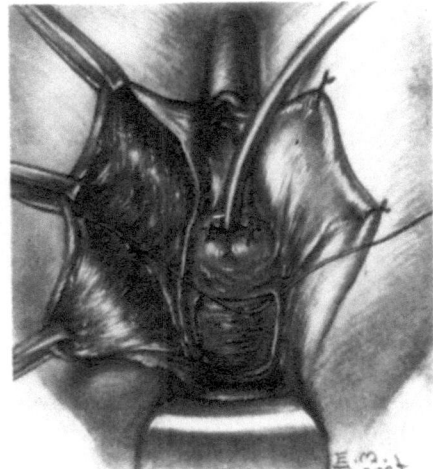

Figure 108 d

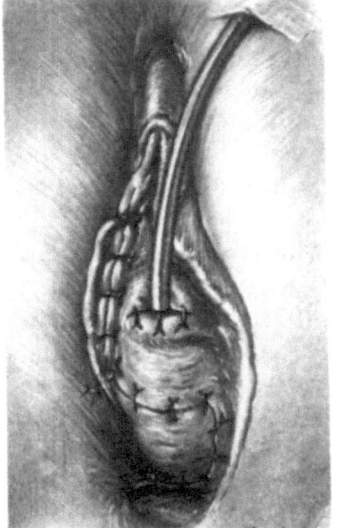

Figure 108 e

Figures 108 c–e. Labial skin flap closes the defect.
(From Gray Ward)

labial skin flap to cover the denuded vaginal area at the bladder base
(Figs 108 c–e). Closure was achieved together with continence due he believed to "some reinforcing sutures placed at the neck of the bladder at its
junction with the new urethra". McGlinn (1932) discussing difficulties of
curing simple vesico-vaginal fistula, reiterated past advice exclaiming "the

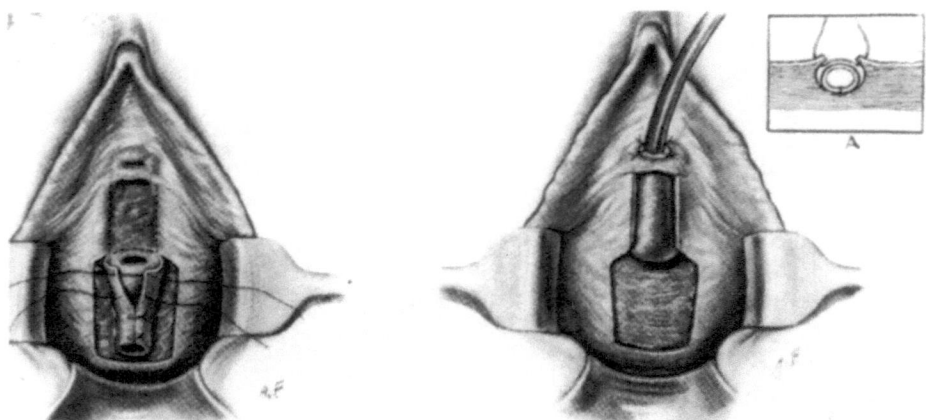

Figure 109. The Farrar-Ward technique converting the Ward flap to a tube. (From Gray Ward)

additional complication of partial or complete absence of the urethra, would present a condition so formidable as to deter a surgeon from attempting to correct the defect by plastic surgery". He gave precedence to Lamballe (1849) Baker Brown (1863) and Lawson Tait (1878) as originators of techniques to deal with the absent urethra and agreed that whilst anatomy often was corrected, incontinence remained, improved a little only by the urethral length. Taussig (1918) transplanted some levator ani fibers on one side only, to reinforce the new urethra and gained excellent control, sufficient to continue through a following pregnancy. Since that turning point, there have been many similar attempts to restore urinary control (Marion Douglass 1931). Nevertheless, Taussig (McGlinn 1931, personal communication), stated none of his results had been more than partly successful, the best outlook following urethral reconstruction after urethral excision for carcinoma where some sphincter could be preserved—the difficulty was "partial dribbling through the nozzle when the kettle fills up". Following the successful case reported by Gray Ward (1923), Lillian Farrar in the discussion which followed the paper, suggested widening the flap so the lateral edges could be united forming a tube and this tube rather than a tongue of tissue would become the new urethra (Fig. 109). McGlinn reported two successes using the Gray Ward-Farrar technique with a minor variant in that the urethral tube was made from a vaginal wall flap with the incision beginning at the anterior fistula margin rather than the posterior. The tube with an inserted catheter was drawn through the tunnel

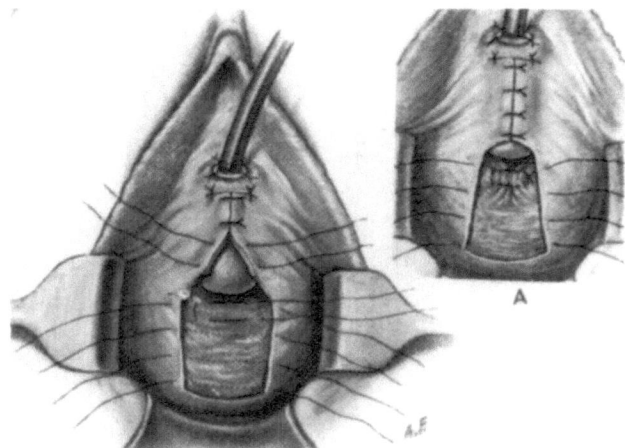

Figure 110. The buried neo-urethra with Kelly bladder neck buttressing sutures in place. (From Gray Ward)

and anchored at either end. At the vesical end, the new urethra was encircled by a constricting band of tissue—the most important step to promote continence. The denuded vaginal area was covered by a labial flap and of three cases reported, the first failed and underwent ureteric transplant; but the second and third healed with good control. In time the continence of the third patient deteriorated; but was restored by passing a flap of rectus abdominus muscle behind the pubis to be split and encircle the urethra. Gray Ward (1934) reported a further improvement burying the neo-urethra in a deep groove rather than a tunnel at the site of the former urethra, inserting Kelly mattress sutures at the new bladder neck, then closing the vaginal defects (Fig. 110). However he resorted to a vaginal pessary to produce pressure on the urethra in an endeavor to prevent leakage. Mahfouz (1930) with a wide surgical experience stated "all fistula patients should be operated upon—I reject only those cases in which the urethra and sphincter are totally destroyed and cases where insufficient bladder remains to form a sufficient bladder". However in 1938 he advocated the Ward-Farrar technique; but in 1957 indicated he had seldom effected a cure with the procedure and suggested the Couvelaire procedure in which a neo-urethra was connected to the bladder via a puncture wound produced by a trocar, then a catheter passed into the bladder to await healing.

Benion Thomas (1947) referred to the difficulty of closing a juxta-urethral vesico-vaginal fistula when bladder and the top of the urethra

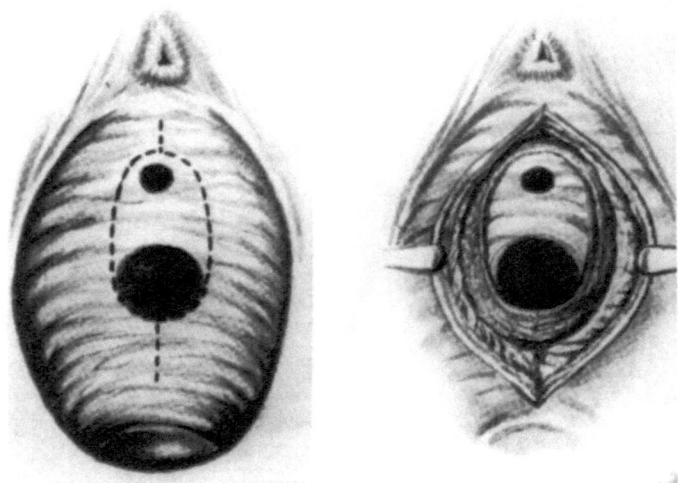

Figure 111 a. The incision indicated, flaps elevated and bladder mobilized

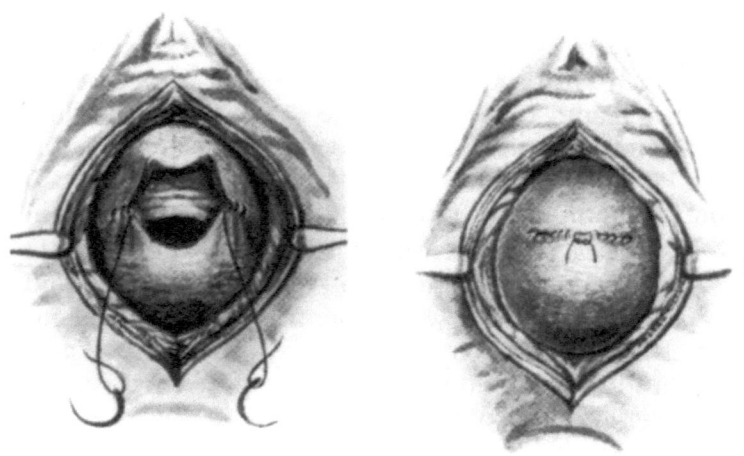

Figure 111 b. Suturing begins at each side, approximating the upper edge of the bladder fistula to the lower edge of the urethral defect. (From Benion Thomas)

opened separately into the vagina. Frequently the urethra was about 1 "long before it opened into the vagina, and the lower border of the fistula could be $^1/_2$" above the bladder fistula with the intervening space continuous with vaginal skin. The problem was anastomosing the large bladder fistula to the small urethral fistula and since the urethra was so thin-walled, sutures usually cut out, and suturing a large hole to a small hole meant puckering with probably a urine leak. Benion Thomas' solution was as follows: An oval incision included both fistulae, and through the incision the bladder was mobilized freely particularly from the cervix, until the upper fistula border could be drawn to the piece of vaginal skin surrounding the urethra, and until this was possible without any tension, suturing would be futile. Suturing began at the center of the long side of the oval; but often it was advantageous to commence a continous center stitch from each side later to meet in the midline (Fig. 111 a, b). So an area of vaginal skin remained enclosed and in contact with the urine, the lateral vaginal flaps closed over the repair and the bladder drained as usual. He reported five such fistulae all closed at the first attempt.

Barnes and Wilson (1949) suggested urethral reconstruction with a tube made from a flap of bladder wall, a technique proven successful in ureteric restoration. The bladder was exposed through an extraperitoneal suprapubic approach and the entire bladder dome freed by moving the peritoneal

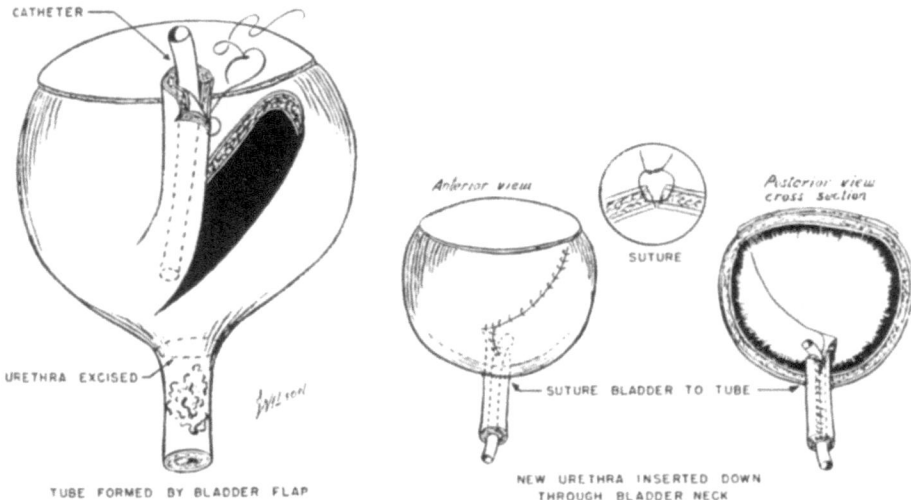

Figure 112. Detail of urethral reconstruction using a bladder flap. (From Barnes and Wilson)

attachment. Two oblique incisions in the bladder wall 3 cm apart passed from the dome nearly to the bladder neck with the lower ends about two centimeters lateral to the midline, enabling a flap to be raised and converted to a tube with which to replace the urethra. This "urethra" was buried beneath the vaginal mucosa and the new external meatus sutured to the vaginal epithelium (Fig. 112). They used the technique following urethral excision for carcinoma which left the patient fair control. Studdiford (1954) believed problems associated with surgical correction of bladder neck and upper urethral fistulae were the difficulty of exposure and the use of a urethral catheter for postoperative drainage, which produced tension on the sutures and was in direct contact with the repair. To obviate these objections, he used the prone position with the operating table broken at the hip, depressing both the trunk and legs (Kraske position) and suprapubic bladder drainage.

Chassar Moir (1954) reported 12 patients with complete urethral destruction in whom anatomical continuity was restored but not continence, although two were helped by a special vaginal pessary which pressed on the lower urethra, and four others improved with an Aldridge suburethral sling. A later report (1956) attributed improved control to a more thorough tissue build-up near the bladder neck. By 1961, Moir had discarded the Ward-Farrar technique because of the risk of flap sloughing and preferred to create a simple tunnel made from residual tissues at the site of the absent urethra. The new urethral tube was outlined as a flap by two deep incisions lateral to the midline, and the area depicted was sufficient to permit construction of a tube without tension over a catheter. Incisions in the vaginal wall extended down to the bladder defect merging over the bladder neck. Bladder fistula closure and urethral reconstruction proceeded together inverting the bladder mucosa, and the bladder neck area was buttressed by Kelly-type sutures. Lawson (1978) advocated the Moir technique of urethral reconstruction.

Shirodkar (1960) offered a radical approach to the problem of urethral damage putting the patient into a plaster cast encasing the pelvis, but open anteriorly. Bilateral pubiotomy with upward reflection of the symphysis pubis exposed the entire urethral area, scar tissue was excised easily, and mobilizing the bladder neck, it was joined to the urethra. The bone flap was returned and fixed to adjacent bone by silver wire sutures passed through drill holes. He recommended median pubiotomy for all difficult vesico-vaginal fistulae.

Symmonds (1969) reiterated past conclusions stating that anatomical closure although successful, was not associated necessarily with restoration of urinary control, and believed that although bladder neck and urethral defects might appear extensive, actual tissue loss was much less due to retraction of undamaged urethral muscle. The muscle remnant could be identified as a red line distinct from pink vaginal epithelium and if that remnant could be fashioned into a urethra so urethral muscle could function once more, even though the urethra would be narrowed continence might be restored. He reported 20 patients and in all, three-quarters of the urethra had been destroyed associated with bladder neck and trigone defects. Four degrees of damage were recognized, and four principles of operative correction stated:

1. Adequate mobilization to allow tension-free closure of the new urethra.

2. Bladder neck plication with midline approximation of lateral tissues giving a second tension-free suture line.

3. Vaginal wall closure without tension using a labial skin and fat flap if necessary.

4. Second stage retro-pubic urethro-vesical suspension for persisting incontinence after successful closure.

A vaginal pack for 48 hours helped bed-down tissues minimizing hematoma, and open suprapubic cystotomy was the preferred method of urinary drainage. Symmonds (1978, 1984) again noted the problem of incontinence after successful closure, listing various tissues used to replace the urethra—ileum, appendix and Fallopian tube, and levator ani, pubococcygeus and gracilis muscles used in an attempt to produce a urethral sphincter. He favored urethral reconstruction from persisting urethral tissues with reinforcement and replacement of the anterior vaginal wall using a myocutaneous flap, and when required, retropubic bladder neck suspension to correct incontinence. Fifty patients, all with major urethral and bladder neck tissue deficit were reported, and underwent 74 operative procedures, including retropubic suspension in 20. Symmond's technique of closure and reconstruction was as follows:

1. A midline anterior wall incision was extended about the margins of the defect and carried laterally to allow adequate mobilization of the urethral remnant.

2. Wide bladder neck mobilization followed by insertion of sutures in the lateral tissues which when tied later in the procedure, reinforced urethral closure.

3. Urethra reformed about the catheter, followed by approximation of the lateral tissues, so burying the reconstruction (Figs. 113 a–c).

4. A Martius fat graft reinforced the repair then the vaginal epithelium

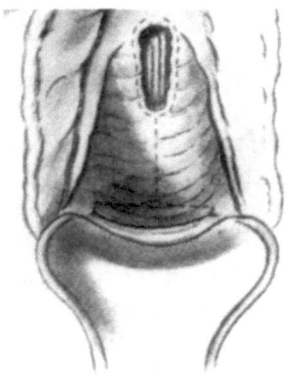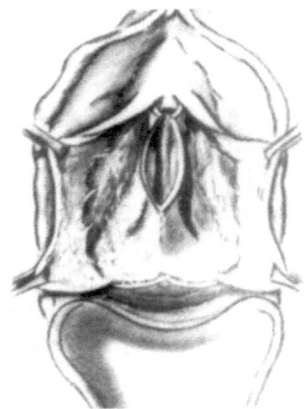

Figure 113 a. Tissue mobilization with urethral roof undermined sufficiently to permit tension-free closure.

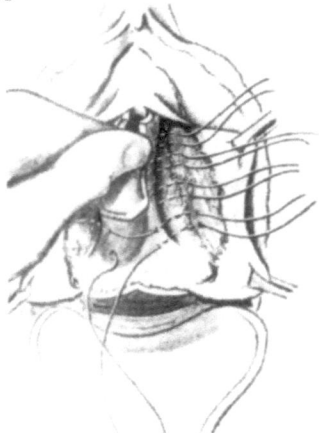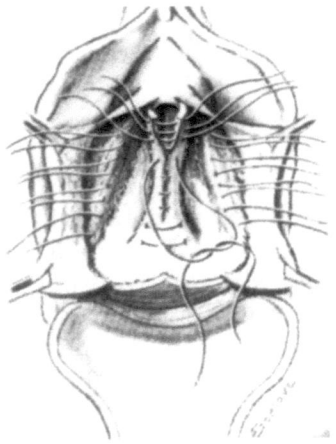

Figure 113 b. Urethral reconstruction followed by bladder neck plication

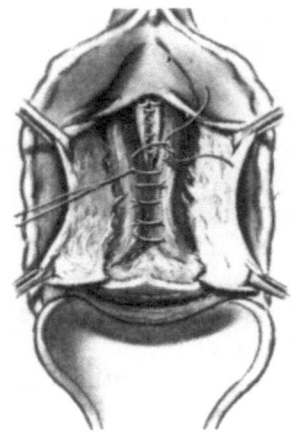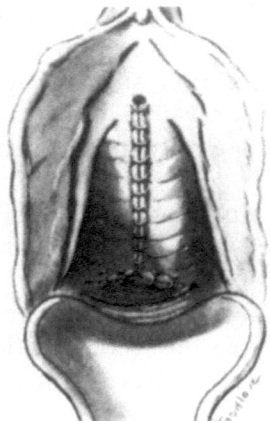

Figure 113 c. Bladder neck and urethral plication, then vaginal closure. (From Symmonds)

was closed; but should closure be difficult without tension, a myocutaneous fat graft was employed (Fig. 59). This graft supported the new urethra and allowed tension-free closure of the vaginal wall with the advantage of minimizing stenosis so allowing better subsequent vaginal function. The point was made with clarity that differentiation of urge and stress incontinence as relative components of postoperative incontinence, no matter what method of investigations was employed, was fraught with difficulty especially since many patients suffered both types of incontinence prior to the development of the fistula. Long-term (15 years) follow-up showed excellent results with 75% cured. Morgan et al. (1978) reported success in terms of closure and restoration of continence in eight of nine patients, using a synchronous-combined abdomino-vaginal approach. The principle involved were:

1. Urethral reconstruction from wide mobilization of vaginal tissue.
2. Improved blood supply and support from a Martius graft.
3. Marlex suburethral sling placed over the fat graft.
4. Labial skin flap where vaginal epithelium was deficient.

Tehan et al. (1980) dissatisfied with disappointing results from vaginal repair of an absent urethra, returned to the suprapubic bladder flap technique; but encountered complications of fistula recurrence, urethral shortening and retraction, reflux, calculi and even malignancy. Davis et al. (1980) and Webster et al. (1984) again emphasized the importance of the Martius graft in reinforcing the urethral repair, and the use of myocutaneous flaps for associated defects in the vaginal epithelium. They recommended the technique for all patients and àttributed improved continence to its use.

Hanash and Sieck (1983) described typical large obstetric fistulae with urethral loss in Saudi Arabia. They favored the use of an anterior bladder flap rolled into a tube and sutured to the distal urethral remnant to restore urethral continuity. An omental pedicle flap interposed between the neo-urethra and vagina completed the procedure. This one case was successful both in terms of reconstruction and continence, and followed a large series of failures using vaginal techniques alone. With more recent and increased experience, they were able to recommend the anterior bladder flap technique strongly for that select group of patients in whom a large circumferential vesico-vaginal fistula was associated with urethral loss.

Hamlin and Nicholson (1969), drawing on their extensive experience with difficult fistulae, described their technique for the reconstruction of the urethra totally destroyed in labor. Their detailed procedure included many contributions from earlier publications notably by Martius, Chassar

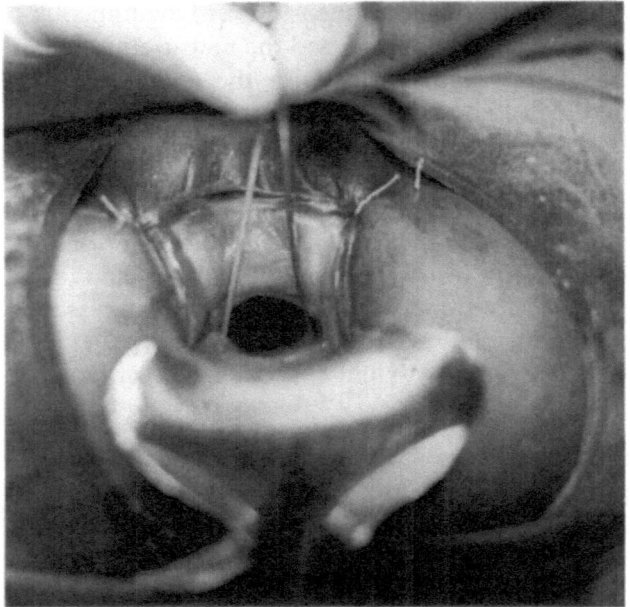

Figure 114. Complete urethral absence, ureteric catheters in place

Moir and Ingelman-Sundberg. The principles of closure for their type six, or difficult urinary fistula are as follows:

1. Lithotomy position with steep Trendelenburg tilt.

2. Postero-lateral introital incision to open the stenosed vagina.

3. The vesical defect was such that usually ureteric orifices could be identified easily and catheterized, but if not, then along with mobilization of tissues to be used in constructing the neo-urethra, bladder mobilization commenced laterally and centrally, avoiding the ureteric areas. The ureters were identified and catheterized.

4. Remains of the external urethral meatus were seen as two small epithelial elevations adherent anteriorly to the pubic bone, while the site of the absent urethra was marked by tough scar tissue which joined urethral remnants to the ischiopubic rami and the anterior edge of the bladder defect (Figs. 76 c,114).

5. Deep "para-urethral" incisions were made demarcating tissue to be used in forming the new urethra. Extending the incisions deeply allowed adequate mobilization of this tissue which was rolled over a Foley 12 catheter to form the new urethra (Fig. 115).

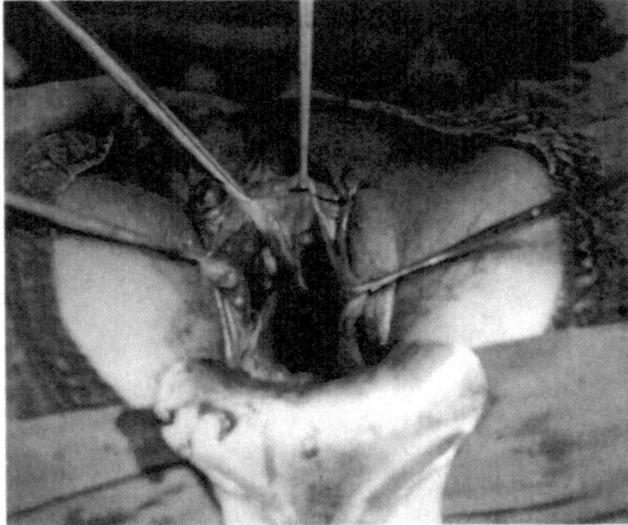

Figure 115. "Paraurethral" incision outlining new urethra

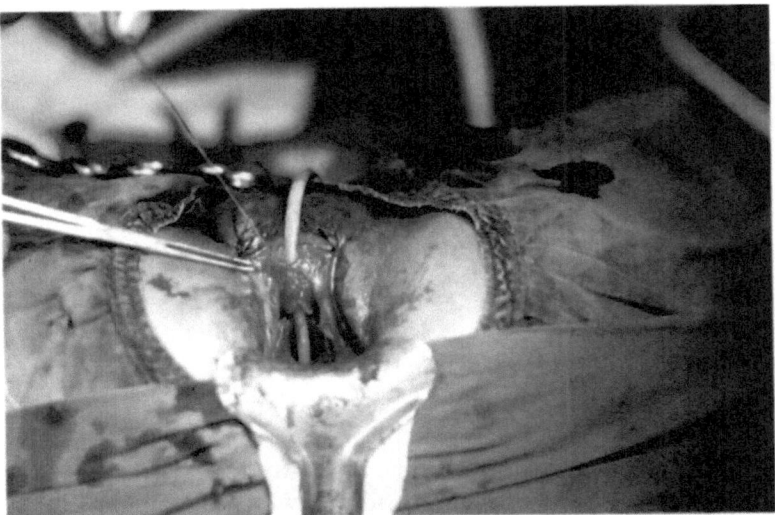

Figure 116 a

Figures 116 a, b. Urethral reconstruction

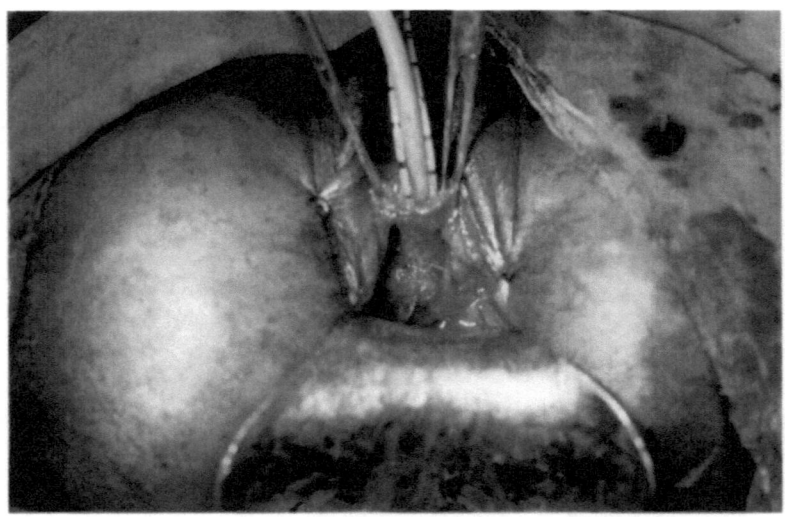

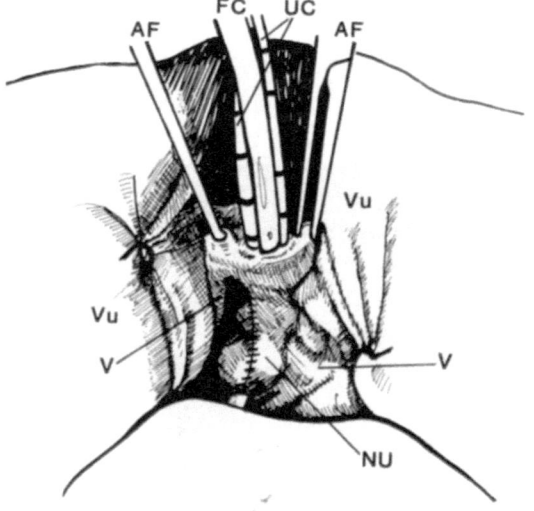

Figure 116 b

6. The bladder was mobilized widely with special attention given to bony adhesion.

7. Before beginning urethral closure, the Foley and two ureteric catheters were held in place against the new urethral roof whilst the first inverting suture of "00" chromic catgut was placed, then the urethral tube transmitting the three catheters was completed to the bladder defect with a series of mattress sutures—not too many, and not too tight. During urethral

reconstruction, the danger point at the urethro-vesical junction was reinforced with extra sutures, which drew bladder muscle over this junctional zone both to invert the join, and minimize the risk of later stress incontinence (Figs. 116 a, b).

8. The bladder was closed, rolling in the mucosa with the contained ureteric orifices and catheters—often the bladder defect because of its size was closed transversely and it was important to insert the anchor sutures which stabilized the bladder wall laterally, against the ischio-pubic rami. The closure then was tested with dye.

9. The repair was reinforced with a gracilis muscle graft and in some cases a Martius fat graft was also used. Passing the gracilis muscle beneath the labial tissues into the vagina was used first in this fashion in 1962. It was anchored to the anterior lip of the cervix and covered the new urethra and repaired bladder. When the Martius graft was used in addition, it lay between the gracilis muscle graft and the vaginal epithelium.

10. The anterior vaginal wall was closed if necessary using a labial flap graft, the incision of access in the introitus was repaired, and a firm vaginal pack inserted.

11. Postoperative management of packs and catheters followed details outlined already. In 1969, the Hamlins reported 50 cases of urethral reconstruction with good results apart from incontinence in 16%. Minor problems dealt with subsequently were residual pin-hole urethro-vaginal fistula and urethral stricture. Now in 1986, their series includes a very large number of patients, and their technique is the standard method for dealing with the problem of urethral destruction following obstructed labor.

Vesico-Cervico-Vaginal Fistula

Vesico-uterine fistula whether involving cervix or lower uterine segment is a complication of lower uterine segment Cesarian section or ruptured uterus. The ruptured lower segment may involve the bladder, its vitality already compromised by the prolonged obstruction. It is more likely in both instances, where there has been a pre-existing lower uterine segment scar present, due to adhesion between uterus and bladder at this site. Comparatively, it is a rare condition. Macknight (1962) could find only three cases in 30 years in a large obstetric institution. Fistula between bladder and uterus follows an unrecognized bladder perforation or inclusion of the bladder wall with the uterine closure, necrosis following the latter error, producing a communication in 7–10 days. The earliest sign of damage is hematuria, which settles gradually following catheter drainage, only to be followed some days later by a urine leak from the vagina, and examination with Sims speculum will show urine escaping through the cervix, and when menstruation is re-established monthly hematuria occurs. Lawson (1977) noted that fistulae following lower uterine segment Cesarian section, whilst commonly vesico-cervico-vaginal, might in fact open into the anterior vaginal fornix.

Three types of clinical presentation of such a fistula are recognized:

1. Amenorrhoea and cyclic hematuria—the "menouria" described by Youssef (1957).

2. Urinary leak through the cervix.

3. A combination of cyclic hematuria with urinary incontinence.

Variation in symptomatology depends upon the size of the communication and the mechanics of the situation. Macknight reported two of three vesico-uterine fistulae in which there was no vaginal leak of urine, only cyclic hematuria despite an obvious fistula and a patent cervical canal. In both patients the uterus was acutely retroflexed at the site of the fistula, and this was considered to permit easy passage forwards from uterus to bladder; but not in the reverse direction because of the acute angle at the cervix. It was suggested this angulation was produced by unopposed muscular action of the intact posterior uterine wall, for in both patients, the anterior wall gap measured one centimeter. Furthermore when the anterior deficiency was repaired, the uterus straightened and corrected the retroflexion.

Diagnosis:

The history and findings are typical—the past Cesarian section or uterine rupture, hematuria, vaginal urine leak and the demonstration of urine trickling through the cervix. Investigations may include:

(a) Injection of dye into the uterus via a Rubins cannula and its appearance in the bladder.

(b) Injection of dye into the bladder and its appearance in the vagina. Ward (1980) stated that in some utero-vaginal fistulae, it was necessary to apply traction to the cervix to observe leakage of the dye.

(c) Hysterogram.

(d) Cystoscopy—the common site is just behind the inter-ureteric bar and the usual features of fistula diagnosis must be sought.

(e) Cytological examination of urine may reveal endometrial cells.

Management

A) Prophylaxis

At repeat Cesesarian section, the surgeon should be aware of the problems of bladder mobilization and take adequate precautions. In particular the bladder should be freed by sharp dissection, putting the bladder on stretch with fine-toothed forceps. In addition to central bladder mobilization, lateral bladder mobilization also is important to avoid ureteric damage. Should the bladder be damaged inadvertently, the defect must be defined carefully and closed with a double layer of mucosal inverting "00" chromic catgut sutures. Postoperatively adequate bladder drainage and antibiotics usually will ensure success.

B) Conservative

Prolonged catheter drainage may be successful; but this can only be anticipated with small defects. If the fistula has not closed, then the catheter should be removed since its presence will not prevent incontinence, and prolonged use may damage the urethra. Graziotti et al. (1978) reported an unusual case of spontaneous healing with a vesico-uterine fistula following Cesesarian section after the diagnosis had been confirmed by a cervical urine leak, cystography and cystoscopy. Clearly the fistula must have been very small; but nonetheless they used this case to emphasize the importance of delay in intervention. Rubino (1980) reported two patients with cyclic hematuria and amenorrhea; but no urinary leak. In both, closure of the confirmed utero-vesical fistula was effected following induction of amenorrhea using continuous administration of an estrogen/progesterone combination for six months. These successes were attributed to cessation of menstruation which prevented the menstrual discharge flowing through the fistula, hence encouraging healing. Such a regime prior to thoughts of surgical intervention has a place in patiens with proven utero-vesical fistula without urinary leakage.

C) Operative

Choices of technique depend upon whether or not the uterus is to be retained.

    1. Should there be a valid reason for hysterectomy at the time of fistula repair, the easiest procedure is transperitoneal total abdominal hysterectomy, bladder mobilization and fistula identification. After adequate mobilisation the fistula is closed with a double layer of "00" chromic catgut suture inverting the mucosa.

    2. If the uterus is to be retained the choices are:

    (a) intraperitoneal approach separating uterus and bladder,

    (b) extraperitoneal cystotomy,

    (c) intraperitoneal cystotomy with bladder splitting.

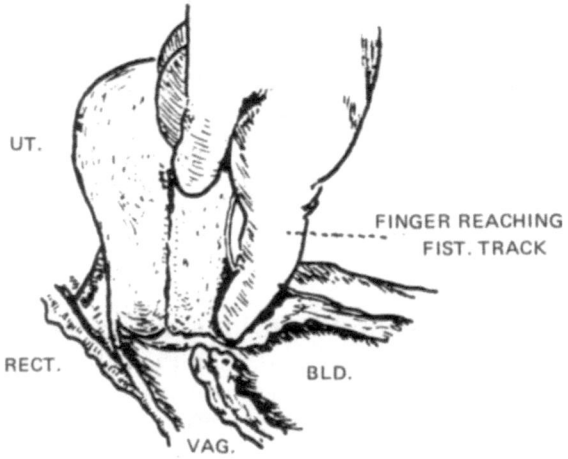

Figure 117. Intraperitoneal approach separating bladder and cervix. (From Foda)

(a) Intrapertioneal approach: Whilst avoiding bladder entry, this approach entails reopening the plane between bladder and uterus, exposing the communication between them and closing each defect separately (Fig. 117). Chassar Moir described this simple approach as a theoretical concept rather than a practical reality, for the bladder was densely adherent to the uterus and vagina, attempted separation might result in tearing of its wall and also the ureters were at considerable risk during dissection. Adequate closure also can be difficult due to the limited access. However, should such an approach be chosen, following wide mobilization of bladder from uterus, both defects are closed and the suture lines separated by using either a peritoneal or omental graft. Macknight facilitated separation of uterus and bladder by performing cystotomy and placing a finger inside the bladder against the fistula.

(b) Extraperitoneal cystotomy: Advocated by Lawson (1972) this approach offers several very real advantages. The adherent bladder and cervix are avoided and the ureters may be catheterized prior to fistula closure. The bladder and uterus are mobilized widely about the fistula and closed separately—the uterus with interrupted chromic catgut sutures and the bladder in two layers—the first in the muscle and the second to oppose the bladder mucosa so minimizing intravesical bleeding from the cut edges. Again however there is the problem of access especially with overweight patients and there can be technical difficulties gaining watertight closure.

(c) Intraperitoneal cystotomy with bladder splitting: This technique suggested originally by von Dittel (1893) and revived in 1914 by Legueu (Legueu 1929) offers excellent access to the fistula and permits accurate closure, which can be reinforced by omental grafting. In principle, the posterior bladder wall is split to the fistula site, allowing accurate identification of ureters and their catheterization if necessary, then the uterus and bladder are separated widely and closed independently. Additions to the technique include excision of the fistula track, bladder flap techniques to close the bladder defect and interposition of either peritoneum or omentum between bladder and uterus.

Postoperative care is the same with all techniques, the important principles being:

(i) continued catheter drainage using a Foley 12 catheter for at least 14 days—Ward (1980) commented that catheter blockage after transvesical fistula closure was common due to clumps of tissue debris, so careful catheter management in this group of patients was especially important,

(ii) appropriate antibiotics,

(iii) abdominal suction drainage to the site of bladder closure.

Association of Spontaneous Vesico-Vaginal Fistula with Recto-Vaginal Fistula

Technically it is more efficient to deal with the vesico-vaginal fistula first for should the recto-vaginal fistula be repaired first, vaginal access will be further restricted. A low recto-vaginal fistula can be closed subsequently once the vesico-vaginal fistula has been closed; but higher recto-vaginal fistulae and those with much tissue loss will require special grafting techniques and a preliminary colostomy to defunction the lower large bowel and rectum. The colostomy may be performed at the time of vesico-vaginal fistula closure.

Long-Term Management

It should be standard practice for any female cured of obstetric fistula never again to risk vaginal delivery and usually this ideal can be attained. At the Fistula Hospital Addis Ababa, cured patients are given a stout cardboard card with relevant details and told emphatically of the need for elective Cesesarian section in the next pregnancy, and asked to report to a health care center early in that pregnancy. Of the large number of successful patients managed by the Hamlins, more than 2,000 young women have had successful delivery in the next pregnancy. Believing as they do that a significant part of the pathological process was acute retention of urine, in selected cases, while they remained in charge of the obstetrical patients at Princess Tsahai Hospital, they delivered many vaginally without any fistula recurrence merely by keeping the bladder empty and following the course of labor with great skill and care.

Presently, with their time committed fully at the Fistula Hospital, they advise elective Cesarian setion for such women.

Complications

Early Complications

Important early complications are hemorrhage, ureteric obstruction, and failed healing with recurrence of urinary leakage. Hemorrhage should be controlled during the surgery and spill into the bladder minimized by suction. After bladder closure and the Martius graft in place, little dead space should remain and this is minimized further by a firm vaginal pack. Following abdominal closure of a fistula, hemorrhage into the bladder is more likely often occurring from the access incision into the bladder wall; but evacuation by reopening the bladder is required only rarely. Ureteric obstruction should be a rare accident for ureters are likely to be damaged only when a fistula is large and in such cases, ureteric identification before completing bladder mobilization, and then their catheterization, is absolutely essential. Ojo (1967) reported 34 ureteric injuries following obstetric and gynecological procdures and noted that in 50% of the patients, repair of high juxta-cervical or vesico-cervico-vaginal fistulae had been the primary procedure. It was reiterated that such fistulae were formidable and associated often with enormous destruction of vaginal and vesical tissues. In addition there was commonly poor access, excessive scarring and difficulty locating the ureteric orifices so without ureteric catheterization, even a most careful and experienced surgeon might injure the ureter. Ojo concluded "a careful preoperative appraisal of the urinary tract is necessary and in the repair of vesico-vaginal fistula, identification and catheterization of ureters is imperative.".

Breakdown of a fistula repair may follow an over-distended bladder and means mismanagement, the over-distension causing bleeding between layers of the repair with infection as a secondary phenomenon. Ward (1980) comments that patients who have had repair by the abdominal approach and patients who have had prolapse of the bladder mucosa, give most trouble postoperatively due to clumps of tissue debris blocking the catheter as a result of friction to the bladder mucosa. Failure to close the fistula may occur for a variety of reasons either technical or as a direct effect of poor postoperative managment. Once failure has occurred, reinsertion of the catheter to continue bladder drainage is worth trying; but unlikely to be successful except with tiny defects. After an initial 14 days drainage, a further 10–12 days might be useful; but if incontinence still occurs, the catheter should be removed. Most often the recurrence is much smaller than the original defect and with time will shrink even further; but if further reparative surgery is contemplated, a time lapse of 10–12 weeks is essential to allow proper tissue healing and scar contraction.

Late Complications

The most important late complication is recurrence of incontinence, careful evaluation being required to distinguish the true incontinence of fistula recurrence from stress incontinence and urge incontinence. Stress incontinence is more likely to be a post-fistula closure problem when the fistula involves the urethro-vesical junction. A preoperative tendency towards stress incontinence possibly would be masked by true incontinence produced by the fistula, then the scarring following fistula closure, draws the upper urethra away from its normal supports producing or accentuating the situation. Abdomino-perineal urethral suspension (Zacharin, 1983) has proven successful in such patients for suburethral dissection is not worth the risk, and the Marshall-Marchetti-Krantz procedure is much too unreliable. Parke Gray (1970) noted in all cases with residual stress incontinence, both bladder and vagina had been closed horizontally because of dense scarring at the fistula angles, and whilst there were patients without stress incontinence whose bladder had been closed horizontally, it was significant that when closure had been effected vertically, no patient developed stress incontinence. Total continence following fistula repair correlated with the location of the fistula, and to a lesser extent the degree of scarring, maximum incidence of stress incontinence following large fistulae involving the urethro-vesical junction. Hassim and Lucas (1974) believed their low incidence of postoperative stress incontinence followed a meticulous technique which combined the initial flap-splitting procedure to close the fistula with an appropriate operation for bladder neck reinforcement. Stress incontinence following fistula repair presented a formidable problem and all their cases had been associated with repair of fistulae involving bladder neck, so whenever possible they attempted fistula closure in the long axis of the vagina and reinforced the bladder neck (87 cases) either with a muscular fascial buttressing, a pubococcygeal sling, a Martius graft or a Hamlin-Nicholson gracilis graft, the latter graft being highly successful in 4 cases. With increasing experience, they advocated a combined technique—flap-splitting closure with bladder neck reinforcement—at the primary repair to reduce the incidence of stress incontinence.

True Incontinence

With large fistulae when combined with total or partial uethral loss, tissue deficit is great involving important sphincteric musculature and bladder wall. Simple closure even with bladder neck bolstering is most unlikely to restore continence control due to an inability to reconstitute sphincters, and the unavoidably low bladder capacity. For this reason many experienced fistula surgeons regard a huge bladder fistula with total urethral loss as inoperable, and advise ureteric transplantation. Undoubtedly the degree of continence may be greatly improved following successful closure of such a fistula, and might be aceptable to the patient in many societies as a very reasonable alternative to her former state, whilst avoiding the hazards of ureteric transplantation. Ward (1985) believes bladder drill is a vital part of postoperative management in patients with lowered bladder capacity, to minimize urgency and incontinence; but unfortunately this can be difficult and discouraging due to language problems, illiteracy and the lack of patient cooperation. Moir (1955) noted that no matter how long the fistula had been present, when the bladder was closed, bladder capacity returned to a reasonable level. However with underlying bladder damage, e.g. bilharzia (Hassim and Lucas 1974) the bladder capacity in such patients can be between 35–95 ml, with some showing radiological calcification of the bladder wall. Remodelling the urinary tract utilizing an isolated segment of bowel, offers obvious advantages over ureteric transplantation and they performed ilio-cystoplasty twice, and sigmoido-cystoplasty on five patients with pleasing results in terms of continence control in six of the seven patients.

Other Complications

Naidu (1963) reported on 40 women pregnant after fistula repair indicating that loss of tissue in some cases had an untoward influence on the course of pregnancy and the nature of labor, and routine vaginal examination enabled the nature of labor to be predicted. After very large fistula repair, shortening of the anterior vaginal wall was appreciated easily with the anterior cervical lip considerably distorted often as early as 30 weeks, and pulled toward the symphysis causing the cervix to gape as widely as 3 cm. Repeatedly such women could not recognize early labor symptoms and in some, experiencing painless labor, it was not surprising they could develop obstruction and fetal anoxia rapidly. He stressed the need for routine Cesarian section in all patients at 34–35 weeks when scar distortion was severe about the site of previous repair. Hamlin and Nicholson on the other hand, selected women pregnant after fistula closure who could be delivered safely by the vaginal route since already it had been shown in over 50% of such patients, the fistula might well have been prevented if the bladder had been kept empty. Careful hospital management of their patients, regular and careful assessment in labor and most importantly, keeping the bladder empty, enabled them to achieve a high rate of vaginal delivery.

Dick and Strover (1971) achieved satisfactory results with vaginoplasty using full thickness labial skin flaps in women with vaginal stenosis and severe dyspareunia or apareunia following repair of large vesico-vaginal fistulae. Simply dividing thick bands of scar tissue or repeated stretching did not help, and full thickness skin graft or flaps interposed between the divided fibrosed areas, meant contracture did not reform. They incised the scar at 4 o'clock and 8 o'clock, allowing it to fall backwards, then placed a full thickness flap of labia minora into the defects. The incisions were deepened to healthy muscle and widened producing large defects carefully protecting the rectum and the flaps were marked on the labia minora with the base of each of adequate width and situated level with the fourchette. The flap was sutured into position with interrupted atraumatic "000" chromic catgut, the donor area closed and a Foley catheter inserted (Figs. 118 a–c).

Evoh and Akinla (1978) reported 162 patients in whom a success rate of 91% with fistula closure was achieved; but after repair, the degree of integration into family and society depended not only on urinary continence, but how well she performed reproductively, the yard stick of success being measured by regular menstruation, satisfactory coitus and child-bearing. Sixty-six patients suffered secondary amenorrhea lasting four months to 15 years with menstruation returning in 38 women, within six months of repair. Thirty-one patients had 38 pregnancies, a majority being delivered by Cesarian section; but five had unplanned vaginal deliveries because they came too late into hospital presumably to avoid an operation. Kelly (1967) reported painless labor in many Nigerian women after a vesico-vaginal fistula believing pressure necrosis damaged the paracervical plexus so the patient would be unaware of the onset of labor and perhaps explain late attendance at hospital. Evoh and Akinla concluded that a combination of malnutrition, anemia, endometritis, psychological upsets and endocrine malfunction due to anterior pituitary necrosis were likely reasons for the

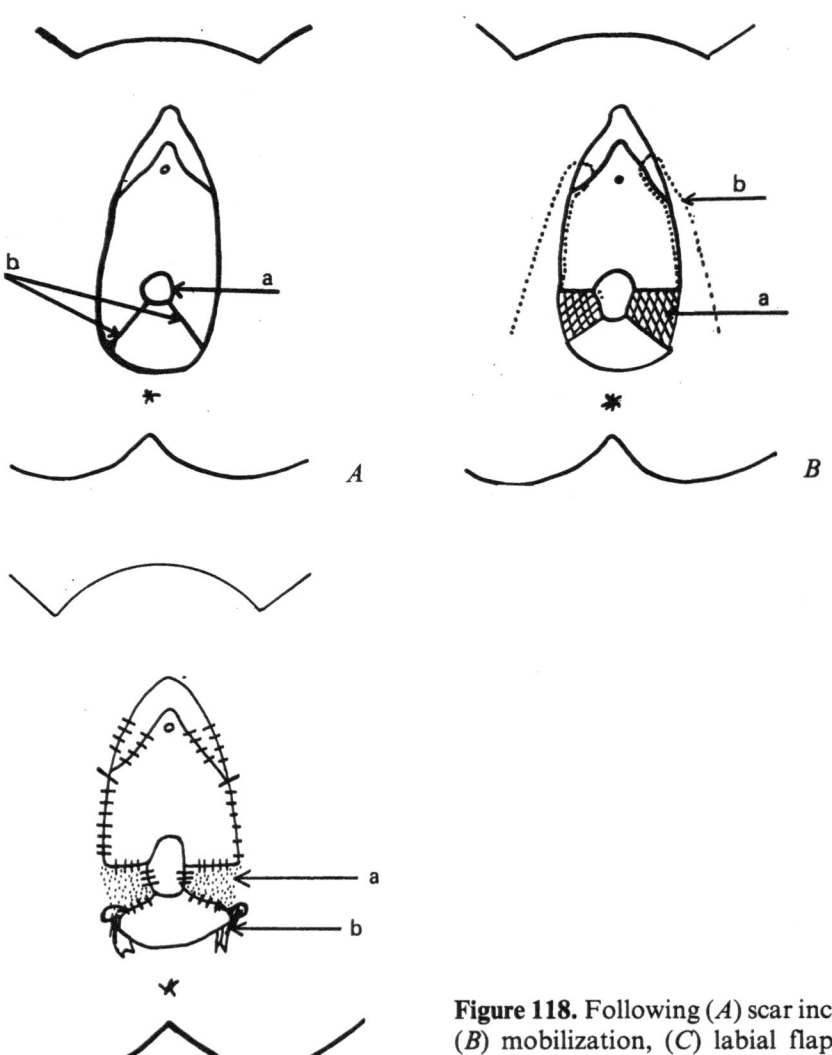

Figure 118. Following (*A*) scar incision and (*B*) mobilization, (*C*) labial flaps fill the defects. (From Dick and Strover)

high incidence of secondary amenorrhea, and advocated attempts to limit sepsis with antibiotics at the time the fistula occurred to minimize vaginal stenosis and hasten the resolution of endometritis. Bieler and Schnabel (1976) studied 11 patients with menstrual disorders dating from an obstructed prolonged labor which resulted in a vesico-vaginal fistula, and concluded that the disorders followed upset of different hypophyseotrophic areas of the hypothalamus.

8

Recto-Vaginal Fistula

Introduction

While the occurrence of recto-vaginal fistula due to an obstetric cause is less frequent than vesico-vaginal fistula, nevertheless those same factors which cause vesico-vaginal fistula are responsible for recto-vaginal fistula.

Etiology

Pressure necrosis caused by long continued impaction of the presenting part accounts for the majority of urinary fistulae, yet less often causes fecal fistula. This apparent anomaly occurs because the sigmoid colon enters the pelvis but evades pressure by passing over the pelvic brim related to the left sacro-iliac joint, not the promontory. Rectal fistulae are classified best as superior and inferior, the superior fistula involving the upper half of the vagina at or near the vault, while the inferior lies in the lower half. On rare occasions a superior fistula is produced by pressure necrosis; but in such females always there is associated a marked pelvic contraction with irregularity of the inlet and a long period of impaction. More usual is a large third degree defect involving the posterior vaginal wall and extending to the cervix following difficult forceps delivery or efforts at embryotomy (Fig. 119).

Inferior recto-vaginal fistula, the common type, follows perineal rupture at the time of delivery, a tear extending through the vaginal wall and perineal body into the anal canal, splitting the external anal sphincter. In some patients with a lesser degree of damage, a lower vaginal split can extend and involve the anal canal associated with marked bruising of the external anal sphincter, yet without its disruption. Third degree tear is more common with large babies, posterior position of the occiput, rapid or precipitate delivery, and forceps delivery with a small episiotomy. A sudden push or pull can extend a small episiotomy quickly, and involve anal sphincter and anal canal. In some countries, vulvo-vaginal trauma of tra-

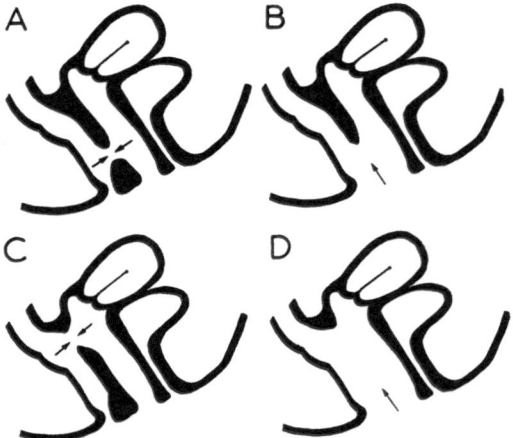

Figure 119. Sites of recto-vaginal defects (*A*) low fistula (*B*) third degree tear (*C*) high fistula (*D*) massive third degree tear. (From Lawson)

ditional origin—female circumcision of Pharaonic type and insertion of caustics—produces marked stenosis of the lower genital tract due to introital and vaginal wall fibrosis. Such tissues are more likely to damage during delivery, and in the Sudan it is usual for anterior episiotomy to be required in addition to large para-rectal episiotomy. Even with such a safeguard, the patient pushing suddenly to deliver the fetal head, may split the scarred tissues and tear the anal canal. After delivery in the Sudan, patients usually demand restoration of the introital tightness. While a majority of rectal damage in obstetrics is third degree tear and relatively easily corrected, high recto-vaginal fistula opening into the posterior fornix is a vastly different problem. When rectal fistula occurs combined with bladder fistula, the general view accepts that the bladder defect should be repaired first, since preliminary posterior repair would narrow the vagina limiting access to the anterior vaginal wall. Lawson (1978) advised that bladder fistula should be dealt with first to gain the best chance of success, then the rectal defect could be repaired about a month later providing examination under anesthesia showed the bladder fistula healed. If this were not so, further bladder surgery could be attempted in three months, however until the bladder fistula was corrected, rectal repair should be deferred. As mentioned already, it is the usual practice at the Fistula Hospital, Addis Ababa to close both fistulae at the one operation.

Clinical Features

Common symptoms produced by low recto-vaginal fistula or third degree tear are incontinence of flatus and/or feces, with the problem worsening during episodes of diarrhea. Since the fistula lies below the puborectalis sling, solid faeces usually are retained.

A third degree tear sustained some years previously may cause minor incontinence problems although accentuated by diarrhoea, so often the condition remains uncorrected. However, with advancing years and diminishing levator efficiency, the situation deteriorates and help is sought.

The size of the defect usually determines the degree of incontinence, and in an unsophistocated community, patients may seek help only because of difficulty with bowel evacuation should a rectal stricture be present above the fistula site (Hudson 1970). On the other hand, high vault fistula lies above levator ani so persistent fecal loss occurs.

Diagnosis

Large recto-vaginal fistula and third degree tear are easy visual diagnoses. With division of the external anal sphincter, the cessation of anal skin rugae due to the corrugator cutis ani muscle marks the ends of the retracted sphincter. Restoration of the "anal crinkle" signifies adequate sphincter reconstruction has been achieved. Smaller fistulae above an intact sphincter must be sought carefully, for usually they lie in scar tissue at or just above the fourchette, the scar resulting from obstetric damage or previous attempts at surgical repair. Palpation of the recto-vaginal septum between an index finger in the rectum and the thumb in the vagina often pin-points a defect, and all such suspicious folds and depressions, or areas showing loss of mucosal mobility must be probed from the vaginal side. Passage of the probe into the anal confirms the track; but great care must be exercised not to push the probe through a thinned and scarred yet intact recto-vaginal septum. Occasionally the use of rectal dye or an opaque enema may help, or even filling the vagina with radio-opaque fluid might demonstrate a track.

Management

Prophylaxis

Prevention entails careful antenatal screening of patients to remove those in whom obstructed labor is likely. Following third degree tear at delivery, immediate surgical correction is required, ideally not in the labor ward; but under proper operating theater conditions. Under anesthesia the tear is defined and hemostasis secured. The anal canal rent is repaired by continuous "00" chromic catgut suture beginning above the defect, continuing to the anal verge, locking and returning, so a double layer closure is effected. Closure should invert the anal mucosa and the stitch does not enter the bowel lumen. The ends of the external sphincter are picked up with Allis forceps and approximated in the midline with "0" "Vicryl to produce a lumen sufficient to admit the little finger. The vaginal wall is reconstituted with "00" chromic catgut as a running locking suture to the fourchette, and the perineal wound closed with horizontal mattress sutures. A short penrose drain is placed between vagina and anal canal for 48 hours. Postoperative care must include appropriate antibiotics and bowel confinement. Should primary closure fail and fistula result, no further surgery should be considered until tissues have healed and scar contraction ceased. As with vesico-vaginal fistula, this time rarely can be less than eight to ten weeks, and for the same reasons earlier intervention is fraught with risk.

Surgical Correction

Perineal Approach

As might be expected, the history of attempts to close recto-vaginal fistula has paralleled closely that of vesico-vaginal fistula, but in the main there are two specific difficulties associated with recto-vaginal fistula which have been the major problems, namely dealing with the fecal stream and with flatus. Early on, attempts to correct recto-vaginal fistula were confined to the superficial type lying below the external sphincter and consisted of splitting the fistula and cauterizing the base. Successes encouraged surgeons to extend the practice to fistulae above the sphincter splitting the perineum vertically to the level of the fistula, and allowing the wound to heal by granulation. So began the era of modern surgery converting a recto-vaginal fistula to a complete tear. Guillemeau, a student and contemporary of Ambrose Pare (1510–1590) probably was first to attempt surgical union of a completely ruptured perineum and later Mauriceau (1637–1709) and Smellie (1697–1763) recommended operation and suturing; but there was no evidence to show they ever performed restoration by this method. General acceptance of suturing was inevitable but slow. Nicolas Sebastian Saucerotte (1798) attempted repair of a recto-vaginal fistula three and a half months after it had occurred, and Titius (1794) gave a case report of recto-vaginal fistula. Nadel (1801) described freshening and approximating the edges of perineal rupture, and also recommended fat and oil applications with soft massaging to make the perineum more yielding and less likely to tear. Wendelstadt (1803) described cleansing the wound and tying the legs together; but because of exhaustion from sleeplessness and constant irritation due to diarrhoea, the legs had to be loosened and the form of treatment abandoned. Later he pared the edges of the wound and approximated them with strong wax thread. Even as late as 1840, Payan, Paris recommended confinement to bed for six weeks with the patient kept on her side and the legs tied together. Isolated reports in which the recto-vaginal fistula was converted to a complete tear to be dealt with a later period, were given by Ricord (1841), France, Baker Brown (1864), England and Simon (1867), Germany; but complete control of feces and gas after such surgery seldom wa attained (Figs. 120 a–c). However better results occurred with the adoption of Lawson Tait's technique of complete perineorrhaphy which corrected fistulae just above the sphincter; but when the fistula was situated at a distance from the perineum, dividing the sphincter caused more harm than good, and accordingly attempts to close such fistulae were made in a different manner and the flap-splitting procedure employed in the cure of vesico-vaginal fistula, was adopted. The rectal and vaginal walls were separated one from the other by dissection, and united separately by two layers of sutures. Sanger (1888) modified the technique further by suturing the mucus membrane of the rectum with a third and additional layer of interrupted sutures applied from inside the rectum after gradual dilatation of the sphincter. He used Chinese silk in preference to catgut which was considered unsafe because of too rapid absorption. Warren (1882) described a new procedure performed first in 1878 and intended chiefly for the most serious cases of perineal rupture where the sphincter muscle and also part of the anterior rectal wall had been damaged (Fig. 121 a). He believed the weak point of each previous operation lay in management of the rectal wound and emphasized that the perineal body was situated not in front of the rectum; but formed the floor of the cavity, which at that point took a sudden curve backward to reach the anal orifice. So a freshly united linear rectal wound at that point would present itself at right angles to the rectal axis, and sustain the full force of

---

Historical references are taken mainly from:

    1. Mahfouz (1934) "A new technique in dealing with superior recto-vaginal fistulae."

    2. Miller and Brown (1937) "The surgical treatment of complete perineal tears in the female."

    3. Eden (1914) "A case of superior recto-vaginal fistula dealt with by the abdominal route after preliminary colostomy."

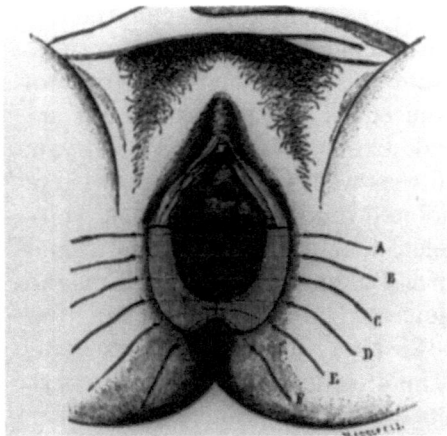

Figure 120 a

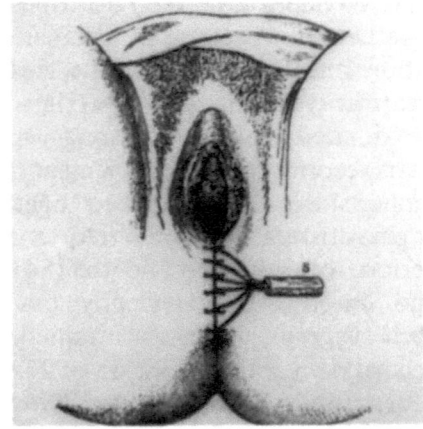

Figure 120 b

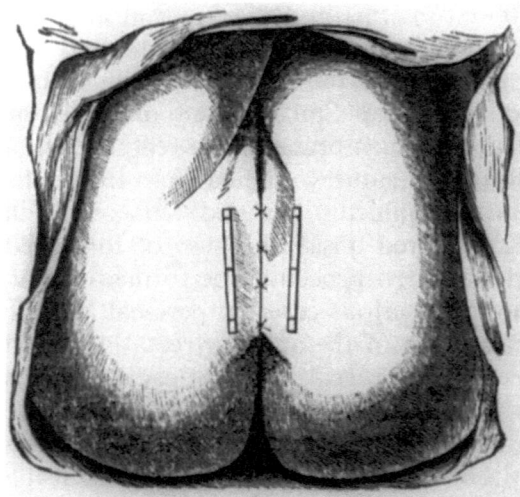

Figure 120 c

Figures 120 a–c. Early attempts at perineal repair. (From Miller and Willis-Brown)

a column of gas or bowel content coming from above. If the rectal wound were long and the perineal body not thick, the point of least resistance would be in the direction of the vagina and recto-vaginal fistula may result. He believed Emmet, who had done more than any other surgeon to date to place this operation on its present comparatively firm basis, sought to overcome the danger by drawing down the edge of the recto-vaginal septum

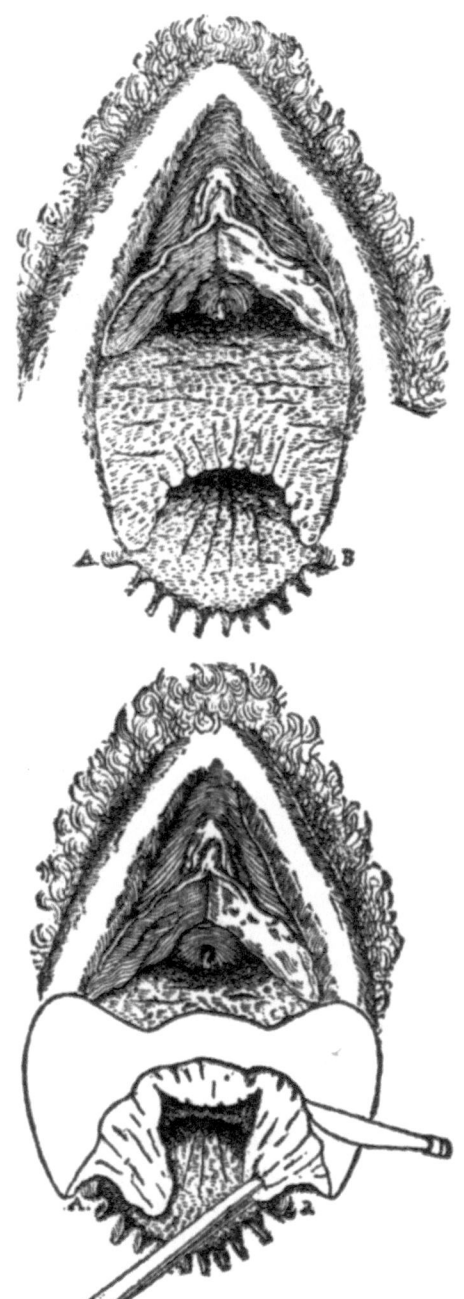

Figure 121 a. Warren's third degree tear—the posterior rectal wall displayed between (*A*) and (*B*)

Figure 121 b. Butterfly flap of "vaginal and vulvar mucous membrane"

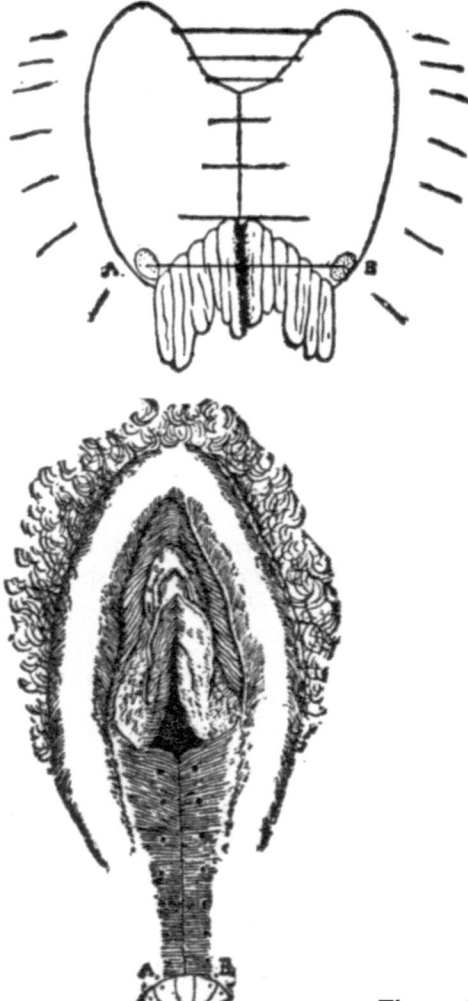

Figure 121 c. Flap fully developed with exposure of the ends of the ruptured sphincter

Figure 121 d. Sphincter reconstituted over the flap. (From Warren)

to the sphincter muscle, and do away with a rectal wound as completely as possible. However tension of the recto-vaginal septum under these conditions was increased greatly, so the rectal wall could retract leaving an open wound in the rectum. Warren's contribution was "to shut the rectum out entirely, using a flap so it could no longer enter as an element to be considered in the healing process". He devised a butterfly incision to elevate a flap of vaginal and vulval mucous membrane, including a certain amount of cicatricial tissue found at the margin of the rent. The flap was elevated in a continuous mass carefully avoiding a button-hole (Fig. 121 b). At the sides, dissection was carried down sufficiently to expose the ends of the ruptured sphincter muscle, and the flap hung downward, becoming portion of and continuous with the anterior rectal mucus membrane (Fig. 121 c). The bowel terminated in a sort of fimbriated extremity, and twisting the first sphincter stitch pulled the divided ends together over it. After remaining stitches had been inserted, the flap projected at the anterior margin of the anus, and if the portion of flap projecting was unnecessarily long, it could be trimmed and the raw edges sewn together apearing as a small hemorrhoid (Fig. 121 d). In the after treatment, a special diet was emphasized in which milk was rigidly excluded to avoid a large accumulation of feces, and this regimen began the day before operation and for the first 24 hours following, when little else other than cracked ice and small doses of beef fluid extract were given, avoiding discomforts and dangers of flatus. Principles of the procedure were "restoration of the recto-vaginal septum by a flap doing away with the rectal wound, and selection of an appropriate diet so the character of fecal discharges could be controlled". Fritsch (1888) and Le Dentu (1890) suggested dissecting a flap of vaginal tissue from below the fistula, then carrying it beyond the upper edge after which the fistula was freed on all sides and closed; but on the whole results were unsatisfactory. Emmet (1868), following surgery for lacerated perineum, indicated that "it was customary and following the practice of Dr. Sims to always retain in the rectum, a straight catheter tube about four inches in length with a view of allowing flatus to have a free escape".

The next attempts to gain access to the fistula adopted the incision used by Lawson Tait, although the perineum was split transversely using a crescentic incision sited midway between anus and vulva, and vaginal wall was separated from rectum by carrying the dissection well above the upper limit of the fistula, so both fistulous openings could be sutured separately, and the perineum reconstructed. Extensive operations have been performed by the perineal route, and even with fistulae situated in the middle third of the vagina, free access can be obtained through a transverse crescentic incision midway between vulva and anus. By displacing peritoneum upward, the anterior and lateral aspects of the rectum can be freed almost to any required height without opening the peritoneal sac, and a point of great practical importance was to carry the dissection well above the level of the fistula, so the edges might be brought together without tension. An important modification to the perineal operation was introduced by Segond (1895) Paris, and although similar procedures were being performed independently by van Noorden (1895), Munich, Dudley (1902), New York and Legueu (1903), Paris, Segond's case presented several interesting features. Aged 31 years and married, when 15 years old she and an older girl each had introduced an ointment pot into the vagina. The elder girl became ill and died of peritonitis, whilst the younger initially suffered a great deal of pain, but married four years later. Ultimately when the foreign body was discovered embedded in the posterior vaginal wall, it was removed with great difficulty since a mass of granulation tissue had filled the cavity of the pot, and after removal, the posterior fornix opened directly into the rectum. Operation consisted in excising the lower rectum including the fistula, then stitching the cut edge of the upper segment to the skin of the anal margin. The aperture in the posterior vaginal wall was closed by catgut sutures with a perfectly satisfactory final result. Legueu recommended splitting the detached vaginal wall in the middle line up to the fistula to gain additional access at the deeper level. Dudley (1902) modified the Segond procedure, "in my judgement in a case of high fistula it would not be necessary to resect to the level of the fistula, but only such portion of the bowel as would be sufficient to change the position of the rectal opening with that of the vaginal, so as to flap each fistulous membrane against unbroken structure, and then sewing the parts carefully together with whatever suture you deem best suited to the occasion." Von Herff (1907) modified Dudley's technique even further by freeing the rectum in front and at the sides; but not posteriorly until the level of the fistula had been passed. For the fistula situated high in the vaginal vault involving the cervix and the pouch of Douglas, it was almost impossible to adopt the foregoing techniques since freeing the lower sigmoid from the pelvic peritoneum was extremely difficult if not impossible, and moreover the blood supply of the rectal tube was uncertain. Nearly all writers deprecated opening the peritoneal cavity when dealing with recto-vaginal fistula; but Freund (1902) published the following interesting operation: He opened the posterior fornix and retroverted the uterine body completely into the vagina, then stitched the uterus to the freshened edges of a large fistula in the posterior vaginal wall. The procedure concluded by making a permanent opening into the uterine fundus to allow menstrual fluid to escape into the vagina, and gradually the uterus atrophied to assume the characters of vaginal mucus membrane. He advised the operation should be restricted to elderly women past the climacteric, and even then should any other procedure be practicable, it should be done in preference.

Abdominal Approach

Whilst correction of third degree tear was now reasonably standard, problems of the superior fistula remained unsolved. Simon (1867) reported a case in which the anterior lip of the cervix was sutured to the lower pole of the fistula after denuding their mucus membranes, so the external os opened into the rectal cavity; but not surprisingly the operation received little support. Eden (1914) made an historic departure in the management of superior recto-vaginal fistula in a patient with an inaccessible fistula involving the posterior cervical lip. Examination showed an aperture in the posterior fornix through which two finger tips could be passed and when exposed with the speculum, only the anterior cervical wall was present. The posterior wall was absent, replaced by a large aperture opening into the rectum and because of its size and position and the certain difficulty of accurate suturing, Eden decided upon preliminary colostomy believing with so large a fistula, healing would be aided if the fecal stream were diverted. Later a rectal bougie was passed above the fistula to aid identification, then the abdomen was opened through a paramedian incision. The floor of the pouch of Douglas was obscured by extensive adhesions uniting rectum to cervix and vagina; but the upper third of the rectum was free. Following hysterectomy, the next step was separation of rectum from cervix above the fistula, which required time and patience. When the upper fistula margin had been laid open, the lower margin was dealt with by separating rectum from vagina below the level of the fistula with scissors and finger, then cutting through the intervening bridge of tissue to leave most of the scar tissue attached to the vagina (Fig. 122). The rectal wall was now free about one inch below the fistula. Interrupted thread sutures taking all layers were introduced so the scar in the rectum was transverse. The vagina was divided at each side to form a flap of the posterior wall, and this was stitched to the rectal wall over the fistula, covering it completely. The vagina was left open and the anterior peritoneal flap brought over and sewn to rectum and peritoneum on each side, completely covering the pelvic floor with peritoneum. Eden found mention of only one previous case in which an abdominal operation had been undertaken for recto-vaginal fistula and even this was not recorded in full, but mentioned in a case discussion by Legueu (1903) and described in only a few words as "union with two layers of silk suture; closure of the abdomen without drainage and recovery of the patient". Eden could not find any case recorded in the literature in which preliminary colostomy had been performed, and decided on an abdominal approach because of the unusually

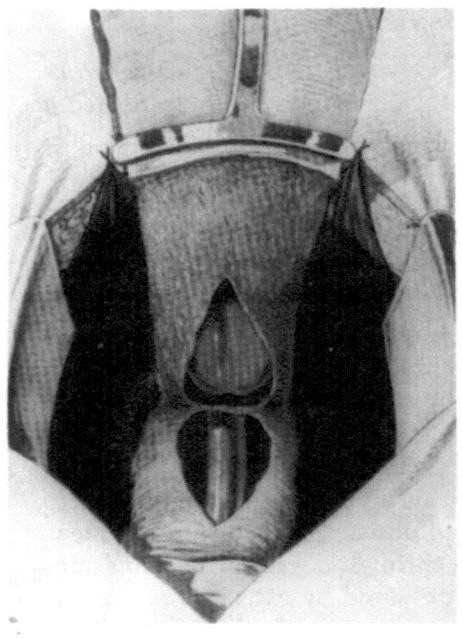

Figure 122. Separation of rectum from vagina below the level of the fistula—rectal bougie in situ. (From Eden)

high level of the fistula and complete immobilization of the cervix which formed its upper border. He did not believe fears of former writers regarding septic complications were justified in view of favorable results of intestinal surgery at that time, and also it was comparatively easy to isolate the pelvic cavity from the upper abdomen during surgery and drain it efficiently afterwards. Preliminary colostomy was of greatest importance, with clear advantages allowing the operation area to be prepared by irrigation, the bowel rested following surgery minimizing risk of reinfection, and finally the absence of flatus and feces favored wound healing. Unaware of Eden's technique, Mahfouz (1929) adopted the transperitoneal abdominal route in dealing with an inaccessible fecal fistula of the vault, when he found it impossible to close the fistula by the vaginal route. Preliminary colostomy was not used, the uterus was drawn up to the wound and the rectum and uterus separated so that the rent in the rectum could be closed in two layers, whilst the vaginal tear was left open to allow for drainage. The wound healed by first intention and recovery was uneventful. It occurred to Mahfouz that the difficulty in dealing with such fistulae by the vaginal route could be overcome to a great extent if the peritoneum was opened in the posterior vaginal fornix as a preliminary step. Separating the upper edge of the fistula from the cervix beginning at the sides where the tissues

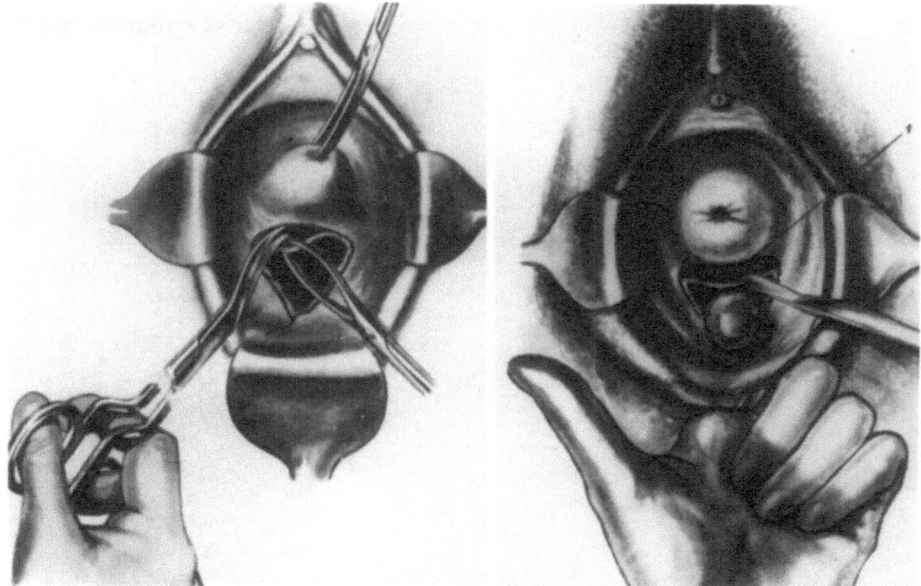

Figure 123 a   **Figure 123 b**

Figure 123 a. Fistula mobilized from cervix and peritoneum opened
Figure 123 b. Finger in rectum exerting traction on the fistula

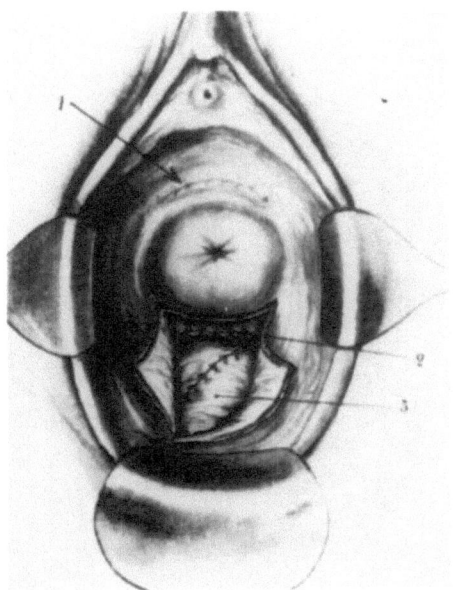

Figure 123 c. Closure of Peritoneum and rectal defect (*2*) and (*3*). (*1*) shows a
previously healed vesico-vaginal fistula. (From Mahfouz)

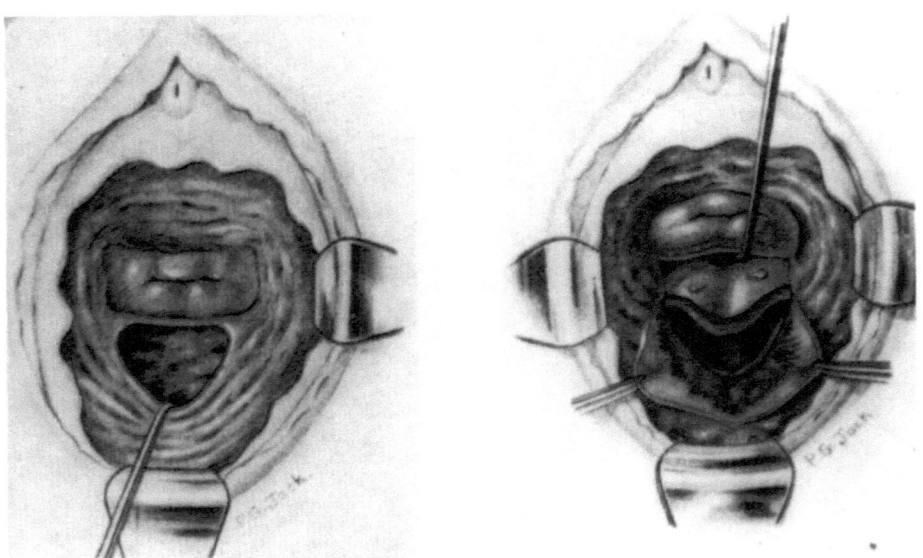

Figure 124 a. High recto-vaginal fistula accessible after traction on the posterior margin. Pouch of Douglas opened mobilizing upper fistula margin

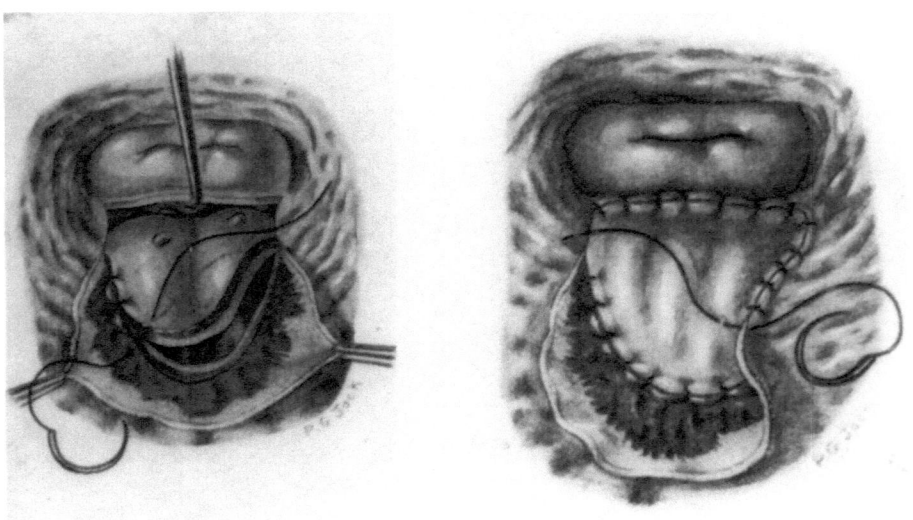

Figure 124 b. Rectal defect repaired, and rectal wall above the closure sutured to the cervix. (From Lawson)

were found to be more mobile the peritoneal cavity was then opened deliberately (Fig. 123 a). Following this step, the liberated upper edge of the fistula could be drawn sufficiently low to complete separation of the tissues with much more ease. Additional help was gained inserting a finger into the rectum hooking down the lower edge (Fig. 123 b). Finally, protecting the peritoneal cavity with a gauze pack, the rectum was separated from vagina on the lateral and inferior aspects, and it was Mahfouz who emphasized how much easier it was to gain wide rectal mobilization, than to mobilize a bladder with a vesico-vaginal fistula. In addition, once freed from the scarred vagina, the soft and yielding rectum was easily closed without tension (Fig. 123 c).

Opening the pouch of Douglas to facilitate fistula surgery was described first by Howard Kelly (1902) and initially used to aid separation of the bladder on all sides before attempting closure of a large vesico-vaginal fistula. The technique was applicable with even greater satisfaction to recto-vaginal fistula situated high in the vagina, and if the cul-de-sac was opened widely behind the cervix from side to side and down the sides of the rectum, a great advantage of increased bowel mobility was gained, including the area above the fistula which could then be turned in by sutures to cover the upper angle of the opening. Kelly closed the bowel with fine silk sutures in one or two layers but not the vaginal wound, putting an iodoform gauze drain between the edges of the vaginal opening, allowing the wound to close by granulation. In addition an opening was left in the peritoneum wide enough to admit a small iodoform drain. Lawson (1977) modified this transperitoneal technique by deliberately suturing the rectum to the back of the cervix so the serous rectal coat formed a new posterior fornix (Figs. 124 a, b).

Development of Surgical Techniques

A. Layered Repair

Miller and Brown (1937) reported 182, third degree tears, indicating that most had been repaired by the flap procedure described initially by Warren (1882) and later by Noble (1902). Preoperative treatment included castor oil daily for three days prior to surgery, an enema on the day prior to operation and again on the morning of operation, repeated until the return was clear with finally a low residue diet begun three days before surgery. This treatment represented efforts to minimize dangers of infection, and reduce bowel peristalsis during convalescence. An important feature of the surgery was subcutaneous sphincter division in the posterior quadrant,

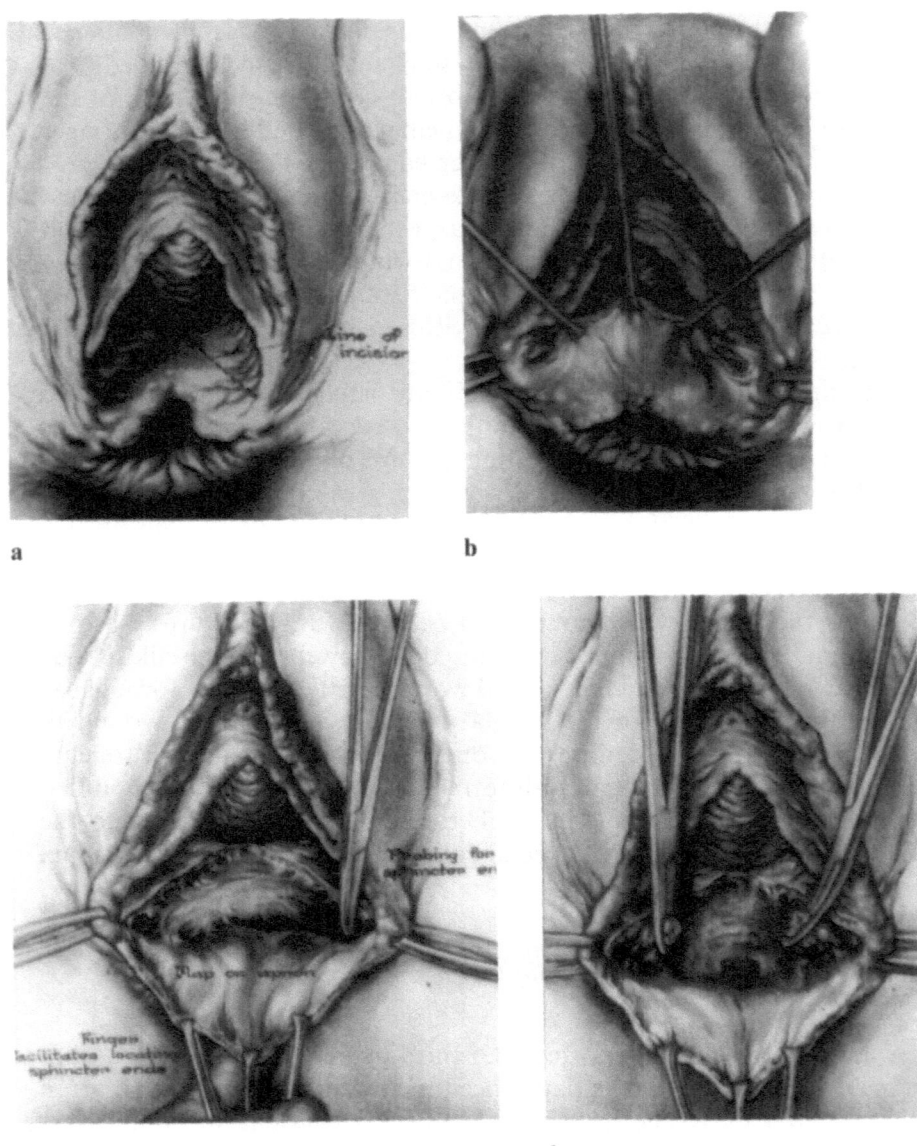

a

b

c

d

Figure 125 a–g. a Incision defined. — **b** Flap elevated. — **c** Flap completed. — **d** Sphincter ends identified.
— **e, f** Sphincter reconstitution associated with — **g** Subcutaneous sphincter division. (From Miller and Willis-Brown)

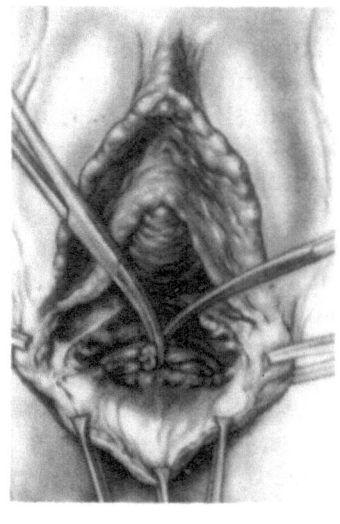

e

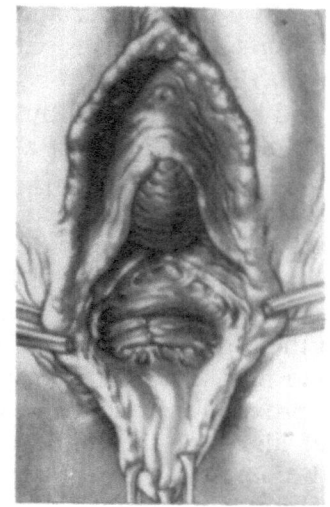

f

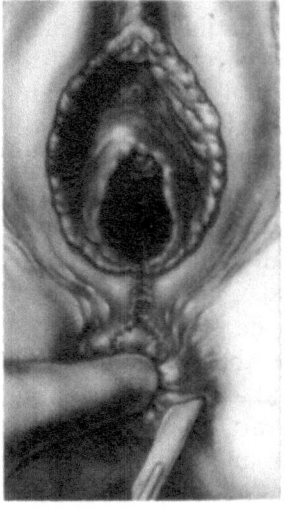

g

following reunion of a divided sphincter anteriorly, and if any difficulty was noted approximating sphincter ends, early cutting of the sphincter facilitated the procedure (Figs. 125 a–g). They pointed out this technique of sphincter division had been performed by Saucerotte (1798) and again by Baker Brown (1860). Saucerotte and his assistants Castera and Rousel (1798) were confronted by a patient 40 days postpartum, who demanded something be done for unbearable fecal incontinence. "Posture and other traditional remedies had proved valueless and a first fruitless attempt with the then almost unheard of suture method had failed. Impelled by the undaunted spirit of their patient these courageous pioneers again undertook repair but this time at the suggestion of one of the assistants, the sphincter was divided in order to release tension. There followed days of anxious waiting needless as it proved for the patient was cured." Saucerotte and his assistants were far ahead of their time, and the real value of their contribution did not become known until popularized by such illustrious men as Baker Brown who attributed much of his success in 75 cases reported in 1860, to the practice of cutting the sphincter (Miller and Brown 1937).

Shirodkar (1960) concerned with management of combined vesico-vagina and recto-vaginal fistulae, often found it impossible to repair the bladder fistula because of its position, extent and surrounding scar tissue, and also impossible to perform ureteric transplantation because of a recto-vaginal fistula irreparable by known methods. Accordingly, he devised an operation for this condition and three weeks after preliminary colostomy, the coccyx was removed exposing the posterior rectal wall which was incised to reveal the fistula in the anterior wall. Now the rectal wall could be mobilized sufficiently all around the fistula, and the fistula closed followed by closure of the posterior wall. When the posterior wall had healed firmly, the colostomy was closed and the ureters transplanted.

Fistulae in the middle third of the vagina may be treated without sphincter division, incising the vagina in the midline, then extending an inch above and below the fistula. Separation of vaginal and rectal walls is followed by closure of both defects. Lescher and Pratt (1967) believed principles of cure for simple recto-vaginal fistula were removal of the entire track, then maximum strength repair without tension. With any doubt in diagnosis, proctoscopic examination was performed and methylene blue injected into the rectum after a pack had been applied to the recto-vaginal septum. Preoperative colon preparation was employed, the track was demonstrated by passing curved forceps into the anal canal and out through the fistula, then the fistula edges and vagina were grasped by Allis forceps and a long elliptical incision made around the fistula. Vaginal and rectal walls were mobilized, care being taken to remove enough rectal wall about the fistulous track to eliminate dense scar tissue, yet conserve as much tissue as possible enabling closure without tension. Although this seems a contradiction in terms, generally speaking when there was any doubt, they suggested that the more tissue removed, the better! Given (1970) reported 38 cases treated by converting the fistula to a third degree tear then excision of the fistula edges using a sphincterotomy incision recommended by many surgeons including Telinde, to enhance success of recto-vaginal fistula repair.

B. Rectal Wall Advancement

In 1902, G. H. Noble described, "a new operation for complete laceration of the perineum designed for the purpose of eliminating danger of infection from the rectum." The procedure consisted of "splitting the recto-vaginal septum, mobilizing the lower end of the rectum from the vagina and drawing the anterior wall down and through the anus". Mengert and Fish (1955) rediscovered the procedure and reported results of its use in 26 patients with complete perineal laceration, and 9 with recto-vaginal fistula. The technique was termed anterior rectal wall advancement. Preoperative care included a low residue diet for two or three days, and bowel preparation with antibiotics and cleansing enemas. Rectum and vagina were separated to the level of the cervix avoiding wide lateral mobilization to minimize bleeding, and once accomplished, the anterior rectal wall would stretch easily and without tension outside the torn sphincter, lengthening the anterior portion of the rectal tube and eliminating a suture line in the rectum. After reuniting the divided sphincter, the perineal body was reformed and excess vaginal mucosa excised (Fig. 126). Gallagher and Scarborough (1962) indicated the principle of using a tissue flap for repair of recto-vaginal fistula was not new, and attributed its introduction to Noble (1902), Elting (1912) and Laird (1948). An essential part of the procedure was good preoperative bowel preparation, then mobilization of a full thickness of the anterior rectal wall. Complete mobilization was tested by applying gentle traction on the flap to draw it down below the point of origin of the fistula. Anterior rectal wall was separated from the track by sharp dissection and the rectal opening together with adjacent scar tissue, included in the flap to be removed. Belt and Belt (1969) favored anterior rectal wall advancement as the best means to correct low recto-vaginal fistula and emphasized the considerable degree of rectal mobilization required to minimize the risk of flap retraction. Segmental advancement of the internal

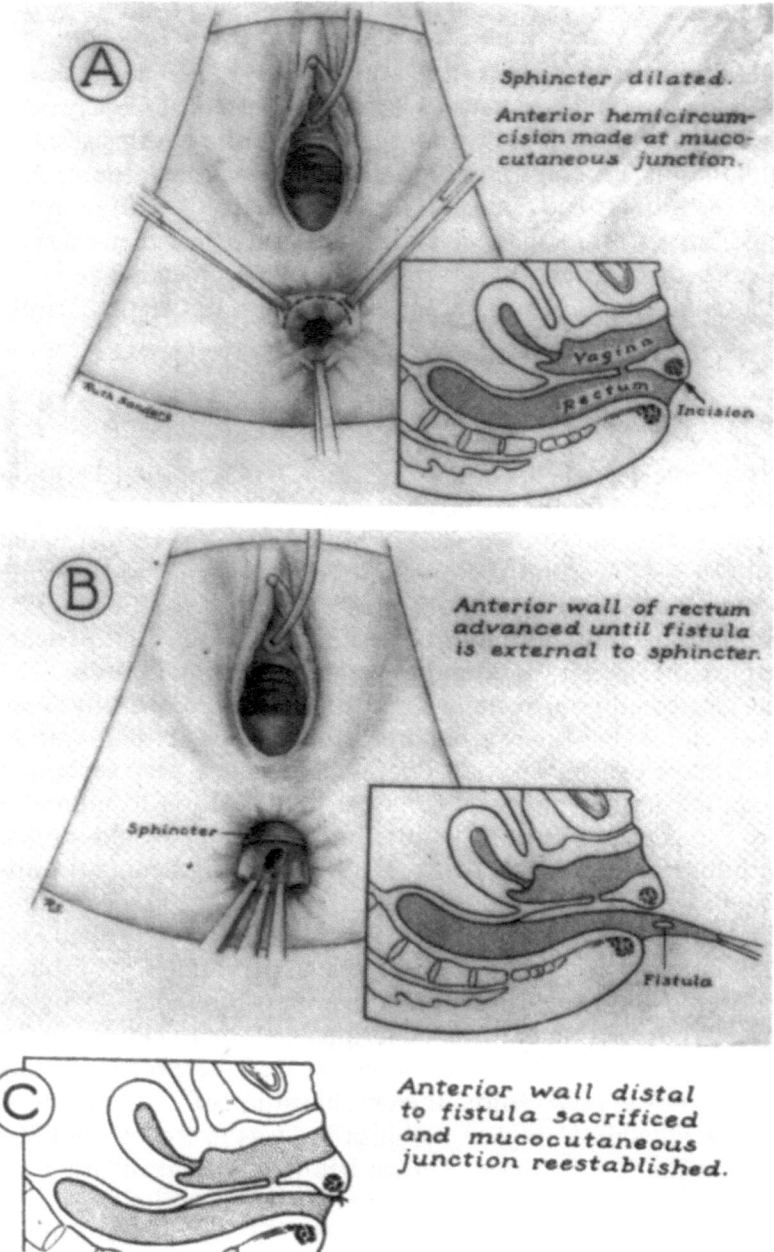

Figure 126. Anal dilatation followed by mobilization of anterior rectal wall inside the sphincter, then advancement external to the sphincter. (From Mengert and Fish)

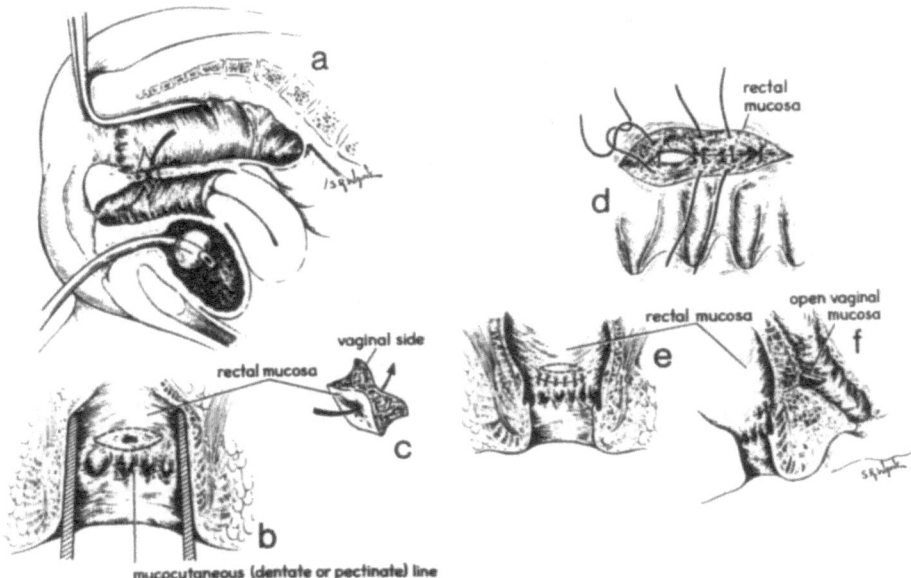

Figure 127. Fistula track excision followed by repair of recto-vaginal septum and rectal wall advancement with closure of the rectal defect. The vaginal defect remains open. (From Greenwald and Hoexter)

sphincter muscle was practiced, together with the overlying attached mucosa and internal or primary fistula opening. Advancement of this portion of the muscle only, lessened the need for wide mobilization and retraction, and the technique could be employed providing the internal fistula opening lay at the dentate line. Russell and Gallagher (1977) enumerated important surgical principles for closure of recto-vaginal fistulae and advocated fistula exposure in the recto-vaginal septum without dividing the external sphincter, then completing closure by anterior rectal wall advancement. Hibbard (1978) made the comment, that on many occasions in repair of low recto-vaginal fistula by standard three layer closure, much time was wasted in unsuccessful attempts to mobilize the fistula before resorting to sphincter division. Also, he advocated the use of a Martius graft at the time of secondary repair, rather than preliminary colostomy. Greenwald and Hoexter (1978) approached the fistula through the anal canal, placing the patient in a jack-knife position and inserted a large retractor into the anal canal to expose anterior rectal wall and fistula. If necessary a posterior or lateral sphincterotomy was performed allowing introduction of the retractor, then a transverse elliptical incision encircled the fistula extending through the entire septum and vaginal mucosa. The rectal mucosa was mobilized exposing the attenuated recto-vaginal septum and the septal defect closed longitudinally or transversely to avoid tension, then the rectal mucosa was advanced over the repair and sutured distal to it, with interrupted "000" chromic catgut sutures (Fig. 127). The vaginal mucosa remained open for drainage, and any sign of outlet obstruction of the anal canal was corrected by dilatation from the retractor or by sphincterotomy. They reported 20 patients with no recurrence between three and twelve years. Recto-vaginal fistula was regarded as a shunt between high and low pressure systems, normal rectal pressures being between 25–85 cm of water whilst the vagina was atmospheric. Frequently, with anorectal disease, there might be increased rectal pressure which could exaggerate this pressure differential, and they believed a trans-anal approach was superior to the vaginal approach since it allowed better access to the rectum, the high pressure side of the fistula. Rothenberger and Goldberg (1983) reviewed managment of recto-vaginal fistula with details of an approach to the simple fistula in which endo-rectal advancement of an anorectal flap of mucosa, submucosa and circular muscle was employed. The fistula was exposed with an anoscope, and the rectal flap of mucosa, submucosa and circular muscle outlined around the fistula basing this flap at least 4 cm above the fistula. The base was twice the width of the flap apex to ensure adequate blood supply and raised from apex to base exposing attenuated septum and perineal body. The sphincter ends were overlapped to decrease the anal aperture, until it fitted snugly over the index finger (Fig. 128 a). Then the rectal flap was advanced over the repaired area and sutured in place at its apex and along the sides, leaving the vaginal mucosa open for drainage. Excess flap including the fistula was then removed and they achieved an 88% cure rate (Fig. 128 b).

Present Surgical Practice

The precise method of operative repair depends upon location, size and cause of the fistula, the number and type of repairs and especially the presence of sphincter damage or a coexistent vesico-vaginal fistula. The surgeon's experience is of particular importance in choosing an appropriate procedure to employ, but regardless of the approach selected, many surgeons advocate interposing a vascularized pedicle between rectum and vagina. Many tissues have been used including omentum, Martius graft, and the gracilis, rectus abdominus, adductor longus, sartorius and gluteus maximus muscles.

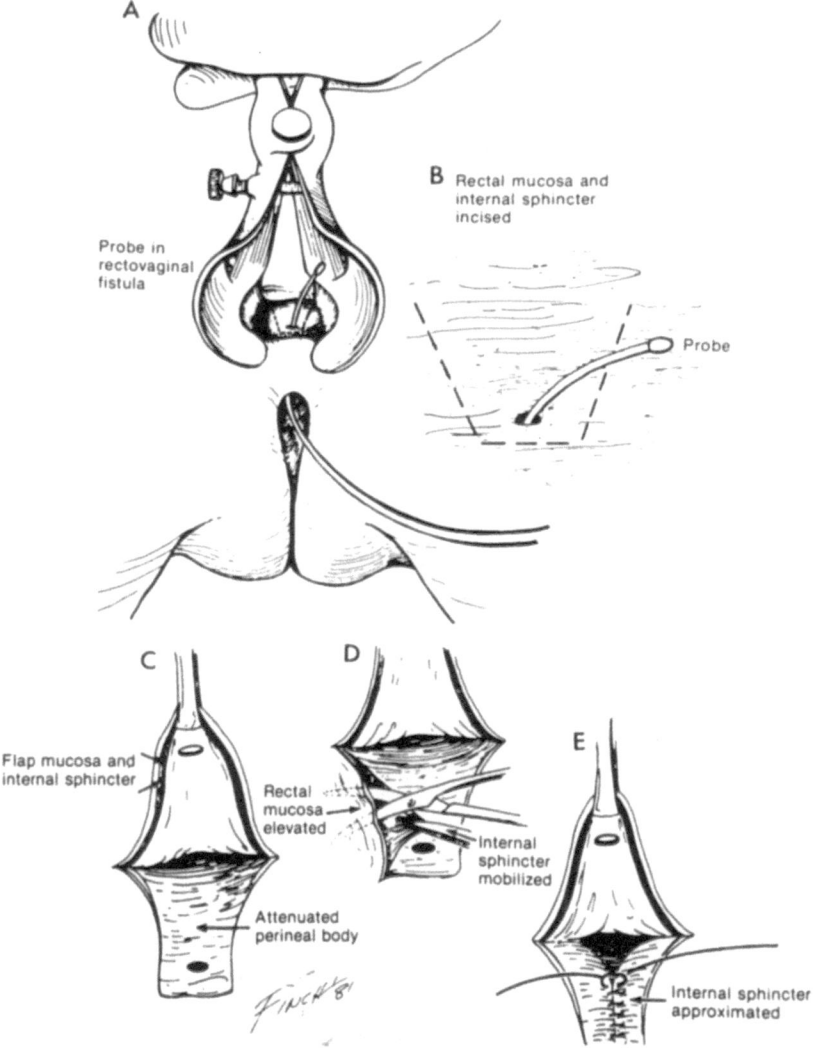

Figure 128 a. Probe identifies the fistula, rectal flap elevated and external sphincter and perineal body reconstituted

Obstetric Recto-Vaginal Fistula and Old Third Degree Tear

Whilst preoperative preparation for vesico-vaginal fistula repair is minimal, it is most important in the management of recto-vaginal fistula. Timing of intervention in both instances is governed by the same features partic-

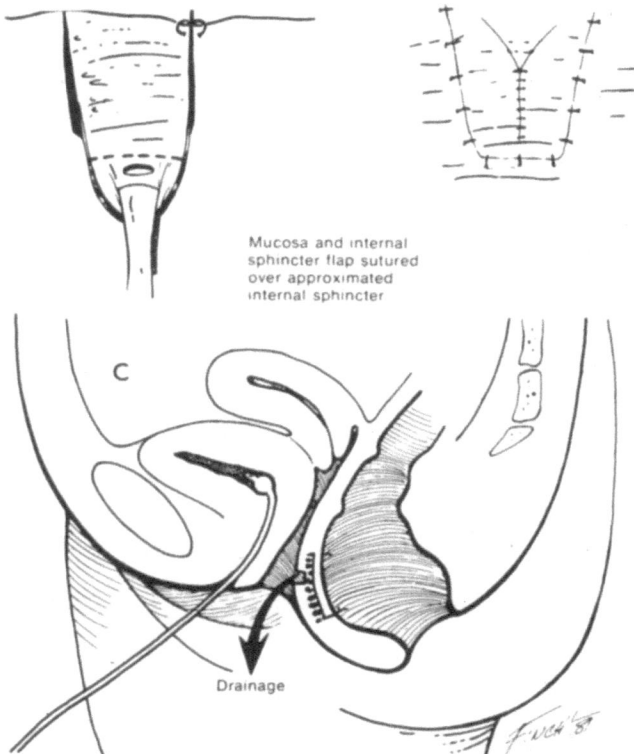

Mucosa and internal
sphincter flap sutured
over approximated
internal sphincter

Drainage

Figure 128 b. The advanced rectal flap fixed over the repaired perineum. (From Rothenberger and Goldberg)

ularly tissue normality, menstruation, and the use of oral contraceptives. Scarred tissues about a fistula are difficult to deal with, and technical problems of dissection and mobilization increase during menstruction or in women using oral contraceptives, because of greater tissue friability and venous engorgement. Initially, difficulties during menstruation were noted by Atlee (1860) and Milton (1887). Oral contraception should cease until the normal menstrual pattern emerges, when plans can be finalized for surgery at midcycle. Should such calculations come to nought and the patient commence menstruating after admissing to hospital, surgery should be deferred and a new time selected. There is wide divergence of opinion about the need for preliminary defunctioning colostomy; but for most simple fistulae, it is unnecessary. However, colostomy is indicated after two or more failures at closure, particularly if grafting has been employed;

but if a graft has not been included in previous attempts, one further attempt with a graft is reasonable. Colostomy is a big step, but if required, fistula closure can proceed 10–12 weeks after the last attempt and three months later, when examination under anesthesia shows success has been achieved, the colostomy can be closed.

Low Recto-Vaginal Fistula

Recto-vaginal fistula poses more difficult problems with healing than vesico-vaginal fistula, all other things being equal, due first to gas pressure in the bowel with the likelihood it might produce a microscopic fistula during early healing phase, and secondly because of solid and infected bowel contents. The worst thing that can happen in the early postoperative phase is a large mass of feces descending upon the reconstructed rectum, so preoperative preparation must be efficient and meticulous. Milton (1887) presenting results on 60 cases of vesico-vaginal and recto-vaginal fistula treated at the Cairo Civil Hospital, commented that whilst most authors agree that recto-vaginal fistulae was easier to operate upon, they were much more difficult to cure than vesico-vaginal. This statement was corroborated by his results where failures apparently were due to the difficulty of preventing rectal gas passing between the edges of the closed fistula.

Preoperative preparation

One cannot be too careful with this phase of management, and everything must be right if final success is to be achieved. One week prior to admission, a low residue diet is commenced, and the patient enters hospital four days before contemplated surgery. In hospital the regime to empty and sterilize her bowel continues with a non-residue diet, an enema given on admission and repeated 24 hours later, and low pressure saline bowel washouts administered twice daily for two days prior to surgery. Metronidazole 200 mg is prescribed eight hourly until normal bowel function is resumed post-operatively, and gentamycin 80 mg intramuscularly is given with the pre-medication and repeated once, six hours later. An important practical point in the patient with a long standing third degree tear is that all bowel preparation including enemas may not be as effective as anticipated, because of the large defect in the anal canal which does not allow an enema to be retained properly. Rectal examination during preoperative preparation is necessary, and occasionally manual disimpaction may be required in such patients to ensure an essential empty rectum and lower large bowel. An alternative method of bowel cleansing using Golytely (Davis et al. 1980),

is useful in preparing the large bowel for diagnostic studies and may su-
percede standard bowel preparation prior to fistula surgery. Golytely is an
orally administered colon electrolyte lavage solution, isotonic with respect
to bowel contents and due to the inclusion of polyethylene glycol which
acts as an osmotic agent, ion absorption or loss is almost nil.

Surgical Correction

(a) Exaggerated lithotomy position with slight Trendelenburg tilt, the buttocks being placed well over the table edge, and the drapes arranged to
allow the whole perineum to be exposed.

With a Third Degree Tear

(b) The skin dimples indicating the divided ends of the external sphincter
are picked up with Allis forceps, and the muco-cutaneous junction put on
the stretch and incised from side to side. Vaginal skin is elevated with three
fine short artery forceps—three to minimize tearing—and stretched over
the index finger which pushes the vaginal skin forward. This step facilitates
the sharp dissection necessary to free the underlying anal canal from vaginal
skin. The anal canal always is tissue-paper thin at this level—a result of
the initial trauma—and stretching the vaginal skin diminishes the risk of
perforating this thin structure. A rectal finger may be a useful guide also.

With Recto-Vaginal Fistula

(c) The vaginal introitus is picked up at 5 o'clock and 7 o'clock with Allis
forceps and the fourchette put on the stretch.

(d) The fistula track is identified with a fine probe, the assistant puts
it on tension by drawing forward on both ends of the probe, then a vertical
incision in the line of the probe gradually is deepened until the probe is
reached and released, opening the entire fistula track (Figs. 129 a–c).

(e) It is necessary always with a low fistula to divide the sphincter and
convert the problem to a third degree tear. This ensures good access, and
means that susequent mobilization can be done accurately and widely
without being confined by the intact sphincter. In any case the sphincter
in such women always is damaged, and usually healed incompletely. When
breakdown to a recto-vaginal fistula occurs following attempted repair,
the sphincter always shares in the resulting deficit.

(f) Rapidly the normal anal canal is reached, and mobilization must
proceed well above the defect. Lateral mobilization is effected out to, and
lateral to the ends of the divided sphincter. The degree of mobilization

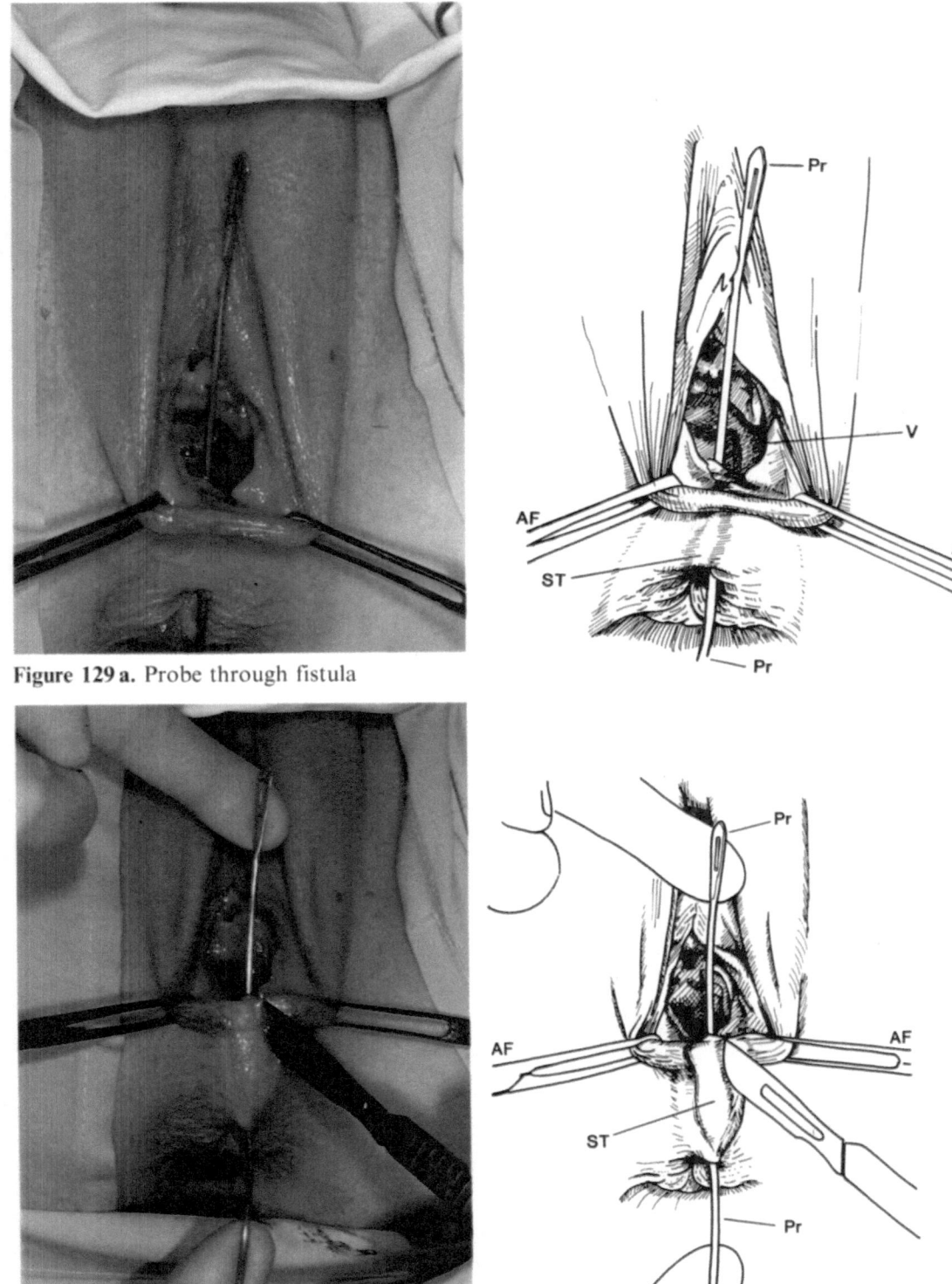

Figure 129 a. Probe through fistula

Figure 129 b. Probe on tension, and incision of scar

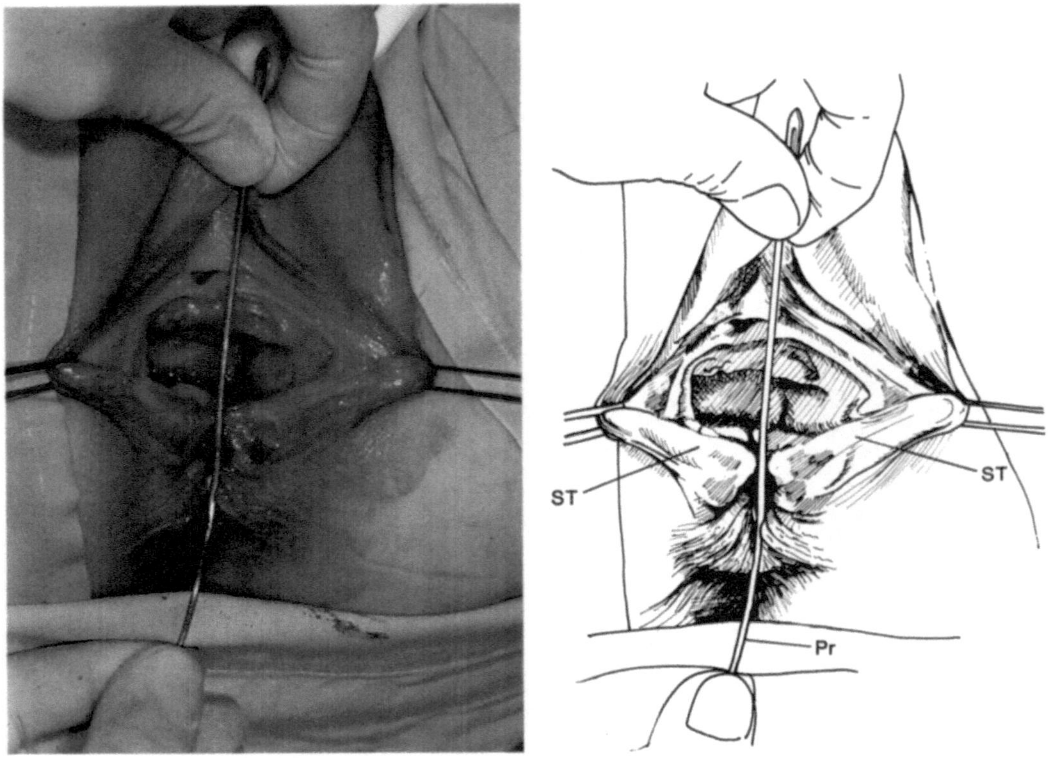

Figure 129 c. Conversion of fistula to third degree tear

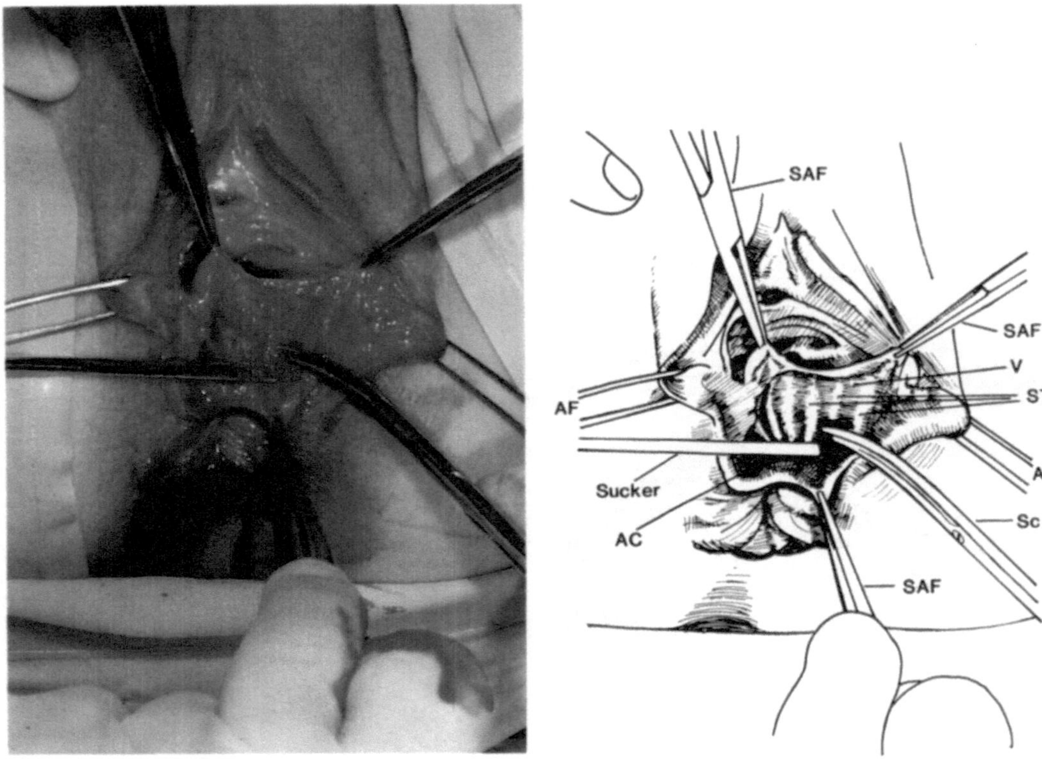

Figure 130 a. Mobilization of anal canal from vagina

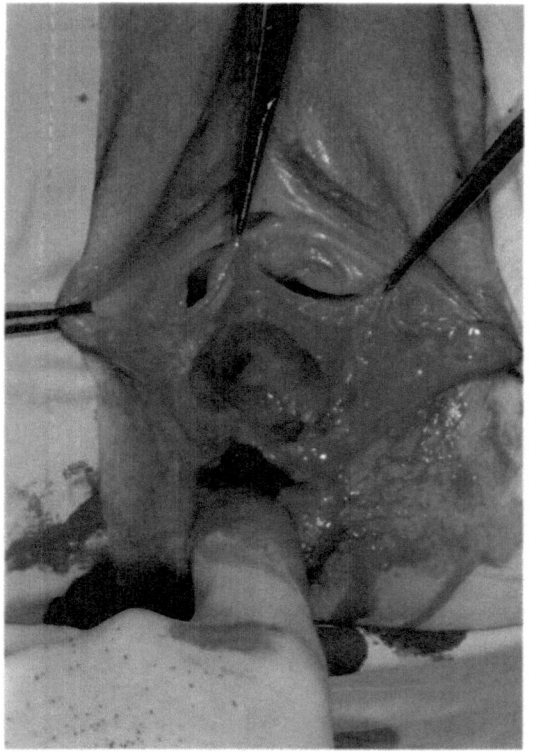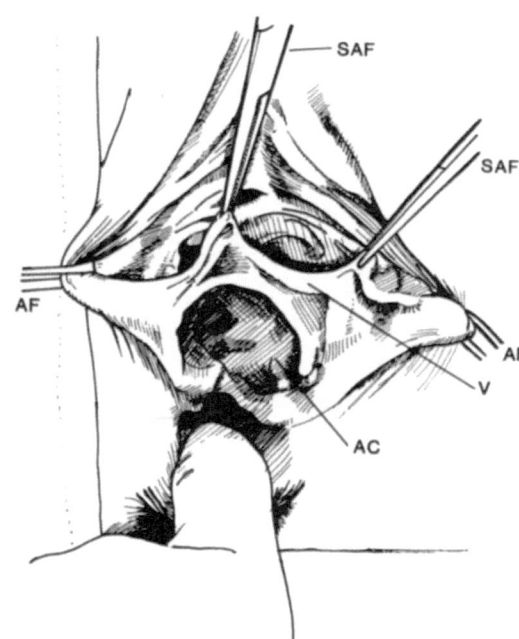

Figure 130 b. Mobilization completed

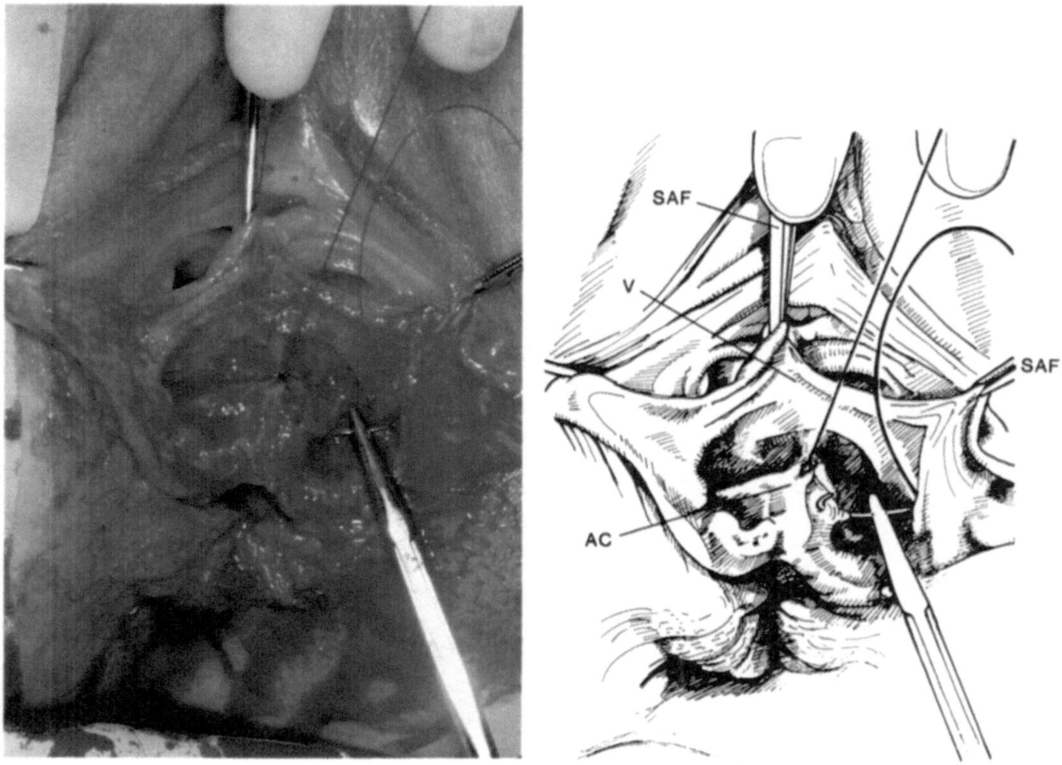

Figure 131 a. Commencement of anal canal closure

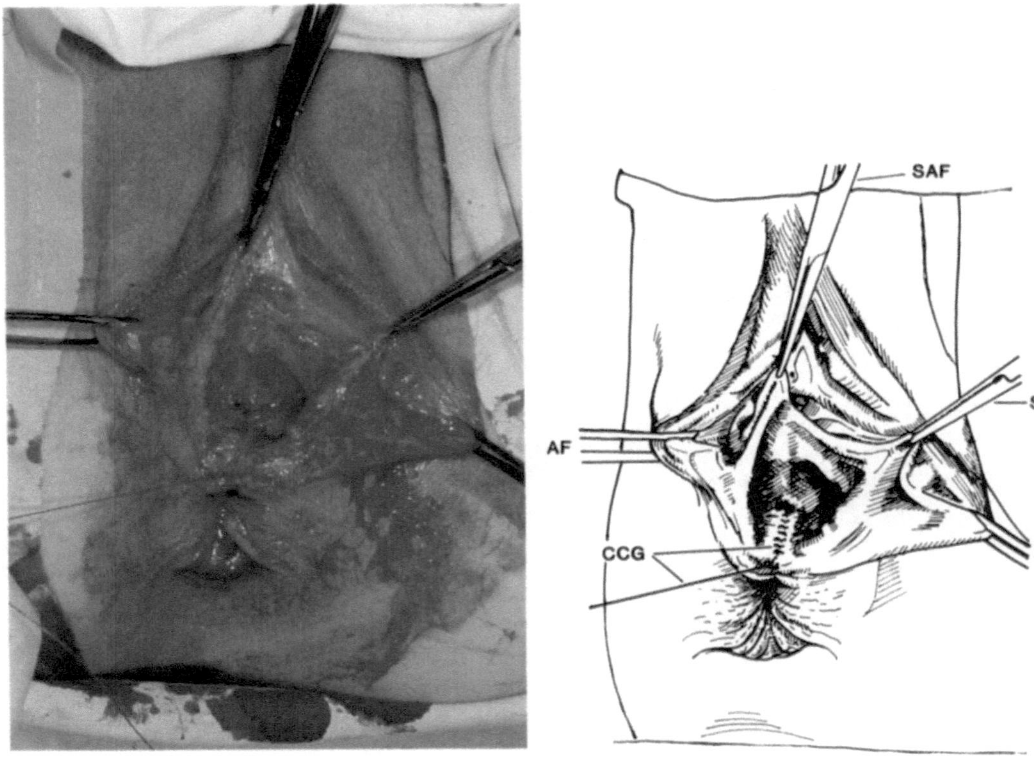

Figure 131 b. Completion of anal canal closure

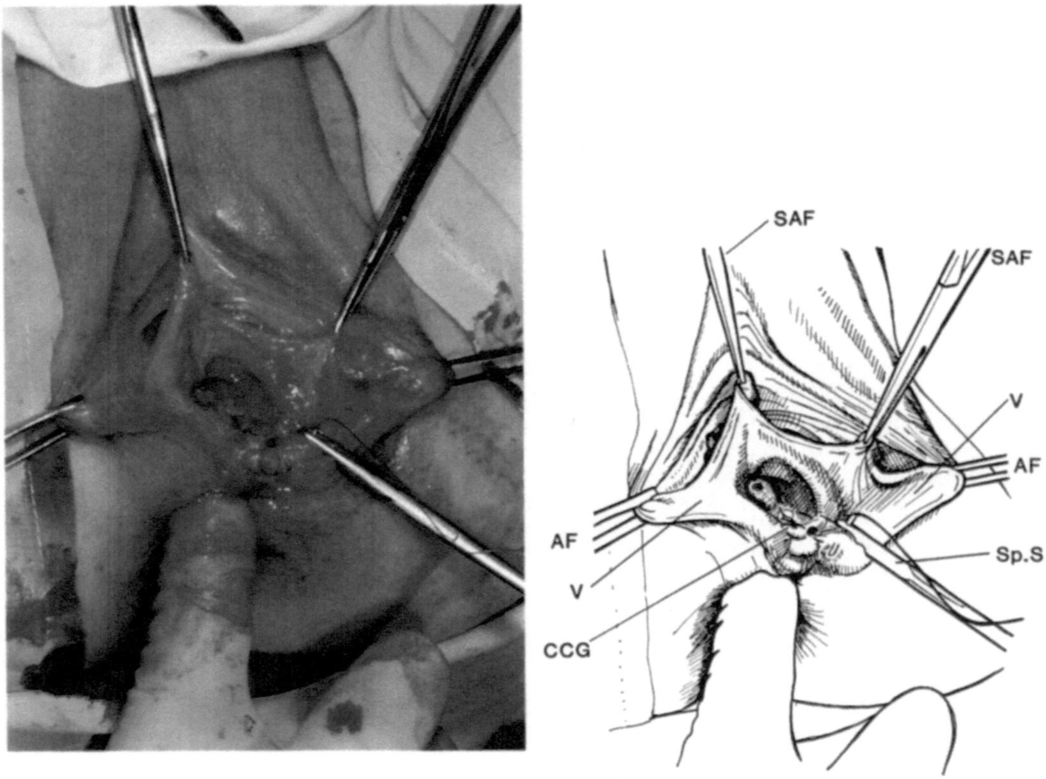

Figure 132 a. Insertion of sphincter sutures

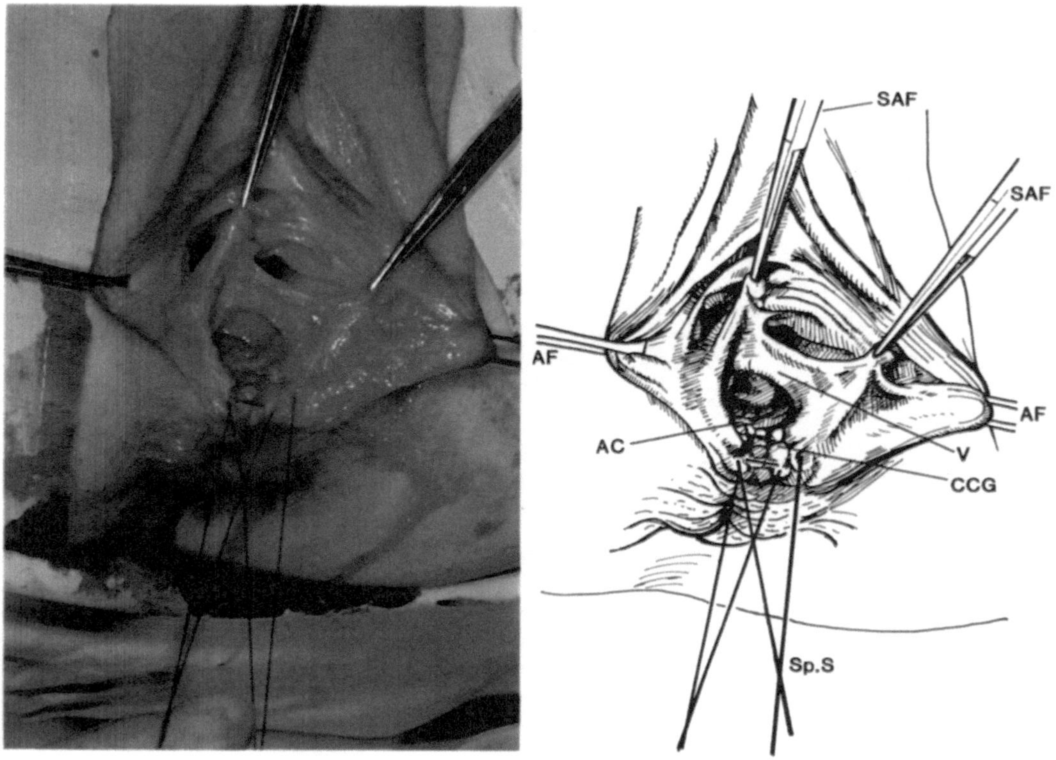

Figure 132 b. Anal canal closure, and sphincter sutures in place

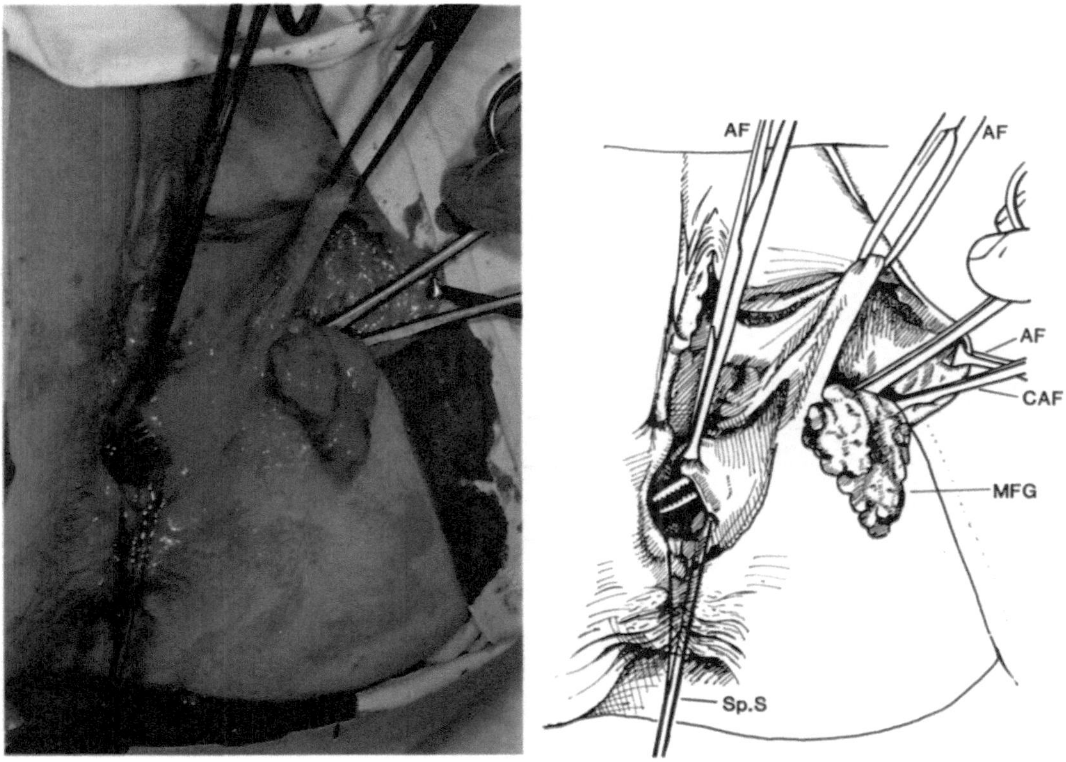

Figure 133 a. Martius graft developed and tunnel created

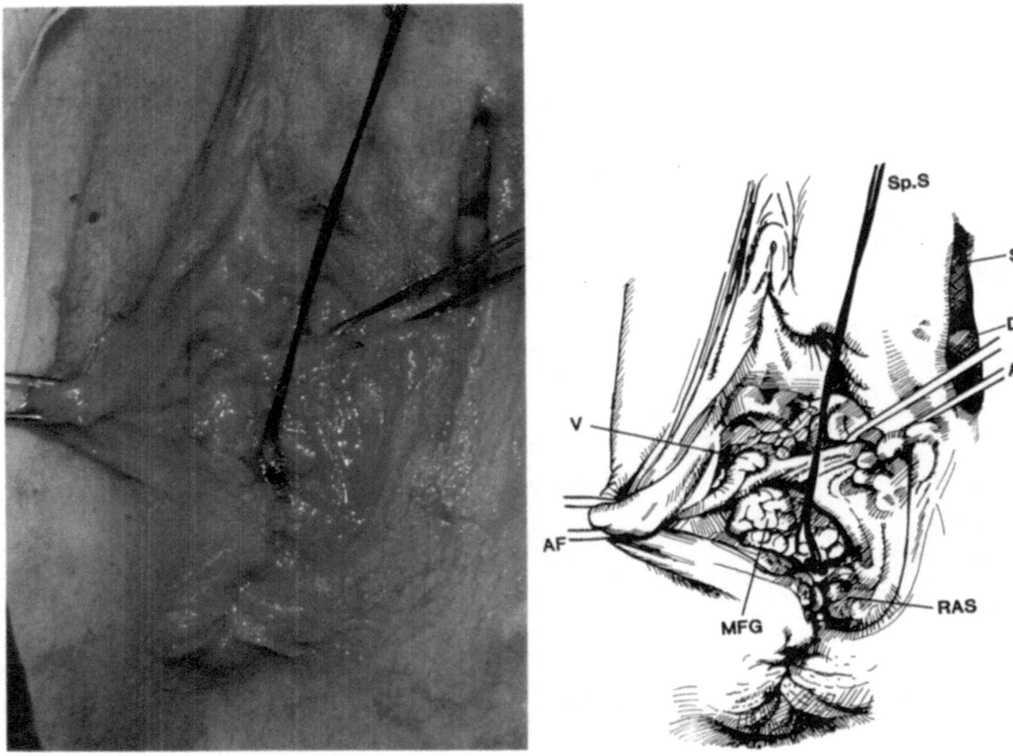

Figure 133 b. Graft fixed with anchor sutures, and sphincter reconstituted

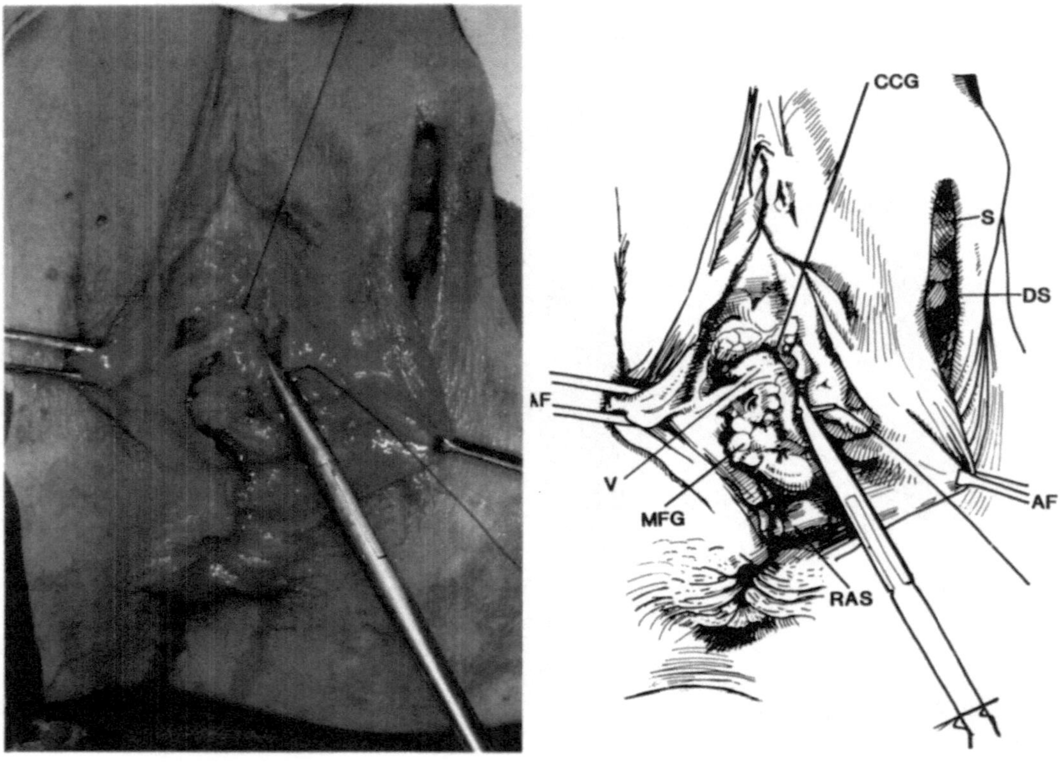

Figure 134 a. Vaginal skin closed incorporating Martius graft

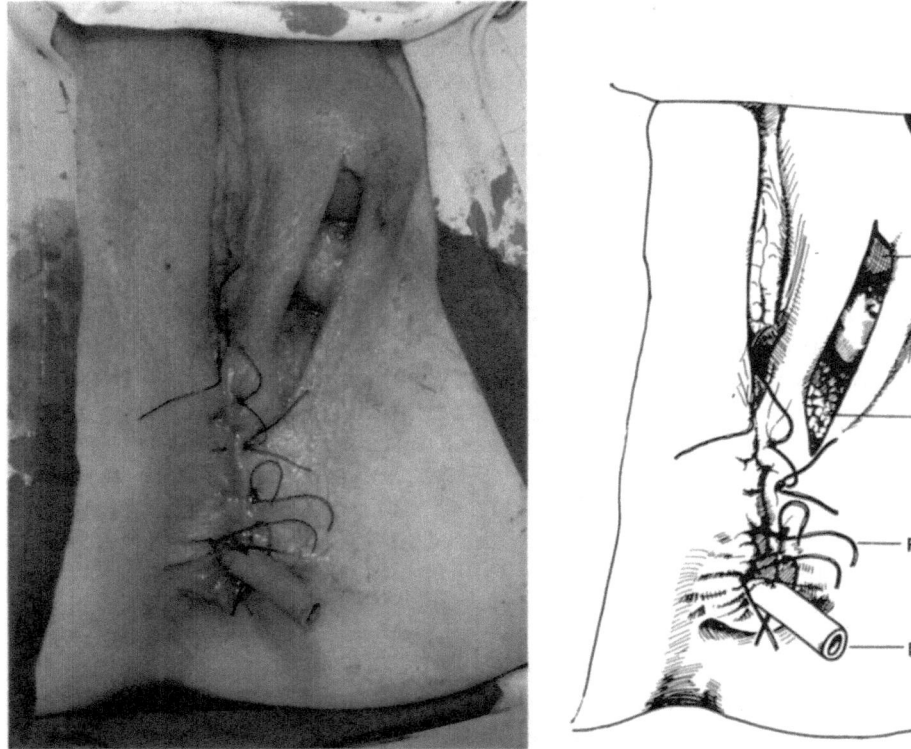

Figure 134 b. Perineum reconstructed, and rectal drain tube inserted

required is determined by the size of the anal canal defect, the ultimate object being double layer closure without tension since the anal canal near a fistula always is very thin, and single layer closure unlikely to be sufficient to ensure an adequate result (Figs. 130 a, b).

(g) Anal Canal Glosure

Using "00" chromic catgut on a fine curved atraumatic needle, closure begins 1 cm proximal to the upper limit of the defect, picking up muscle wall and submucosa; but not entering the anal canal lumen. The suture is running and continuous, terminating at the anal verge near to the skin dimples which indicate the ends of the divided sphincter. Accurate suture placement is facilitated with a finger in the anal canal particularly when the wall is extremely thin, and at the anal verge the suture is locked to return to the beginning as a continual running stitch; but this time picking up more superficial tissues, burying the first suture line. At the upper limit, the suture is tied to the free end of the first suture. Gentle vaginal and rectal examination will demonstrate the integrity of the suture line (Figs. 131 a, b).

(h) With a finger in the anal canal for guidance, a suture of "1" vicryl is passed on a no. 3 Mayo taper needle through the end of the external sphincter on one side, taking a good bite through subcutaneous and para-anal tissues and completed by passage through the other side. Usually two such sutures are required, traction indicating the degree of anal aperture reduction that will follow their ligation—ideally the reconstruction should admit the little finger tip easily (Fig. 132 a, b).

(i) With the anal canal closed and the sphincteric apposition sutures in place, anchor sutures for the Martius graft are placed in three or four convenient positions, then the graft is cut, taken beneath a skin bridge to the closed anal canal and fixed in place by the upper and middle anchor sutures. At this juncture, the sphincter is reconstituted, the anal aperture is checked gently, then the inferior edge of the Martius graft is anchored to the repaired sphincter. Using the graft in this fashion not only reinforces the anal canal repair; but keeps dead space to a minimum (Figs. 133 a, b).

(j) Hemostasis is secured and the vaginal skin closed with a running locking suture of "0" vicryl on a fine curved cutting edge needle, the suture picking up the vaginal skin of one side, then the graft followed by vaginal skin of the other side. Such a suture ensures skin apposition together with elimination of dead space. The perineal muscles are joined across the midline, and the perineal skin closed with horizontal mattress sutures of "0" vicryl (Figs. 134 a, b).

(k) The donor site is closed and the operation concludes with:

1. A Foley 12 self-retaining catheter.

2. A firm vaginal pack.

3. A small rectal tube whose upper end extends several centimeters above the anal canal. This tube should have two small side vents, and is sutured to the anal verge with fine silk (Figs. 135 a, b).

(1) Postoperative Management

The catheter is inserted merely for patient comfort and ease of nursing, and need stay only 48 hours. At 48 hours, the vaginal pack, the catheter and pressure dressing on the graft site are removed. When flatus is passing freely via the rectal tube, usually by the second or third day, the tube can be removed. A low residue diet commences on the third postoperative day,

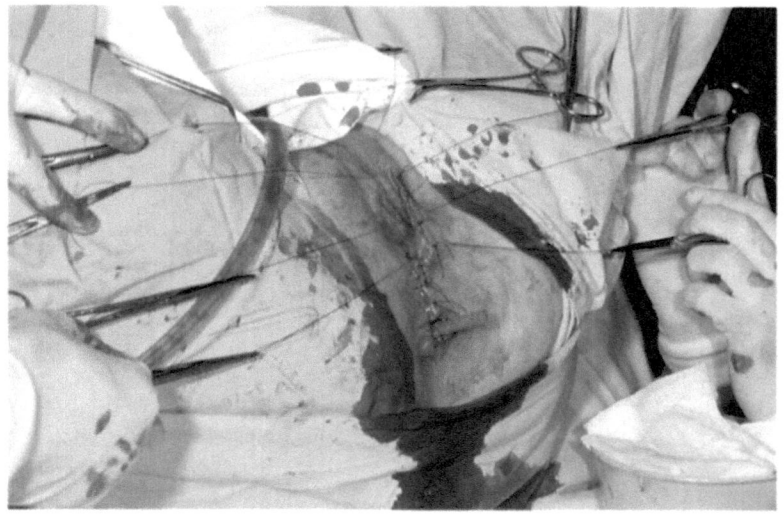

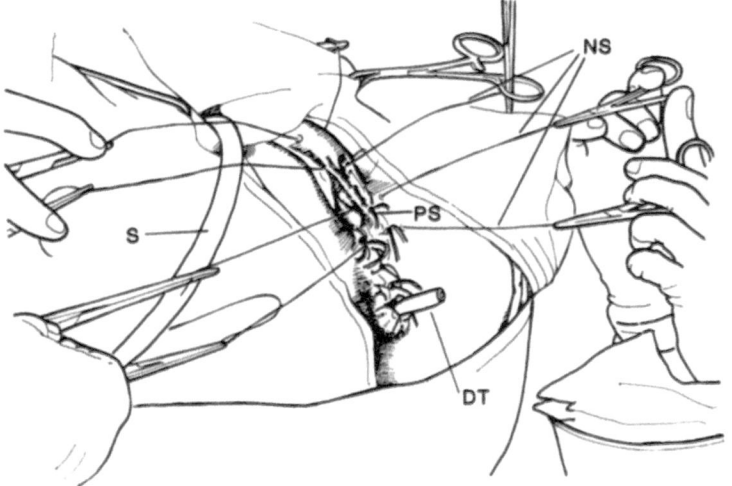

Figure 135 a. Donor site skin closed, and nylon sutures inserted deep to donor site

and by the fifth, full diet can begin with twice daily dosage of milk of magnesia as an aperient. Under no condition should any attempt be made to promote bowel actions by suppositories, enemeta etc., and in particular, rectal examination should be forbidden. Salt baths twice a day and the local application of xylocaine jelly 2% are instituted from day five, and once normal bowel actions are occurring, the patient may be discharged.

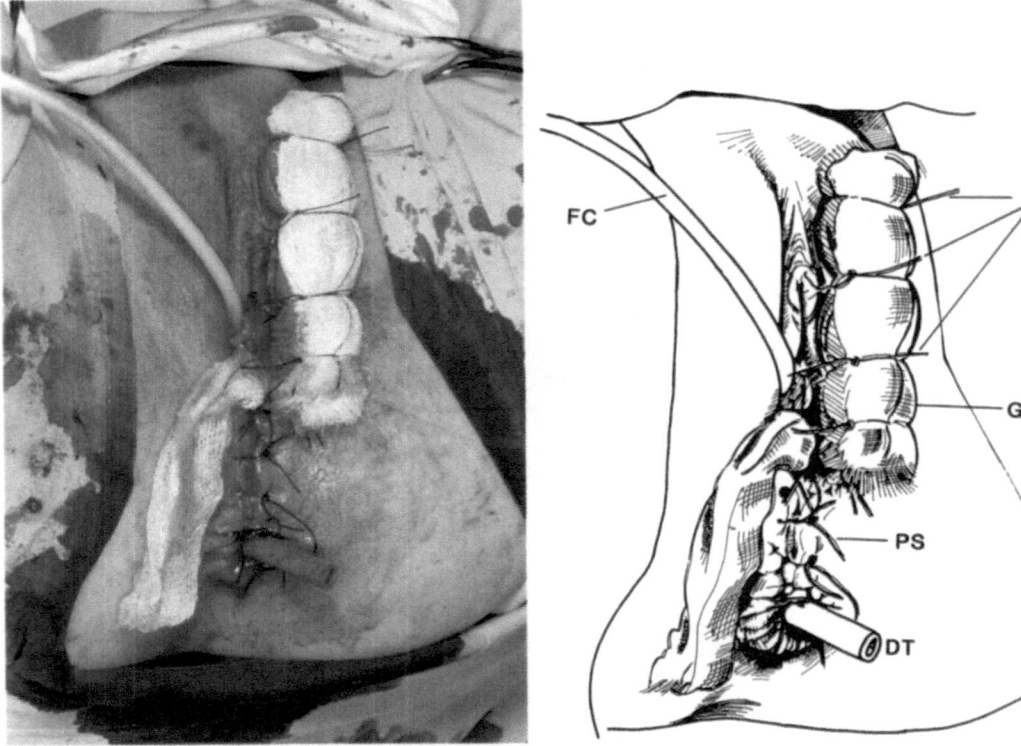

Figure 135 b. Gauze roll compressed against donor site by nylon sutures. Vaginal pack, Foley catheter, and rectal tube in place

Intercourse is prohibited until the postoperative visit in four weeks. During the healing phase it is not unusual for a seemingly purulent discharge to appear from the vagina making both patient and doctor concerned about the integrity of the repair; but usually it is only a discharge of necrotic fat from the Martius graft which settles uneventfully after frequent salt baths.

High Recto-Vaginal Fistula

High rectal fistula may be symptomless arising usually after tissue necrosis, so severe stricture formation is the rule, often forming a flap over a slit-like fistula and creating a rigid posterior horseshoe below it. Such strictures must be divided in order to allow surgical access and division may demonstrate fecal leakage for the first time. At preliminary examination under anesthesia, Lawson (1972) decided whether the fistula should be ap-

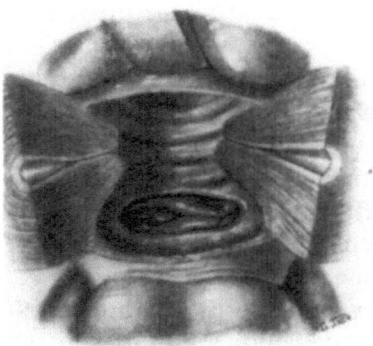 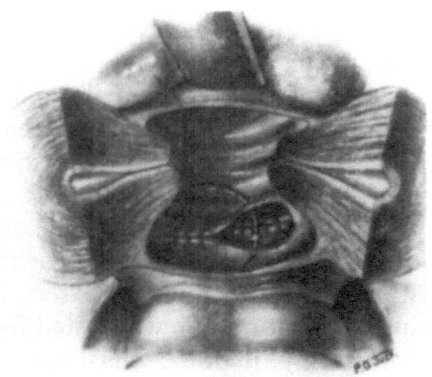

Figure 136. Subtotal hysterectomy, splitting the cervical stump, and the halves retracted, providing access to the recto-vaginal fistula. (From Lawson)

proached through the vagina or abdomen, with the abdominal route indicated when the fistula was tethered so high, its upper edge could not be reached through the vagina. If the vaginal route were chosen for a high recto-vaginal fistula, a deep Schuchardt incision often facilitated the vaginal approach and after opening the pouch of Douglas behind the cervix and drawing the rectum down, the high fistula could be mobilized more readily. Colostomy was advised when a high recto-vaginal fistula of more than 1″ in diameter was to be repaired vaginally, especially if the rectum at the fistula site was stenosed.

Prior to abdominal exploration, preliminary colostomy is required in all cases, with transverse colostomy preferable to iliac colostomy in order not to restrict access during the subsequent surgery. Principles of abdominal recto-vaginal fistula closure enunciated by Lawson, included mobilization of vagina from rectum, closure of both defects and then the interposition of a tissue pedicle between the suture lines. Other options included the pull-through procedure which unfortunately carried the likelihood of incontinence or a low anterior resection using a stapler which allowed resection of the bowel segment containing the fistula. Should the cervix be tethered to the sacral promontory it was possible to release it without too much difficulty and then dissect below the floor of the pouch of Douglas between rectum and vagina to reach the fistula. With dense fibrosis the preliminary hysterectomy of access devised by Eden (1914) could be most difficult, so Lawson (1968) advocated subtotal hysterectomy then splitting the cervical stump in the sagittal plane, enabling vital tissues lateral to the cervix to be moved safely out of danger, allowing access to the posterior vaginal fornix (Fig. 136).

Bentley (1973) reported abdominal repair of high recto-vaginal fistula after mobilizing rectum from vagina, closing the defects, then interposing a pedicle graft of omentum. The mobilized rectum was drawn up and away from the vagina and repaired; but if the vaginal side of the fistula could not be closed, it was left open. The omental graft was sutured to the rectum below the rectal closure as a buttress between rectum and vagina, and peritoneum closed above the rectal suture line. Three weeks following closure, the suture line was tested by running water into the distal end of the colostomy. Bentley, whilst appreciating the difficulties and danger of dense pelvic fibrosis, nevertheless criiticized Lawson's alternative involving subtotal hysterectomy and cervical splitting, since for a young woman in a Moslem community, it was a grave disadvantage to lose her uterus.

Bibliography

Abbott DH (1950) The repair of vesico-vaginal fistulae. East Afr Med J 27: 109–118

Agrawal V, Sapre S, Shrivastava SK, Patil S (1985) Menstrual fistula following Caesarean section. Asia-Oceania J Obstet Gynaecol 11: 325–328

Agnew DH (1873) Lacerations of the female perineum and vesico-vaginal fistula. Lindsay & Blakiston, Philadelphia, pp 57–64

Akasheh F (1966) Vesico-vaginal fistula following the use of vacuum extractor. Postgrad Med J 42: 793–794

Akasheh F (1985) Personal communication

Apajalahti A (1931) Über die Ursachen und die Behandlung der Harnweg-Scheidenfisteln mit besonderer Berücksichtigung der Methode der vierfachen Catgutnaht. Acta Obstet Gynecol 11: 1–34

Atlee WL (1860) Case of successful operation for vesico-vaginal fistula. Am J Med Sci 39: 67–82

Aziz SA (1965) Urinary fistula from obstetrical trauma. J Obstet Gynaecol Br Cwlth 72: 765–768

Aziz FA (1980) Gynecologic and obstetric complications of female circumcision. Int J Gynaecol Obstet 17: 560–563

Bailey H, Bishop WJ (1959) Notable names in medicine and surgery. Lewis, London, p 85–87

Baines REM, Orford HJL, Theron JLL (1976) The repair of vesicovaginal fistula by means of omental slings and grafts. S Afr Med J 50: 959–961

Bandl L (1878) Zur Entstehung und Behandlung der Harnleitenscheidenfisteln, und zur Operation der Blasen-Scheidenfisteln. Cited by: Latzko WA Op cit

Banerji B (1966) Role of musculofascial pedicle grafts in operative repair of vesicovaginal fistulae. Int Surg 45: 391–396

Bardescu N (1900) Ein neues Verfahren für die Operation der tiefen Blasen-Uterus-Scheidenfisteln. Zentralbl Gynak 24: 170–181

Barker-Benfield GJ (1977) The horrors of the half-known life. Harper & Row, New York

Barnes RW, Martin IE (1949) Repair of vesicovaginal fistula. Urol Cutan Rev 53: 67–70

Barnes RW, Wilson WM (1949) Reconstruction of the urethra with a tube from bladder flap. Urol Cutan Rev 53: 604–606

Batayneh A (1985) Personal communication 1985

Belt Jr, RL Belt RL (1969) Repair of anorectal vaginal fistula utilizing segmental advancement of the internal sphincter muscle. Dis Col Rectum 12: 99–104

Bender GA (1961) Great moments in medicine: a collection of the first thirty stories and paintings in the continuing series, A history of medicine in pictures. Parke Davis & Co, Detroit, pp 254–263, J. Marion Sims, gynecologic surgeon

Benson RC, Hinman F JNR (1955) Urinary tract injuries in obstetrics and gynecology. Am J Obstet Gynecol 70: 467–485

Bentley RJ (1973) Abdominal repair of high rectovaginal fistula. J Obstet Gynaecol Br Cwlth 80: 364–367

Betson JR JNR (1961) The bulbocavernosus fat pad transplant for severe stress incontinence and vesicovaginal fistula: rationale of the procedure, indications and technique. Am Surg 27: 129–136

Bickenbach W (1965) Professor Dr. med. et Dr. med. h.c. Heinrich Martius. Zentralbl Gynakol 87: 594–595

Bieler EU, Schnabel T (1976) Pituitary and ovarian function in women with vesicovaginal fistulae after obstructed and prolonged labour. S Afr Med J 50: 257–266

Bird GC (1967) Obstetric vesico-vaginal and allied fistulae: a report on 70 cases. J Obstet Gynaecol Br Cwlth 74: 749–752

Birkhoff JD, Wechsler R, Romas NA (1977) Urinary fistulas: vaginal repair using a labial fat pad. J Urol 117: 595–597

Bishop ES (1897) Vesico-vaginal fistula: with a description of a new method of operation. Trans Med Soc Lond 20: 123–135

Bissel D (1928) Genito-urinary fistula in the female: with an appreciation of Sims and his work. Proc Roy Soc Med 22: 179–196

Bissell D (1929) J. Marion Sims: surgeon and humanitarian. Am J Surg 6: 561–565

Blaikley JB (1965) Colpocleisis for difficult vesicovaginal and rectovaginal fistulas. Am J Obstet Gynecol 91: 589–596

Bland KG, Gelfand M (1970) The influence of urinary bilharziasis on vesico-vaginal fistula in relation to causation and healing. Trans Roy Soc Trop Med Hygiene 64: 588–592

Bohne AW, Osborn RW, Hettle PJ (1955) Regeneration of the urinary bladder in the dog, following total cystectomy. Surg Gynecol Obstet 100: 259–264

Bozeman N (1869) Remarks on the advantages of a supporting and confining apparatus, and a self-retaining speculum in the operation of vesico-vaginal fistule. NY Med J 8: 484–507

Bozeman N (1870) Vesico-vaginal fistules: comparative analysis of different surgical methods. Results, American and European. Am J Med Sci 60: 100–112

Brown IB (1860) Record of nineteen cases of ruptured perineum with practical remarks. Lancet 1: 214–215

Brown IB (1861) On surgical diseases of women. John W. Davies, London, pp 112–177

Brown IB (1864) On vesico-vaginal fistula, the mode of operating and the results obtained in fifty-five cases, at the London Surgical Home. Trans Obstet Soc Lond 5: 25–40

Buxton CL (1968) James Marion Sims. In: Sims JM, The story of my life. Foreword to 1968 edition. Op cit

Carmichael EB (1960) J. Marion Sims: inventor, physician, surgeon. J Int Coll Surg 33: 757–762

Carter B, Palumbo L, Creadick RN, Ross RA (1952) Vesicovaginal fistulas. Am J Obstet Gynecol 63: 479–496

Charlewood GP (1950) A simple and successful technique for the repair of vesico-vaginal fistulae with results on 72 cases. S Afr Med J 24: 232–238

Clark DH, Holland JB (1975) Repair of vesicovaginal fistulas: simultaneous trans-vaginal-transvesical approach. South Med J 68: 1410–1413

Clegg DR (1979) Vaginal repair of obstetric vesico vaginal fistulae. Cent Afr J Med 25: 67–71

Cockshott PW (1973) Pubic changes associated with obstetric vesico vaginal fistulae. Clin Radiol 24: 241–247

Coetzee T, Lithgow DM (1966) Obstetric fistulae of the urinary tract. J Obstet Gynaecol Br Cwlth 73: 837–844

Collins CG, Davidson VA, Mathews NM (1952) Use of cortisone in pelvic cellulitis: a preliminary report. New Orleans Surg J 104: 389–394

Collins CG, Jones FB (1957) Preoperative cortisone for vaginal fistulas. Obstet Gynecol 9: 533–537

Collins CG, Collins JH, Harrison BR, et al (1971) Early repair of vesicovaginal fistula. Am J Obstet Gynecol 111: 524–528

Collis MH (1861) Further remarks upon a new and successful mode of treatment for vesico-vaginal fistula. Dublin Quarterly J Med Sci 31: 302–316

Counseller VS, Haigler FH (1956) Management of urinary vaginal fistula in 253 cases. Am J Obstet Gynecol 72: 367–376

Cutner LP (1985) Female genital mutilation. Obstet Gynecol Surv 40: 437–443

Cutter IS (1928) J. Marion Sims and vesicovaginal fistula. Int Abstr Surg 47: 173–175

Das K (1928) Remarks on the operability and operative technique of vesico-vaginal fistula. Indian Med Gaz 63: 698–700

Das RK, Sengupta SK (1969) Vesico-vaginal fistula of obstetric origin. J Obstet Gynaecol India 19: 383–389

Davis GR, Santa Ana CA, Morawski SG, Fordtran JS (1980) Development of a lavage solution associated with minimal water and electrolyte absorption or secretion. Gastroenterology 78: 991–995

Davis RS, Linke CA, Kraemer GK (1980) Use of labial tissue in repair of urethrovaginal fistula and injury. Arch Surg 115: 628–630

Derry DE (1935) Note on five pelves of women of the eleventh dynasty in Egypt. J Obstet Gynaecol Br Emp 42: 490–495

Dick JS, Strover RM (1971) Vaginoplasty following vesicovaginal fistula repair: a preliminary report. S Afr Med J 45: 617–620

Dittel L (1893) Abdominale Blasenscheidenfistel-Operation. Wien Klin Wochenschr 6: 449–452

Dorman PF (1985) (Assistant Curator, Metropolitan Museum of Art). Personal communication

Dorsey JW (1960) The repair of vesicovaginal fistula by the transperitoneal, transvesical approach. J Urol 83: 404–408

Douglass M (1931) Reconstruction of the urethra and vesical sphincter by employing the levator ani muscles. Am J Obstet Gynecol 22: 739–790

Dowman CE (1920) The utilization of the transposed uterus for the cure of extensive vesicovaginal fistula. Surg Gynecol Obstet 30: 403–405

Dudley EC (1887) Gynaecological antiseptics, and other means of preventing pelvic inflammations. Chicago Med J Examiner 54: 228–236

Eden TW (1914) A case of superior recto-vaginal fistula dealt with by the abdominal route after preliminary colostomy. J Obstet Gynaecol Br Emp 26: 175–185

Editorial (1969) "Irreparable" vesicovaginal fistula. Br Med J 1: 132–133

Editorial (1981) Obstetric fistula. Lancet 1: 1402–1403

Eisen M, Jurkovic K, Altwein JE, Schreiter F, Hohenfellner R (1974) Management of vesicovaginal fistulas with peritoneal flap interposition. J Urol 112: 195–198

Elting AW (1912) The treatment of fistula in ano: with especial reference to the Whitehead operation. Ann Surg 56: 744–752

Emmet TA (1868) Vesico-vaginal fistula from parturition and other causes with cases of recto-vaginal fistula. William Wood & Co, New York

Emmet TA (1879) The principles and practice of gynaecology. H. C. Lea, Philadelphia, p 614

Emmet TA (1884) A memoir of Dr. James Marion Sims. NY Med J 39: 1–5

Emmet TA (1895) Incurable vesico-vaginal fistula: a new method of treatment by suprapubic cystotomy. Am J Obstet Dis Women Childr 31: 593–603

Englebach R, Derry DE (1942) Mummification. Ann du Service des Antiquités de l'Egypte 41: 233–265

Evoh NJ, Akinla O (1978) Reproductive performance after the repair of obstetric vesico-vaginal fistulae. Ann Clin Res 10: 303–306

Falk HC, Tancer ML (1957) Vaginal cystostomy. Obstet Gynecol 9: 86–88

Falk HC, Kurman M (1963) Repair of vesicovaginal fistula: report of 140 cases. J Urol 89: 226–231

Falk HC, Tancer ML (1969) Urethrovesicovaginal fistula. Obstet Gynecol 33: 422–431

Fearl CL, Keizur LW (1969) Optimum time interval from occurrence to repair of vesicovaginal fistula. Am J Obstet Gynecol 104: 205–208

Foda MS (1959) Evaluation of methods of treatment of urinary fistulae in women. J Obstet Gynaecol Br Emp 66: 372–381

Freund WA (1912) Eine neue Operation 2 Schlies gewisse Harnfisteln beim Weibe. Cited by: Kelly HA. Op cit

Frith K (1960) Vaginal atresia of Arabia. J Obstet Gynaecol Br Emp 67: 82–85

Gallagher DM, Scarborough RA (1962) Repair of low rectovaginal fistula. Dis Colon Rectum 5: 193–195

Garlock JH (1928) The cure of an intractable vesicovaginal fistula by the use of a pedicled muscle graft. Surg Gynecol Obstet 47: 255–260

Given Jr FT (1970) Rectovaginal fistula: a review of 20 years experience in a community hospital. Am J Obstet Gynecol 108: 41–45

Goldstein MB, Dearden LC (1966) Histology of omentoplasty of the urinary bladder in the rabbit. Invest Urol 3: 460–469

Gosset M (1834/35) Calculus in the bladder—incontinence of urine—vesico-vaginal fistula: advantage of the gilt-wire suture. Lancet 1: 345–346

Graham H (1950) Eternal Eve. Heinemann, London

Graham JB (1965) Vaginal fistulas following radiotherapy. Surg Gynecol Obstet 120: 1019–1030

Gray LA (1968) Urethrovaginal fistulas. Am J Obstet Gynecol 101: 28–36

Gray PH (1970) Obstetric vesicovaginal fistulas. Am J Obstet Gynecol 107: 898–901

Graziotti P, Lembo A, Artibani W (1978) Spontaneous closure of vesico-uterine fistula after Cesarean section. J Urol 120: 372

Greenslade NF (1969) Vesico-vaginal fistula: a method of repair. Aust N Z J Surg 38: 283–285

Greenwald JC, Hoexter B (1978) Repair of rectovaginal fistulas. Surg Gynecol Obstet 146: 443–445

Hamlin RHJ, Nicholson EC (1969) Reconstruction of urethra totally destroyed in labour. Br Med J 2: 147–150

Hamlin RHJ, Nicholson EC (1986) Personal communication

Hanash KA, Sieck U (1983) Successful repair of a large vesicovaginal fistula with associated urethral loss using the anterior bladder flap technique. J Urol 130: 775–776

Harer B (1985) Personal communication

Harris JE, Wente EF (1980) An X-ray atlas of the Royal Mummies. University of Chicago Press, Chicago

Harrison KA (1980) Traditional birth attendants. Lancet 2: 43–44

Harrison KA (1983) Obstetric fistula: one social calamity too many. Br J Obstet Gynaecol 90: 385–386

Hartfield VJ (1973) A comparison of the early and late effects of subcutaneous symphysiotomy and of lower segment Caesarean section. J Obstet Gynaecol Br Cwlth 80: 508–514

Hartfield VJ (1975) Late effects of symphysiotomy. Trop Doct 5: 76–78

Hassim AM, Lucas C (1974) Reduction in the incidence of stress incontinence complicating fistula repair. Br J Surg 61: 461–465

Hathout HM (1963) Some aspects of female circumcision. J Obstet Gynaecol Br
    Cwlth 70: 505–507
Hauth JC, Gilstrap III LC, Ward SC, Hankins GDV (1986) Early repair of an
    external sphincter ani muscle and rectal mucosal dehiscence. Obstet Gynecol
    67: 806–809
Hayes SN (1945) The operative technique of complicated vesicovaginal and ure-
    throvesicovaginal fistulas. Surg Gynecol Obstet 81: 346–354
Hayward G (1839) Case of vesico-vaginal fistula, successfully treated by an oper-
    ation. Am J Med Sci 24: 283–288
Hibard LT (1978) Surgical management of rectovaginal fistula and complete
    perineal tears. Am J Obstet Gynecol 130: 139–141
Hoskins WJ, Long R, Artman LE, McMahon EB (1984) Repair of urinary tract
    fistulas with bulbocavernosus myocutaneous flaps. Obstet Gynecol 63: 588–
    593
Huddleston CE (1949) Female circumcision in the Sudan. Lancet 1: 626
Hudson CN (1970) Acquired fistulae between the intestine and the vagina. Ann
    R Coll Surg Engl 46: 20–40
Humphries SV (1961) Transplantation of ureters for vesico-vaginal fistula. S Afr
    Med J 35: 643–646
Hutch JA, Noll LE (1970) Prevention of vesicovaginal fistulas. Obstet Gynecol
    35: 924–927
Ingle KM, Saraf AN, Purandare BN (1969) Vesico-vaginal fistula. J Obstet
    Gynaecol India 18: 189–194
Ingelman-Sundberg A (1948) Transplantation of levator muscles in repair of com-
    plete tear and rectovaginal fistula. Acta Chir Scand 96: 313–316
Ingelman-Sundberg A (1954) Repair of vesicovaginal and rectovaginal fistula
    following fulguration of recurrent cancer of the cervix after radiation. In:
    Meigs JV. Surgical treatment of cancer of the cervix. New York: Grune &
    Stratton 419–422
Ingelman-Sundberg A (1960) Pathogenesis and operative treatment of urinary
    fistula in irradiated tissue. In: Youssef AF, Gynaecological urology. Charles
    C. Thomas, Springfield, Ill. pp 263–279
Jaya Rao KS (1979) Attitudes to women and nutrition programmes in India.
    Lancet 2: 1357–1358
Joyner A (1982) Symphysiotomy and vesico-vaginal fistula. Midwives Chronicle
    95: 331–332
Judd ES (1920) The operative treatment of vesicovaginal fistulae. Surg Gynecol
    Obstet 30: 447–453
Kaiser IH (1978) Reappraisals of J. Marion Sims. Am J Obstet Gynecol 132: 878–
    884
Kelly HA (1896) The treatment of large vesico-vaginal fistulae. Johns Hopkins
    Hosp Bull 7: 29–31
Kelly HA (1902) The treatment of vesico-vaginal and recto-vaginal fistulae high
    up in the vagina. Johns Hopkins Hosp Bull 13: 73–74

Kelly HA (1906) The suprapubic route in operating for vesical fistulae. Trans Am Gynecol Soc 31: 225–253

Kelly HA (1912) The history of vesicovaginal fistula. Trans Am Gynecol Soc 37: 3–29

Kelly HA (1912) James Marion Sims. In: A cyclopedia of American medical biography. Saunders, Philadelphia 2: 374–377

Kelly J (1979) Vesicovaginal fistulae. Br J Urol 51: 208–210

Kelly J (1986) Personal communication

Kelly JV (1967) The influence of native customs in obstetrics in Nigeria. Obstet Gynecol 30: 608–612

Kingston AE (1957) The vaginal atresia of Arabia. J Obstet Gynaecol Br Emp 64: 836–839

Kiricuta I, Goldstein AMB (1972) The repair of extensive vesicovaginal fistulas with pedicled omentum: a review of 27 cases. J Urol 108: 724–727

Kirwin TJ, Lowsley OS (1935) Radical relief of vesico-vaginal fistula: report of an unusual case of eversion of the bladder through the fistulous opening, and a review of sixty cases seen at New York Hospital during the past ninety years. J Urol 33: 51–63

Krishnan RG (1949) A review of a series of 100 cases of vesicovaginal fistulae. J Obstet Gynaecol Br Emp 56: 22–27

LH (1866) Ode to Dr Marion Sims. Med Times Gaz 1: 216

Laffont MA (1946) Graves fistules vesico-vaginal traitees par la greffe placentaire. Gynecol Obstet 45: 540–541

Lagundoye SB, Bell D, Gill G, Ogunbode O (1976) Urinary tract changes in obstetric vesico-vaginal fistulae: a report of 216 cases studied by intravenous urography. Clin Radiol 27: 531–539

Laird DR (1948) Procedures used in treatment of complicated fistulas. Am J Surg 76: 701–708

Last M (1976) The presentation of sickness in a community of non-Muslim Hausa. In: Loudon JB, Social anthropology and medicine. Academic Press, London, pp 104–149

Latzko W (1942) Postoperative vesicovaginal fistulas: genesis and therapy. Am J Surg 58: 211–228

Lavery DWP (1955) Vesico-vaginal fistulae: a report on the vaginal repair of 160 cases. J Obstet Gynaecol Br Emp 62: 530–539

Lawson JB (1968) Birth-canal injuries. Proc Roy Soc Med 61: 368–370

Lawson JB (1972) Rectovaginal fistula following difficult labour. Proc Roy Soc Med 65: 283–286

Lawson JB (1972) Vesical fistulae into the vaginal vault. Br J Urol 44: 623–631

Lawson JB (1977) Vesico-vaginal fistulae. In: Proceedings of the 1st International Conference of the Faculty of Gynaecology and Obstetrics, Nigeria, Ibadan, pp 323–329

Lawson JB (1978) The management of genito-urinary fistulae. Clin Obstet Gynaecol 5: 209–236

Lawson JB (1985) The vesico-vaginal fistula—a continuing problem. J. Y. Simpson oration. Roy Coll Obstet Gynaecol, London

Legueu F (1929) The transperitoneal closure of vesicovaginal fistulae. Surg Gynecol Obstet 48: 796–798

Lescher TC, Pratt JH (1967) Vaginal repair of the simple rectovaginal fistula. Surg Gynecol Obstet 124: 1317–1321

Levert HS (1829) experiments on the use of metallic ligatures, as applied to arteries. Am J Med Sci 4: 17–23

Linke CA, Linke CL, Worden AC (1971) Bladder and urethral injuries following prolonged labor. J Urol 105: 679–682

Lister U (1975) Vesico-vaginal fistulae in Zaria. Personal communication

Lister U (1986) Personal communication

Longaker D, Harriman WF (1927) Kielland forceps and vesicovaginal fistula. Int Clinics 37: 224–229

Longo LD (1964) Postobstetric genitourinary tract fistula. Obstet Gynecol 23: 768–773

Macalpine JB (1940) The repair of a vesico-vaginal fistula by a new technique. Br Med J 2: 778–779

Mack WS (1966) The vesical fistula high in the vagina (discussion). Proc Roy Soc Med 59: 1024

Mackenrodt A (1894) Die operative Heilung grosser Blasenscheidenfisteln. Zentralbl Gynakol 8: 180–184

Macknight E (1962) Report of three cases of vesicocervical fistula. Aust NZ J Obstet Gynaecol 4: 179–180

Maglacas AM, Simons J (1986) The potential of the traditional birth attendant. WHO Offset Publications, no. 95

Mahfouz Bey N (1929) Urinary and recto-vaginal fistulae in women. J Obstet Gynaecol Br Emp 36: 581–589

Mahfouz Bey N (1930) Urinary fistulae in women. J Obstet Gynaecol Br Emp 37: 566–576

Mahfouz Bey N (1934) A new technique in dealing with superior rectovaginal fistula. J Obstet Gynaecol Br Emp 41: 579–587

Mahfouz Bey N (1938) Urinary and faecal fistulae. J Obstet Gynaecol Br Emp 45: 405–424

Mahfouz Bey N (1957) Urinary fistulae in women. J Obstet Gynaecol Br Emp 64: 23–34

Mahfouz N (1966) The life of an Egyptian doctor. Livingstone, Edinburgh

el-Mahgoub S, el-Zeniny A (1971) Ureterouterine fistula after Cesarian section. Am J Obstet Gynecol 110: 881–882

Mahran M (1985) Personal communication

Maisoneuve JG (1942) Cited by Latzko WA. Op cit

Marr JP (1949) James Marion Sims, founder of the Woman's Hospital in the State of New York. the author, New York

Marshall VF (1979) Vesciovaginal fistulas on one urological service. J Urol 121: 25–29

Martius H (1928) Die operative Wiederherstellung der vollkommen fehlenden Harnröhre und des Schließmuskels derselben. Zentralbl Gynakol 8: 480–486

Martius H (1932) Über die Behandlung von Blasenscheidenfisteln, insbesondere mit Hilfe einer Lappenplastik. Geburtsh Gynäkol 103: 22–34

Martius H (1942) Zur Auswahl der Harnfistel- und Inkontinenzoperation. Zentralbl Gynäkol 32: 1250–1256

Massee JS, Welch JS, Pratt JH, Symmonds RE (1964) Management of urinary-vaginal fistula. JAMA 190: 902–906

Massoudnia N (1973) Surgical treatment of vesicovaginal fistulas. Int Surg 58: 128

Maughs GM (1884) What the ancients knew concerning obstetrics and gynaecology. JAMA 2: 225–233

Mayo Ch (1916) Repair of small vesicovaginal fistula. Ann Surg 63: 106–107

McAdory Owen T (1921) Dictionary of Alabama biography, Thos Clarke Publ Co, Chicago, Vol III, p 1564

McCall ML, Bolten KA (1957) Martius' Gynecological operations, with emphasis on topographical anatomy. J & A Churchill, London, pp 311–315

McConnachie ELF (1958) Fistulae of the urinary tract in the female. S Afr Med J 32: 524–527

McGill AF (1890) An operation for vesico-vaginal fistula through a suprapubic opening in the bladder. Lancet 2: 966–976

McGlinn JA (1932) Reconstruction of the urethra. Am J Obstet Gynecol 24: 262–266, 292–293

Mengert WF, Fish SA (1955) Anterior rectal wall advancement: technic for repair of complete perineal laceration and rectovaginal fistula. Obstet Gynecol 5: 262–267

Mettauer JP (1840) Vesico-vaginal fistula. Boston Med Sur J 22: 154–155

Mettauer JP (1847) On vesico-vaginal fistula. Am J Med Sci 14: 117–121

Miller NF (1935) Treatment of vesicovaginal fistulas. Am J Obstet Gynecol 30: 675–695

Miller NF, Brown W (1937) The surgical treatment of complete perineal tears in the female. Am J Obstet Gynecol 34: 196–209

Milton H (1887) Sixty cases of vesico-vaginal and recto-vaginal fistulae treated in the Cairo Civil Hospital. St. Thomas' Hosp Rpts 17: 19–37

Moerman M La V (1982) Growth of the birth canal in adolescent girls. Am J Obstet Gynecol 143: 528–532

Moir JC (1940) J. Marion Sims and the vesico-vaginal fistula: then and now. Br Med J 2: 773–778

Moir JC (1947) Urinary incontinence following childbirth, including vesico-vaginal fistulae. Edinb Med J 45: 368–381

Moir JC (1954) Vesicovaginal fistulae: review of 100 consecutive cases. Lancet 1: 57–61

Moir JC (1955) Personal experiences in the treatment of vesicovaginal fistulas. Am J Obstet Gynecol 71: 476–491

Moir JC (1961) The vesico-vaginal fistula. Bailliere, Tindall & Co. London

Moir JC (1964) Reconstruction of the urethra. J Obstet Gynaecol Br Cwlth 71: 349–359

Moir JC (1965) The "circumferential" vesico-vaginal fistula. J Obstet Gynaecol India 15: 441–448

Moir JC (1966) Vesicovaginal fistula: thoughts on treatment of 350 cases. Proc Roy Soc Med. 59: 1019–1022

Moir JC (1977) Obituary. Br Med J 2: 1551

Moir JC (1977) Obituary. Lancet 2: 1240

Montie J (1977) Bladder injuries. Urol Clin North Am 4: 59–67

Morgan JE, Farrow GA, Sims RH (1978) The sloughed urethra syndrome. Am J Obstet Gynecol 130: 521–524

Morton JH (1962) Cesarean hysterectomy. Am J Obstet Gynecol 83: 1422–1432

Munde PF (1894) Dr J. Marion Sims—the father of modern gynecology. Med Record 46: 514–515

Murphy M (1981) Social consequences of vesico-vaginal fistula in northern Nigeria. J Biosoc Sci 13: 139–150

Murphy M, Baba TM (1981) Rural dwellers and health care in northern Nigeria. Soc Sci Med 15A: 265–271

Mustafa AZ (1966) Female circumcision and infibulation in the Sudan. J Obstet Gynaecol Br Cwlth 73: 302–306

Mustafa AZ, Rushwan HME (1971) Acquired genito-urinary fistula in the Sudan. J Obstet Gynaecol Br Cwlth 78: 1039–1043

Nadel SF (1947) The Nuba, Cited by: Huddleson CE, 1949. Op cit

Naidu PM (1962) Vesico-vaginal fistulae: an experience with 208 cases. J Obstet Gynaecol Br Cwlth 69: 311–316

Naidu PM, Krishna S (1963) Vesico-vaginal fistulae and certain obstetric problems arising subsequent to repair. J Obstet Gynaecol Br Cwlth 70: 473–475

Naim A, Fahmy K (1965) Vagina fistula complicating salt atresia in Arabia. Alexandria Med J 11: 218–226

Noble CP (1901) The new formation fo the female urethra, with report of a case. Am J Obstet Gynecol 43: 170–178

Noble GH (1902) A new operation for complete laceration of the perineum, designed for the purpose of eliminating danger of infection from the rectum. JAMA 39: 302–304

O'Conor VJ (1957) Suprapubic closure of vesico-vaginal fistula. Charles C Thomas, Springfield, Illinois

O'Conor VJ, Sokol JK, Bulkley GJ, Nanninga JB (1973) Suprapubic closure of vesico-vaginal fistula. J Urol 109: 51–54

Ojo OA (1967) Ureteric injury in obstetric and gynaecological operations. West Afr Med J 16: 81–85

O'Leary JA, Steer CM (1964) A ten year review of Cesarean hysterectomy. Am
    J Obstet Gynecol 90: 227–231
Orford HJL, Theron JLL (1985) The repair of vesicovaginal fistulas with omentum:
    a review of fifty-nine cases. S Afr Med J 67: 143–144
Patil U, Waterhouse K, Laungani G (1980) Management of 18 difficult vesico-
    vaginal and urethrovaginal fistulas with modified Ingelman-Sundberg and
    Martius operations. J Urol 123: 653–656
Persky L, Herman G, Guerrier K (1979) Nondelay in vesicovaginal fistula repair.
    Urology 13: 273–275
Phaneuf LE, Graves RC (1949) Vesicovaginal fistula and its management. Surg
    Gynecol Obstet 88: 155–169
Quartey JKM (1972) Bladder rotation flap for repair of difficult vesicovaginal
    fistulas. J Urol 107: 60–62
Radman HM (1961) Vesicovaginal fistula. Am J Obstet Gynecol 82: 1238–1242
Ricci JV (1943) The genealogy of gynaecology: history of the development of
    gynaecology throughout the ages, 2000 BC—1800 AD. Blakiston Co, Phila-
    delphia
Roen PR (1960) Combined vaginal and transvesical approach in successful repair
    of vesicovaginal fistula. Arch Surg 80: 628–632
Rothenberger DA, Goldberg SM (1983) The management of rectovaginal fistula.
    Surg Clin North Am 63: 61–79
Royster HA (1922) James Marion Sims. Surg Gynecol Obstet 35: 237–239
Rubino SM (1980) Vesico-uterine fistula treated by amenorrhoea induced with
    contraceptive steroids: two case reports. Br J Obstet Gynaecol 87: 343–344
Rushwan H (1982) Female circumcision: present position and future outlook.
    Singapore J Obstet Gynaecol 13: 3–6
Russell CS (1956) Urinary fistulae and their management. J Obstet Gynaecol Br
    Emp 63: 481–493
Russell CS (1966) The vesical fistula high in the vagina. Proc Roy Soc Med. 59:
    1022–1024
Russell TR, Gallagher DM (1977) Low rectovaginal fistulas. Am J Surg 134: 13–
    18
Sargent JC (1955) Vesicovaginal fistula: an effective technique of repair. J Urol
    73: 520–524
Savage H (1870) The surgery, surgical pathology, and surgical anatomy of the
    female pelvic organs. Churchill & Sons, London
Schuchardt K (1893) Eine neue Methode der Gebärmutterexstirpation. Zentralbl
    Chir 20: 1121–1126
Schuchardt K (1942) Über die paravaginale Methode der Uterusexstirpation.
    Verhandlung der Deutschen Gesellschaft f. Chirurgie. Cited by: Latzko WA,
    Op cit
Shaw W (1949) The Martius bulbocavernosus interposition operation. Br Med J
    2: 1261–1264

Shepherd JA (1980) Lawson Tait—the rebellious surgeon (1845–1899). Coronado Press, Lawrence, Kansas

el-Sherbani A (1985) Personal communication

Shirodkar VN (1960) Contributions to obstetrics and gynaecology. E & S Livingstone, Edinburgh, pp 113–114

Shorter E (1984) A history of women's bodies. Penguin Books Ltd. Harmondsworth, Middlesex

Shrady GF (1894) Dr. J. Marion Sims—surgeon and philanthropist. Med Record 46: 513–514

Simon G (1942) Fälle von Operation bei Urinfisteln am Weibe, Beobachtung einer Harnleiter- Scheidenfistel, 1856. Cited by: Latzko WA, Op cit

Sims JM (1852) On the treatment of vesico-vaginal fistula. Am J Med Sci 23: 59–82

Sims JM (1873) Ovariotomy. D. Appleton & Co, New York

Sims JM (1884) The story of my life. D. Appleton & Co, New York (Reprinted, Da Capo Press, New York 1968)

(Sims JM) (1894) The Sims memorial statue. Am J Obstet Gynecol 30: 712–720

Sinclair R StC (1952) Maternal obstetric palsy. S Afr Med J 26: 708–714

Solms E (1920) Blasenfisteloperation mittels uterovaginaler Interposition der Plica. Zentralbl Gynäk 44: 1022–1027

Souchon E (1894) Reminiscences of Dr. J. Marion Sims in Paris. Med Record 46: 705–708

Souchon E (1895/96) Places rendered famous by Dr. J. Marion Sims in Montgomery Alabama. New Orleans Med Surg J 23: 455–460

Sparkman RS (1975) J. Marion Sims: woman's surgeon and more. Bull Am Coll Surg 60(3) 7–11

Speert H (1958) Obstetric and gynecologic milestones: essays in eponymy. Macmillan, New York

Spencer HR (1925) On some unusual vaginal fistulae. Am J Obstet Gynecol 10: 365–370

St George J (1969) Factors in the prediction of successful vaginal repair of vesico-vaginal fistulae. J Obstet Gynaecol Br Cwlth 76: 741–745

Stephen GM (1978) Difficult obstetric vesicovaginal fistula: a report on 12 cases. Int J Gynaecol Obstet 15: 310–312

Stevens JM (1975) Gynaecology from ancient Egypt: the papyrus Kahun: a treatise of gynaecology that has survived from the ancient world. Med J Aust 2: 949–952

Stewart DB (1967) Unorthodox repair of vesico-cervical fistula. J Obstet Gynaecol Br Cwlth 74: 122–124

Studdiford WE (1954) Vesicovaginal fistulas involving the bladder neck and upper urethra: their surgical management. Surg Clin North Am 34: 293–302

Su CT (1969) A flap technique for repair of vesicovaginal fistula. J Urol 102: 56–59

Symmonds RE (1969) Loss of the urethral floor with total urinary incontinence. Am J Obstet Gynecol 103: 665–678

Symmonds RE, Hill LM (1978) Loss of the urethra: report on 50 patients. Am J Obstet Gynecol 130: 130–138

Symmonds RE (1984) Incontinence: vesical and urethral fistulas. Clinical Obstet Gynecol 27: 499–514

Tahzib F (1983) Epidemiological determinants of vesicovaginal fistulas. Br J Obstet Gynaecol 90: 387–391

Tait L (1871) Operations for vaginal fistulas. Med Times Gaz 1: 332–333

Tait L (1876) Case of vesico-vaginal fistula left fourteen years after lithotomy, cured by a series of plastic operations. Trans Obstet Soc Lond 18: 209–214

Tait L (1878) Two cases of repair of the female bladder and urethra. Trans Obstet Soc Lond 20: 88–96

Tait L (1879) On new methods of operations for repair of the female perineum. Med Times Gaz 2: 597–598

Tait L (1889) The flap splitting operations for lacerated perineum. Am J Obstet Gynecol 22: 1044–1045

Taylor ES, Droegemueller W (1967) Repair of urinary vaginal fistulas. Obstet Gynecol 30: 674–678

Taylor JS, Hewson AD, Rachow P, Tynan P, Ward J (1980) Synchronous combined transvaginal-transvesical repair of vesicovaginal fistulas. Aust NZ J Surg 50: 23–25

Tehan TJ, Nardi JA, Baker R (1980) Complications associated with surgical repair of urethrovaginal fistula. Urology 15: 31–35

Thomas GB (1945) A serie of forty cases of vesicovaginal fistula. J Obstet Gynaecol Br Emp 52: 262–270

Thomas GB (1947) Treatment of a type of juxta-urethral vesicovaginal fistula. J Obstet Gynaecol Br Emp 54: 665–666

Thompson B, Baird D (1967) Some impressions of childbearing in tropical areas, part 1. J Obstet Gynaecol Br Cwlth 74: 329–338

Tozum R, Atasu T, Aksu F (1975) A new approach for treatment of vesicovaginal fistula. Obstet Gynecol 45: 687–688

Trendelenburg F (1890) Über Blasenscheidenfisteloperationen und über Beckenhochlagerung bei Operationen in der Bauchhöhle. Samml Klin Vortr 355 (Chir no 109): 3373–3392

Turner-Warwick R (1976) The use of the omental pedicle graft in urinary tract reconstruction. J Urol 116: 341–347

Twombly GW, Marshall VF (1946) Repair of vesicovaginal fistula caused by radiation. Surg Gynecol Obstet 83: 348–354

Underhill BML (1964) Salt-induced vaginal stenosis of Arabia. J Obstet Gynaecol Br Cwlth 71: 293–298

Vaidyu PR, Jain AB, Thakur SS (1975) Urinary fistula. J Postgrad Med 21: 68–76

Vix VA, Ryu CY (1971) The adult symphysis pubis: normal and abnormal. AJR 112: 517–525

Waghmarae D, Handscomb A (1968) A new method of drainage which has improved the results of repair of vesico-vaginal fistula. J Obstet Gynaecol Br Cwlth 75: 229–230

Walker AHC (1954) The management of urinary fistulas in a primitive population. Surg Gynecol Obstet 99: 301–309

Wangensteen OH, Wangensteen SD (1978) The rise of surgery: from empiric craft to scientific discipline. University of Minnesota Press, Minneapolis, pp 238–245

Wapple CL (1959) Vesico-vaginal fistula: a review of its causes and treatment. West J Obstet Gynecol 67: 227–229

Ward A (1980) Genito-urinary fistulae: a report on 1789 cases. Proceedings of the 2nd International Congress on Obstetrics & Gynaecology, Lagos

Ward A (1986) Personal communication

Ward Jr GG (1917) The operative treatment of inaccessible vesicovaginal fistulae. Surg Gynecol Obstet 25: 126–133

Ward GG (1923) Reconstruction of the urethra after complete loss, complicating an extensive fistula. Surg Gynecol Obstet 37: 678–682

Ward GG (1934) Destruction of the urethra and loss of vesical control associated with vesicovaginal fistula. Surg Gynecol Obstet 58: 67–69

Ward GG (1936) Marion Sims and the origin of modern gynecology. Bull NY Acad Med 12: 93–104

Ward RO (1945) Some surgical aspects of urinary bilharziasis. Proc Roy Soc Med 39: 27–38

Warren JC (1882) A new method of operation for the relief of rupture of the perineum through the sphincter and rectum. Trans Am Gynecol Soc 12: 322–330

Watson-Jones R (1946) Fractures and joint injuries, vol I, p 169. E & S Livingstone, Edinburgh

Webster GD, Sihelnik SA, Stone AR (1984) Urethrovaginal fistula: a review of the surgical management. J Urol 132: 460–462

Weed JC (1967) Management of vesicovaginal fistula: experience with seventy-five cases. Am J Obstet Gynecol 97: 1071–1075

Weyrauch HM, Rous SN (1966) Transvaginal-transvesical approach for surgical repair of vesicovaginal fistula. Surg Gynecol Obstet 123: 121–125

Willis AM (1926) John Peter Mettauer. Surg Gynecol Obstet 43: 235–236

Wolfson JJ (1964) Vaginography for demonstration of ureterovaginal vesicovaginal and rectovaginal fistulas, with case reports. Radiology 83: 438–441

Word SB (1970) Unpublished lecture

Word SB (1972) The father of gynecology (James Marion Sims). Ala J Med Sci 9: 33–39

Yenen A, Babuna C (1965) Genital fistulas: a study based on 197 consecutive cases. Obstet Gynecol 26: 219–224

Youssef AF (1957) "Menouria" following lower segment Cesarean section: a syndrome. Am J Obstet Gynecol 73: 759–767

Zacharin RF (1978) Emigrant eucalypts. Melbourne University Press, Melbourne

Zacharin RF (1980) Grafting as a principle in the surgical management of vesicovaginal and rectovaginal fistulae. Aust NZ J Obstet Gynaecol 20: 10–17

Zacharin RF (1983) Abdominoperineal urethral suspension in the management of recurrent stress incontinence of urine—a fifteen year experience. Obstet Gynecol 62: 644–654

Zimmern PE, Hadley HR, Staskin DR, Raz S (1985) Genitourinary fistulae: vaginal approach for repair of vesicovaginal fistulae. Urol Clin North Am 12: 361–367

Index

Robert F. Zacharin

Pelvic Floor Anatomy
and the Surgery of Pulsion Enterocoele

With a Foreword by **Richard E. Symmonds,** M. D.,
Mayo Clinic, Rochester, Minnesota, USA

1985. 75 partly colored figures. XVI, 170 pages.
Cloth DM 112,—, öS 784,—. ISBN 3-211-81861-8

From the Foreword by Richard E. Symmonds:

At present, for a number of reasons, gynecologic surgical training is most deficient in regard to the surgical correction of severe forms of obstetrically damaged genital tract supports. The operations for prolapse defy standardization
and require great technical individualization; this must be based on the surgeon's
judgment developed through experience, a thorough unterstanding of normal
pelvic anatomy, and recognition of the deficiency responsible for the prolapse in
individual cases.
Over a period of many years, the author of this book, a man of experience, in-
sight, and recognized surgical talents, has reported detailed studies of comparative pelvic anatomy in the female. An understanding of this anatomy is of the utmost importance in any consideration of the etiologic and therapeutic aspects of
prolapse, enterocoele, urinary incontinence, and other gynecologic conditions
that require reconstructive efforts. Included in the monograph is an informative
and remarkably complete historic review of the diverse operative procedures,
largely empirically developed, that have been devised for the correction of prolapse. Careful study and thoughtful consideration of the anatomic concepts proposed and the operative techniques suggested and beautifully illustrated in this
unique volume will be invaluable not only for the resident physician but also for
the specialist-practitioner who performs "routine" operations for prolapse but
may infrequently encounter or not feel qualified to perform the complex operative procedures required for the correction of the unusual, massive and recurrent
forms of pelvic herniations.

Springer-Verlag Wien New York

Moelkerbastei 5, A-1010 Wien · Heidelberger Platz 3, D-1000 Berlin 33 ·
175 Fifth Avenue, New York, NY 10010, USA ·
37-3, Hongo 3-chome, Bunkyo-ku, Tokyo 113, Japan

Peter A. M. Weiss/Donald R. Coustan (Eds.)

Gestational Diabetes

1987. Approx. 50 figures. Approx. 250 pages.
Cloth DM 138,—, öS 960,—. ISBN 3-211-82007-8

Contents: Gestational Diabetes — Survey. — Selected Topics on Gestational Diabetes: The Significance of Gestational Diabetes. On Physiologic and Pathophysiologic Features of Gestational Diabetes. On Screening and Diagnostics in Gestational Diabetes. On Prophylaxis and Therapy in Gestational Diabetes. On the Fetus and Newborn of Gestational Diabetic Women. On Oral Contraception in Gestational Diabetes. On the Further Fate of Women Who Had Gestational Diabetes. — References. — Subject Index.

In developed countries the incidence of gestational diabetes lies between 1 and 8 %. With the general decrease of perinatal mortality and morbidity, the complications arising from gestational diabetes have become more striking and significant. Moreover, impaired maternal carbohydrate metabolism may lead to a non genetic fuel mediated disposition to diabetes in the offspring. The renewed topicality has greatly stimulated research in this field. This book provides both a general survey and the current thinking on special questions of gestational diabetes. It also deals with related topics such as epidemiology, prognosis, follow-up, contraception, etc.
The book is addressed to obstetricians and other physicians engaged in prenatal care as well as to internists and neonatologists.

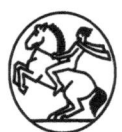

Springer-Verlag Wien New York

Moelkerbastei 5, A-1010 Wien · Heidelberger Platz 3, D-1000 Berlin 33 ·
175 Fifth Avenue, New York, NY 10010, USA ·
37-3, Hongo 3-chome, Bunkyo-ku, Tokyo 113, Japan